SPRINGER PUBLISHING

AF183339

GET THE MOST FROM YOUR BOOK

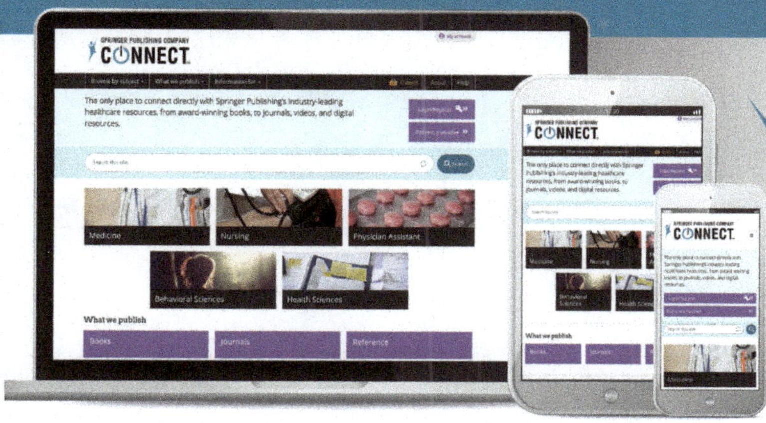

SPRINGER PUBLISHING CONNECT™

VOUCHER CODE:

G3PBGM24

Online Access

Your print purchase of *Sexual Health: Foundations, Treatments, and Resources* includes **online access via Springer Publishing Connect**™ to increase accessibility, portability, and searchability.

Insert the code at http://connect.springerpub.com/content/book/978-0-8261-0041-2 or scan the QR code and insert the voucher code today!

Having trouble? Contact our customer service department at ***cs@springerpub.com***

Instructor Resource Access for Adopters

Let us do some of the heavy lifting to create an engaging classroom experience with a variety of instructor resources included in most textbooks SUCH AS:

INSTRUCTOR MANUAL

POWERPOINTS

TEST BANK

Visit **https://connect.springerpub.com/** and look for the **"Show Supplementary"** button on your **book homepage** to see what is available to instructors! First time using Springer Publishing Connect?

Email **textbook@springerpub.com** to create an account and start unlocking valuable resources.

Sexual Health

Stephanie Baird, LMHC (**she/they**), has provided therapy, assessment, consultation, and educational talks and programming on sexual health, eye movement desensitization and reprocessing (EMDR) therapy, trauma, vicarious traumatization, self-care, burnout, and stress reduction in various mental health settings such as prisons, hospitals, clinics, and private practice, since 1999. Her private practice psychotherapy specialties include sexual health, EMDR therapy, and trauma/posttraumatic stress disorder (PTSD).

Ms. Baird has studied sexual health and human sexuality throughout her entire career, since the early 1990s, attaining an Advancing Clinical Sexuality Excellence certification in 2020. She is trained to teach various OWL (Our Whole Lives) sex education curricula (grades 7 through 12), young adult, adult, and older adult populations). She has taught sexual health and wellness to students at Bard College at Simon's Rock and other institutions. She is a full member of both the Society for Sex Therapy and Research and the Sexual Medicine Society of North America. She is currently teaching at Westfield State University.

Ms. Baird became an EMDR International Association (EMDRIA) approved consultant in 2016 and provides EMDR therapy consultation to clinicians. She has presented regionally, nationally (national EMDRIA conferences), and internationally on integrating EMDR therapy and sexual health. Her first professional book, *EMDR Therapy and Sexual Health: A Clinician's Guide*, originated from these presentations and was published in 2023. She has many other publications on sexual health, as well as vicarious trauma.

Ms. Baird loves bringing sex-positive information and sexual health into her psychotherapy practice and especially loves empowering clients' sexuality using future templates and resources. Furthering her goals of sex-positive and pleasure-positive sexual health education, she has written a monthly column called "Sex Matters" for a newspaper since 2019.

When not writing or working, she volunteers in various capacities at her local Unitarian Universalist (UU) society (including teaching OWL classes), road bicycles, travels with family or friends, and has just completed building a *Wee Lassie* canoe.

Wendy Stock, PhD (**she/her**), completed her undergraduate degree in psychology at the University of California, Berkeley, and earned her doctorate in clinical psychology from State University of New York at Stony Brook. In 2001, she earned a postdoctoral master of science degree in clinical psychopharmacology. Dr. Stock taught in psychology programs for over 20 years, and has over 20 professional publications. Her primary clinical orientation is cognitive-behavioral, and she identifies as a feminist therapist. She has been a licensed clinical psychologist in practice for over 30 years. Dr. Stock specializes in sex therapy, relationship issues, sexual trauma, depression, and anxiety. She is currently based in Berkeley, California. In 2015, Dr. Stock began her teletherapy practice with Doctor On Demand. She is licensed and provides teletherapy to clients in eight western states. She also volunteers with several human rights organizations to provide pro bono psychologic evaluations for survivors of torture seeking asylum, and for the Women's Cancer Resource Center in Oakland, California, in their free therapy program for women cancer survivors.

Katherine Hertlein, PhD (**she/her**), is a professor and associate dean of faculty affairs and professional development at the Boonshoft School of Medicine at Wright State University. She received her master's degree in marriage and family therapy from Purdue University Calumet and her doctorate in human development with a specialization in marriage and family therapy from Virginia Tech. Across her academic career, she has published over 100 articles and book chapters and 12 books. Dr. Hertlein has won numerous awards for research, teaching, mentorship, and supervision across her career including the Nevada System of Higher Education's Regent's Rising Researcher Award and Barrick Scholar Award from UNLV. Dr. Hertlein was also awarded a Fulbright Core Scholar Award (2018–2019) and, in this role, served as a guest lecturer and guest researcher at the University of Salzburg in Salzburg, Austria. Dr. Hertlein is also the editor-in-chief of the *Journal of Couple and Relationship Therapy*. Dr. Hertlein's work has been featured in various media outlets including *Men's Health*, *The APA Monitor*, *The Atlantic*, and *The Huffington Post*. She lectures nationally and internationally on technology, couples, and intimacy. Dr. Hertlein currently maintains a private practice in Las Vegas, Nevada.

Sexual Health

Foundations, Treatments, and Resources

Stephanie Baird, LMHC

Wendy Stock, PhD

Katherine Hertlein, PhD

SPRINGER PUBLISHING

Springer Publishing Company, LLC
902 Carnegie Center/Suite 140, Princeton, NJ 08540
www.springerpub.com
connect.springerpub.com

Acquisitions Editor: Mindy Okura-Marszycki
Production Editor: Susan White
Compositor: Thomson Digital

ISBN: 978-0-8261-8477-1
eBook ISBN: 978-0-8261-0041-2
DOI: 10.1891/9780826100412

SUPPLEMENTS:

SPRINGER PUBLISHING CONNECT™

A robust set of instructor resources designed to supplement this text is located at http://connect.springerpub.com/content/book/978-0-8261-0041-2. Qualifying instructors may request access by emailing textbook@springerpub.com.

Instructor Materials:
LMS Common Cartridge With All Instructor Resources ISBN: 978-0-8261-5383-8
Instructor's Manual ISBN: 978-0-8261-9144-1
Instructor Test Bank ISBN: 978-0-8261-5959-5
Instructor Chapter PowerPoints ISBN: 978-0-8261-6773-6

Student Materials:
Clinician Resources ISBN: 978-0-8261-5507-8

25 26 27 28 / 5 4 3 2 1

Medicine is an ever-changing science. Research and clinical experience are continually expanding our knowledge, in particular our understanding of proper treatment and drug therapy. The authors, editors, and publisher have made every effort to ensure that all information in this book is in accordance with the state of knowledge at the time of production of the book. Nevertheless, the authors, editors, and publisher are not responsible for any errors or omissions or for any consequence from application of the information in this book and make no warranty, expressed or implied, with respect to the content of this publication. Every reader should examine carefully the package inserts accompanying each drug and should carefully check whether the dosage schedules therein or the contraindications stated by the manufacturer differ from the statements made in this book. Such examination is particularly important with drugs that are either rarely used or have been newly released on the market.

Library of Congress Cataloging-in-Publication Data

Names: Baird, Stephanie, author | Stock, Wendy, author | Hertlein, Katherine, author
Title: Sexual health : foundations, treatment, and resources / Stephanie Baird, LMHC, Wendy Stock, PhD, Katherine Hertlein, PhD.
Description: First Springer Publishing edition. | Princeton, NJ : Springer Publishing, [2026] | Includes bibliographical references and index. |
Identifiers: LCCN 2025020334 | ISBN 9780826184771 | ISBN 9780826100412 ebook
Subjects: LCSH: Sexual health
Classification: LCC RA788 .S47835 2026
LC record available at https://lccn.loc.gov/2025020334

***Publisher's Note:* New and used products purchased from third-party sellers are not guaranteed for quality, authenticity, or access to any included digital components.**

Printed in the United States of America.

From Stephanie Baird

This second book is dedicated to my best friend and life partner, Ben, and my daughter, Lyra. Without their support I never could have found and prioritized the time to write this book. It is my hope that books such as these, as well as the entire canon of sex-positive information, will help pave the way for the healthiest, brightest, and most empowered sexual future for Lyra and all children everywhere. Lastly, I also dedicate this book to my stalwart and rallying inquisitive friends, as well as my curious clients, informing my persistent drive to provide positive and empowered sexual health information and encouragement.

From Wendy Stock

My primary motivation as I trained to become a clinical psychologist was, as a feminist, to contribute to the empowerment of women through my research, writing, and clinical work. The opportunity to train as a sex therapist and researcher broadened my understanding of the enormous educational, cultural, and political changes necessary for all individuals to actualize their sexual potential. I am honored to have been a contributor to this book.

I wish to honor my courageous feminist predecessors in this field, my fabulous editor and co-authors, and those who will succeed us in furthering this mission.

From Katherine Hertlein

I dedicate this book to my entire family, with special gratitude and big hugs to my husband, Eric, and our son, Adam. I appreciate their unwavering support as my career has unfolded into magical ways. You are all my favorite people, and I'm thankful for each and every one of you. Thank you to Springer and to my co-authors for allowing me to participate in such an interesting and worthwhile project. There is something to be said about the right time and right people, and I am so glad our paths crossed. I am also grateful for all of my amazing colleagues who over many years have pushed my thinking, creativity, and belief in myself forward. I am especially grateful for Dr. Gerald Weeks, who continues to be a major inspiration and constant source of support in both my personal and professional life.

Contents

PART 3 RESOURCES AND SPECIFIC POPULATIONS

Contributors

Stephanie Baird, MS, LMHC
EMDRIA Approved Consultant, Private Practice, South Hadley, Massachusetts; MaMHCA Certified Clinical Approved Supervisor; EMDR Coach, EMDR Consulting

Kristen Benson, PhD, LMFT
Associate Professor, AAMFT Approved Supervisor, Marriage and Family Therapy Program Director, Department of Human Development and Family Science, Virginia Tech, Blacksburg, Virginia

Sarah Burnham, MSW, LICSW
EMDRIA Certified Therapist, Veterans Administration Medical Center, Northampton, Massachusetts

Nicole Cardarella-Gasper, MA, LPCC
Cardarella Counseling, Minneapolis, Minnesota, LPC & LPCC Supervisor. EMDR Trained

Eterniti Claggett, BS
Human Development, University of Arizona, Tucson, Arizona

Katherine Hertlein, PhD
Professor and Associate Dean of Faculty Affairs and Professional Development, Boonshoft School of Medicine, Wright State University, Fairborn, Ohio

Traccie Hillion, MA, CAGS, LMHC
EMDRIA Certified Therapist, Private Practice, Belchertown, Massachusetts

Elena Isola, MA
Psychotherapist, EMDR Europe Approved Consultant and Facilitator, Clinical Sexologist, Rome, Italy

Ashley L. Mader, PhD, LICSW
Sex Therapist, Consultant and Educator, Founder/Blogger of Ourshine.org, Northampton, Massachusetts

Michelle M. Marchese, LICSW
PhD candidate, Smith School for Social Work, Adjunct Faculty, Smith College, Northampton, Massachusetts; EMDRIA Approved Consultant

Kathy McMahon, PsyD
President, Couples Therapy, Inc, Boston, Massachusetts; Licensed Psychologist AZ, CA, FL, MA; Diplomate of Sex Therapy; Certified Gottman Therapist

Robert Miller, PhD
President, Image Transformation Psychological Institute, Del Mar, California

Sandra Stephenson Murphy, MSW, LICSW
EMDRIA Certified Therapist, Private Practice, Northampton, Massachusetts

Eve Ng, PhD (Communication), PhD (Linguistics)
Associate Professor and Associate Director of Graduate Studies, School of Media Arts and Studies Core Faculty, Women's, Gender, and Sexuality Studies Program, Ohio University Athens, Ohio

Melanie Peele, MA, MEd, LPC
Registered Member MBACP, Private Practice, Scotland, United Kingdom, EMDR Trained

Nicola Pinder, MSc (EMDR Therapy), PhD Researcher
Salomons Institute for Applied Psychology, Psychosexual Therapist AccCOSRT, UKCP reg., EMDR Europe Accredited Consultant, Dip. Supervision AccCOSRT(sup), United Kingdom

Wendy Stock, PhD
Clinical Psychologist, Independent Practice, Berkeley, California

Desia Thrower, MS
Couples and Family Therapy, University of Nevada, Las Vegas, Nevada

Jassy Casella Timberlake, MEd, LMFT, CST
New England Sex Therapy, LLC, South Portland, Maine, AASECT Certified Sex Therapist and Certified Supervisor of Sex Therapy

Jenny Wright, MEd, CAGS
Private Practice, Ludlow, Massachusetts, EMDR Trained

Preface

SNAPSHOT SUMMARY

This new book on sexual health provides comprehensive modern, updated information on sexual health and concerns and addresses the learning needs of upper-level college and graduate-level classes in psychology, psychotherapy, counseling, social work, sexuality, sociology, educational, and nursing programs, as well as new mental health professionals. From a gender-expansive, intersex-inclusive, and nonbinary framework, multiple chapters share foundational information, laying the groundwork for positive and empowered sexual health. Attention to feminist research and intersectionality is included throughout. Case studies include representations of transgender diverse (TGD), neurodivergent, and culturally diverse populations. Information about nonmonogamous relationships (i.e., polyamory and consensual nonmonogamy) is provided. The dual control model of sexual desire and interest is featured in a variety of examples and discussions. Treatment strategies for sexual concerns and difficulties include eye movement desensitization and reprocessing (EMDR) therapy, as well as cognitive behavioral therapy (CBT), psychoeducation, and relational/systemic methods. The potential of trauma impacting sexual health is a running thread throughout this entire book, addressed specifically in the chapter on violence and victimization. This chapter also discusses polyvagal theory and vicarious trauma. Some chapters provide a supplemental section at the end, which contains easy to read questionnaires and handouts for clients, helping to explain vital and useful topics. Many different experts, including international colleagues, contribute case studies and various sections. This book also comes with an accompanying instructor guide, test banks, and PowerPoint presentations.

BOOK AND CHAPTER HIGHLIGHTS

This book is divided into three sections:

Part 1: Foundations for Sexual Health, Part 2: Treatment, and Part 3: Resources and Specific Populations.

Part 1 is the longest section of the book, spanning six chapters. This is due to the need to lay a comprehensive foundation and framework for understanding sexual health. We begin by learning about basic sexual rights and consent, sexual and reproductive anatomy, sexology and sex research, human sexual development, the ubiquitous experience of gender socialization, and the construct of sexual and affectional orientation, along with a range of potential modern relationship statuses, within which humans often locate themselves.

Part 2 contains four chapters devoted to treatment, beginning with a chapter on sex therapy frameworks and basic concepts. The next 3 chapters discuss disorders and difficulties experienced by those with vulvas and related genitals, disorders and difficulties experienced by those with penises and related genitals, and diagnoses, difficulties, and concerns related to sexual violence and the treatment of sexual trauma.

Part 3 includes two chapters on the sexual health of specific populations such as aging adults, BIPOC (Black, Indigenous, and People of Color) communities, individuals with disabilities (including physical or intellectual disabilities), neurodivergent individuals, and erotically marginalized individuals and communities. The final chapter contains information on clinician burnout, vicarious trauma, and recommended self-care, as well as an extensive list of well-vetted sexuality-related resources such as websites, books, media, and educational programs.

To take a closer look at the chapters: Chapter 1, "Sexual Health Frameworks," provides an essential foundational literacy in current sexual health, including concepts of basic sexual rights, sexual rights to pleasure, and sexual consent models and strategies. The widespread problem of cultural and individual erotophobia is discussed. The PLISSIT (Permission, Limited Information, Specific Suggestions, Intensive Therapy) model of sexual health communication is detailed, as well as important foundational elements of sexual health from the longstanding, evidence-based *Our Whole Lives* and Planned Parenthood curricula. Gina Ogden's 4-D Wheel of Sexual Health is explored as a helpful clinical sexual health framework. This chapter also addresses clinicians' own potential discomfort in addressing sexual health with clients, and introduces the idea of the therapists' own sexological worldview.

Chapter 2, "Sexual and Reproductive Anatomy and Health," provides sexual anatomy information written with inclusive (nonbinary) language, specific to the anatomical feature. For instance, "vulvas, clitorises, and related anatomy" are described, as opposed to being worded as "female" anatomy. Intersex development, as a natural biological, chromosomal, and hormonal variation, is also considered. Puberty and menopause are described. Fertility, pregnancy, birth, and pregancy loss are discussed. Essential sexual health information (i.e., sexually transmitted infections [STIs], HIV, pregnancy prevention, abortion access, safer sex) necesasry for sexual health literacy is provided.

In Chapter 3, "Sexology History, Desire and Arousal Models, and Sexual Compatibility," we bring models of sexuality to life by connecting them to contemporary concepts and case examples. Each of the models presented shines a spotlight on the complexity of sexual desire and behavior. We first briefly describe the history of research on human sexuality since the 1940s, beginning with Kinsey, Masters and Johnson, and Kaplan. Information about Basson's concepts of spontaneous desire and responsive desire (desire arising in response to pleasure) and her circular model of sexual response is explained, as well as the willingness model. We are then brought up to date by recent 21st century researchers Jannsen and Bancroft's formuilation of the dual control model of sexual response, consisting of *sexual accelerators* and *sexual brakes*. Important concepts of arousal concordance and nonconcordance, which relate to congruous or incongruous reports of physical sexual arousal and mental and emotional sexual interest, are discussed. This chapter also explores sexual compatibility, a multifaceted construct that involves agreement in behaviors, emotions, and cognitions; sexual personality styles; and erotic and/or sexual arousal templates (which form from birth to the present). The sexual styles questionnaire is provided for clinicians to administer to their clients, helping clients learn about their own sexual style.

Chapter 4, "Human Sexual Development," describes the lessons we learn about sexuality across the life span, both formally and informally, and covers several different kinds of sex education programming. It highlights several of the factors contributing to sexual skill-building including the importance of self-efficacy and self-confidence. The chapter provides discussion on sexual development across the life span, and how sexuality over the life span is regarded over different cultures. Finally, some of the theories of sexual development are explored.

Marchese's Chapter 5, "Considering Genders With All Clients," explores how gender, a social construct, exerts pressure on every individual within their culture. This pressure can take the form of narratives, roles, and expectations. Someone's gender can impact their access to care, how they have learned to express or process emotions, how they react to a variety of situations, and their experience of any potential trauma. This chapter examines some of the ways that gender can impact cisgender and transgender women, cisgender and transgender men, and gender-diverse individuals in the context of mental health treatment, and pertaining to sexual health. While current concepts and language to work with a variety of genders are included within, cultural humility and intersectional understanding are continuously encouraged for every unique therapeutic context.

Chapter 6, "Sexual/Affectional Orientation and Relationship Status," shares current information about sexual/affectional/romantic orientation (including *bisexual, pansexual, asexual, graysexual,* and *demisexual*). Although popular use of "queer" now encompasses a range of nonnormative sexual desires, practices, and identities, one of the most significant contributions of queer theorists, discussed in this chapter, has been to fundamentally challenge assumptions about the categories of "sex," "gender," and "sexuality" themselves. The relationships humans often find themselves in, as a part of sexual expression (e.g., singlehood, monogamy, forms of consensual nonmonogamy, and infidelity) are explored.

Chapter 7, "Sex Therapy Frameworks," describes modern sex therapy frameworks, including historical models, medical models, behavioral models, and feminist approaches. Clinicians learn basic sex therapy information and techniques (i.e., sensate focus, Kegels, mindfulness techniques), learn about commonly reported sexual health problems and misconceptions, debunk sexual myths, and learn accurate, corrective information. Qualities of good, great, and magnificent sex are also discussed. Also included is a resource on "Strengthening a Confident and Joyful Sexual Self" designed to help clients spend more time mindfully and positively developing and experiencing their sexuality.

Chapter 8 "Vulvar, Vaginal, and Pelvic Sexual Dysfunctions, Disorders, and Treatment," focuses on the etiology and treatment strategies for various sexual challenges for people with vulvas and clitorises. The contribution of biology, individual psychology, and relational issues is outlined for arousal and orgasm disorders. The presented treatment approaches reflect attention to the host of factors contributing to and/or maintaining the sexual problems. Case examples are included to illustrate how each factor and element influences the other.

Chapter 9, "Penile and Related Sexual Disorders and Treatment," focus on difficulties and disorders for people with penises. It includes detail and biopsychosocial etiology of the more common disorders, including erectile disorder, delayed ejaculation, and premature ejaculation. The chapter also features case examples detailed in both the scope of the problem and proposed treatment strategies.

Chapter 10, "Sexual Violence, Trauma, and Victimization," explores the high rates and statistics of sexual violence, and the association of PTSD and complex PTSD (CPTSD) with untreated trauma. For trauma survivors seeking sex therapy, it is usually important and more productive to treat trauma first with trauma-informed and focused therapy such as trauma-focused cognitive behavioral therapy (TF-CBT) or EMDR therapy. Information about sex workers, including how the legal system currently does NOT support their full safety and autonomy, is discussed. On the other hand, victims of sex trafficking face difficulties in obtaining justice and treatment. Survivors of sex trafficking benefit from trauma-informed therapy to treat any traumatic symptoms resulting from their experience. Pornography can both positively and negatively impact our clients' sexual health. Exploring this impact can greatly benefit our clients' sexual health and esteem. Treating sex offenders is very complicated and necessitates expert consultation. Many convicted sex offenders report experiencing sexual abuse in their own childhoods.

Chapter 11, "Marginalized Populations and Sexual Health," provides fundamental information about additional culturally and/or erotically marginalized populations and communities. Specifically, this chapter addresses information and clinical considerations regarding the sexual health of BIPOC people. Also included is information about addressing sexual health concerns for folks with disabilities. This chapter shares information about erotically marginalized clients that may engage in kink/bondage and discipline, dominance and submission, sadism, and masochism (BDSM); fetishes; and/or paraphilias. EMDR therapy case studies are provided to illustrate the intersection of sexual health regarding physical disability and kink/BDSM. With regrets, this initial first edition is not able to cover the breadth and depth of all marginalized populations.

Ashley Mader's Chapter 12, "Aging Sexual Health," discusses the needs of older adults. Aging and sexuality is not often considered in the field of mental health, even though aging is something that we are all doing every day. Older adults face menopause, sexual dysfunction/changes, and changes in body functioning and image. Internalized ageist myths and stereotypes can prevent these adults from having a positive outlook on the aging process. It is extremely important that these views do not prohibit older adults from getting help from healthcare providers. All healthcare providers need to be open and comfortable with talking about sex and aging. Clinical and sexual health suggestions are integrated throughout, ending with a case study featuring an older adult, sexual health, and EMDR therapy.

Chapter 13, "Sexual Health Resources for Clinicians and Clients," begins with information about clinician burnout, vicarious trauma, and self-care practices. Sex-positive activism is discussed and encouraged. Helpful sexual health assessments are enumerated. Additionally, this chapter provides a comprehensive, but not exhaustive, list of sexual health resources. As the field of human sexuality continues to expand and interface more positively with mental health, physical health, and our culture at large, increasing numbers of helpful resources are becoming available for sex educators, lay folks, and anyone seeking updated and positive information. This final chapter provides lists (with synopses of the most useful and relevant) essential sexual health-related websites, TED Talks, podcasts, books, television series, and educational resources for clinicians and clients. National and regional sexual health training organizations are listed for further learning. Additionally, although directly addressing children and their sexual health was out of the scope of this book, educational resources for children and teens regarding sexual health are included in this chapter.

Many clients want permission to explore and discuss their sexual health and how their prior history of erotophobic socialization and potentially disturbing events may have negatively impacted their sexual health. Our hope is that this book will help burgeoning clinicians gain updated knowledge and confidence to address current sexual health empowerment and concerns. Please keep in mind that as the field and agents of sexual health continue to expand, these resources may quickly become outdated or replaced by more current versions. Always locate the most current websites and/or editions of the listed resources to learn about updates or revisions.

BOOK ORIGIN

An interest in sexual health and empowerment has been a strong undercurrent throughout Stephanie Baird's entire conscious life, especially since early college, thanks to her first professor of sex education, Dr. Wendy Stock (who has co-authored this book). In Dr. Stock's class, Stephanie's mind was blown nearly every class meeting in "Human Sexuality," circa 1993, at the mostly conservative Texas A&M University. Stephanie never forgot seeing her classmates' stereotypes and myths smashed to smithereens, day by day, very calmly, by the plethora of equalizing, enlightening, and normalizing research and accurate information Dr. Stock shared. That class may have been the first time she heard the word *clitoris*.

Stephanie continued to seek information on sexuality, as well as in women's studies, in upper level classes and took all graduate level sexuality-related classes available at the University of North Texas Counseling Psychology master's program (a whopping two classes). She followed beloved sexuality writers like Betty Dodson and Susie Bright. She also volunteered at rape crisis programs during this time and wrote a thesis on vicarious traumatization of sexual and domestic violence volunteers. This focus turned her attention from pure sexual health to sexual trauma. Everywhere she looked, she encountered and met someone who was a survivor of trauma, fueling an urgency to help this population.

During postgraduate school she worked in prisons with sex offenders, looking at the other side of trauma, then returned to working with sexual violence survivors from 2001 on. Getting trained in EMDR therapy (2009), she fell in love with this highly effective and efficient way of treating sexual trauma survivors.

However, never forgetting her interest in sexual health, she earnestly renewed seeking, obtaining, and integrating fresh sexual health information over a decade ago. During that process

Stephanie became astounded at the continued lack of sexual health discussion and education in public school, college, at psychotherapy conferences and events, and even in graduate level psychotherapy programs. This lack of sexual health discussion within the mental health community is astonishing when one thinks about it, when we consider the high rates of sexual trauma in all genders.

Stephanie jumped in to help fill this sexual health gap by becoming an OWL sex educator for secondary students and adults, initiating an ongoing now 5-year-long monthly newspaper column (*Sex Matters*) and teaching sexual health and wellness adjunct at Bard College at Simon's Rock. This proactive sexual health education, combined with her years as an EMDR therapist and approved consultant, culminated in regional and national presentations integrating EMDR therapy and sexual health and her first book, *EMDR Therapy and Sexual Health: A Clinician's Guide* (2023)—with the goal to bridge a 30-year gap of lack of sexual health for trauma clinicians.

May every reader of this book emerge feeling much more informed, confident, and sex-positive with the integration of sexual health in their own clinical practice.

Gender Terminology: The term *man* generally refers to individuals with a penis, testes, prostate, and so on, and/or socialized into a masculine gender (generally speaking, *cisgender men/cismen*). The term *woman* generally refers to individuals with a vulva, labia, clitoris, vagina, ovaries, and uterus, and/or socialized into a feminine gender (generally speaking, *cisgender women/ciswoman*). This particularly pertains to how researchers have categorized individuals in the studies mentioned throughout and some of the self-identified gender of individuals. However, a transman who may not have all of the biological anatomies generally associated with a cisman (penis, tests, etc.) also receives masculinized gender socialization. This also applies for transwomen. Transgendered individuals are generally referred to as transfemale, transwoman, transmale, and/or transman. *Intersex* refers to individuals with less commonly seen combinations of reproductive organs/anatomy, chromosomes, and/or hormones. *Nonbinary* is another term that may refer to individuals identifying beyond female or male. *Assumed/assigned male at birth* (AMAB) may also be used to describe someone with a penis and testes. *Assumed/assigned female at birth* (AFAB) may be used to describe someone with a clitoris and vulva. Information about *intersex* individuals is included throughout. Case study individuals that identify as *gender nonconforming* and/or *gender nonbinary* are labeled as such. As gender terminology is rapidly (and happily) changing, some of this terminology may be outdated once this book comes out in print.

Case Studies: For case studies, names, ages, and many identifying details have been changed and/or recombined for total anonymity. Many of the case studies feature individuals from non-White identities, and/or LGBTQIA+ individuals.

Working Definition of Sex and Sexual Activity: For the purposes of this book, *sex* and *sexual activity* may refer to any behavior that involves any amount of sexual interest/desire, and/or arousal, among any configuration of consenting individuals and genders. This nonexhaustive list of behaviors includes kissing, deep kissing, making out, outercourse (any nonpenetrative activity), touching sensitive and/or erogenous areas like breasts and genitals, erotic/sensual massage, solo or mutual masturbation, giving and/or receiving oral sex, penis–vagina intercourse, anal sex, manual stimulation, consenting adult kink/BDSM activities, and/or sex toy use with adults of any consenting gender and/or genitalia configuration.

Stephanie Baird
Wendy Stock
Katherine Hertlein

Gender Terminology Statement

The term *man* generally refers to individuals with a penis, testes, prostate, and so on, and/or socialized into a masculine gender (generally speaking, *cisgender men/cismen*). The term *woman* generally refers to individuals with a vulva, labia, clitoris, vagina, ovaries, and uterus, and/or socialized into a feminine gender (generally speaking, *cisgender women/ciswoman*). This particularly pertains to how researchers have categorized individuals in the studies mentioned throughout and some of the self-identified gender of individuals. However, a transman who may not have all of the biological anatomies generally associated with a cisman (penis, tests, etc.) also receives masculinized gender socialization. This also applies for transwomen. Transgendered individuals are generally referred to as transfemale, transwoman, transmale, and/or transman. *Intersex* refers to individuals with less commonly seen combinations of reproductive organs/anatomy, chromosomes, and/or hormones. Nonbinary is another term that may refer to individuals identifying beyond female or male. Assumed/assigned male at birth (AMAB) may also be used to describe someone with a penis and testes. Assumed/assigned female at birth (AFAB) may be used to describe someone with a clitoris and uterus.

Acknowledgments

From Stephanie:

I thank Jassy Casella Timberlake, LMFT, for hosting a sex therapy consultation group at her former group practice Northampton Sex Therapy Associates, which I attended for 3 years. It was at the sex therapy consultation group's suggestion that I present on *Integrating EMDR Therapy and Sexual Concerns*, thus laying the groundwork for regional and national presentations on EMDR therapy and sexual health, culminating in the 2023 book, *EMDR Therapy and Sexual Health: A Clinician's Guide*. I also made several lovely connections within that group, including Dr. Ashley Mader, LICSW, expert on sex and aging, who contributed her expertise with Chapter 12, "Aging Sexual Health." I also thank Jassy Casella Timberlake, LMFT, for providing permission to include the Sexual History Questionnaire. I also thank Dr. Kathy McMahon for providing permission to include the Sexual Styles Survey.

During the last decade of increased focus on sexual health, I was also fortunate to attend many presentations facilitated by the Northeast American Association of Sexuality Educators, Counselors, and Therapists–Northeast. Dr. Jane Fleishman was the regional president during this time and brought many excellent guest speakers including Emily Nagoski (author of *Come as You Are*), Gina Ogden (author of *Expanding the Practice of Sex Therapy*), and Roz Dischiavo (author of *The Deep Yes: The Lost Art of True Receiving*). I owe gratitude to Dr. Fleishman for helping to round out my education with these fascinating and cutting-edge presenters.

I wish to acknowledge and thank Dr. Rosalyn Dischiavo, founder of the Institute for Sexuality, Education, and Enlightenment (ISEE). ISEE offered many classes in my region, including the essential SAR (sexual attitude reassessment) class. It was always an intellectually exciting highlight to take classes from Dr. Dischiavo and her colleagues at ISEE. I was grateful to receive my Advancing Clinical Education in Sexuality (ACES) via ISEE in 2020.

I owe a debt of gratitude to my home Unitarian Universalist society, the Unitarian Society of Northampton and Florence, and Jessica Harwood, director of religious education and faith development. At her suggestion I received the *Our Whole Lives (OWL)* sex educator training in April 2018 (for grades 7 through 12), as well as the adult OWL training (young adult, adult, and older adult) in March 2019. This allowed me to finally enjoy being on the side of prevention.

Teaching and taking so many classes in sexual health gave me the gumption to approach Nina Rossi, features editor at the local *Montague Reporter* newspaper, about writing a sex-positive column on sexual health. I jumped for joy when both Nina and Mike Jackson (editor) loved the column idea, which was one of my lifelong dreams. I have been enthusiastically writing this monthly column since September 2019. Thank you for this fun and meaningful opportunity, Nina and Mike!

I wish to acknowledge the general support of our very vibrant Western Massachusetts EMDR community as well as my EMDR mentors throughout the last couple of decades. Involvement in the Western Massachusetts EMDR Network's board of directors for many years provided lovely connections, including meeting Michele Marchese, LICSW (previous board president), who authored Chapter 5, "Considering Gender With All Clients."

Other EMDR therapy community members—Sandy Murphy, LICSW; Jenny Wright, LMHC; Melanie Peele, LPC; Dr. Robert Miller; and Sarah Burnham, LICSW—contributed important sections and case studies.

I thank Beth Sposito of the Potts Point, Harpswell, Maine waterfront property "Bayberry Ledge" for my many days typing and looking over my laptop at the extraordinary view, affording me precious alone time and mental space to accomplish the bulk of this writing. Also gratitude to my good friends Teddi Olszewski and Denise Fontaine-Pincince for allowing me use of their beautiful homes for quiet writing time. Thank you also to Jamie Sullivan, who provided a flurry of last minute formatting edits before I turned in the manuscript to Springer Publishing Company.

I also wish to thank my editor at Springer Publishing Company, Mindy Okura-Marszycki, for helping to develop and spearhead this new book, and connecting me with the excellent co-author Kat Hertlein, an extremely knowledgeable, hardworking, and responsive collaborator and writer. Kat Hertlein's additional writing and insight greatly enhanced this publication. I thank Wendy Stock for her initial inspirations to my career trajectory back in 1993, her wonderful writing, and our continued collaborations, especially as co-authors.

I hold special appreciation for the clients who brought their sexual health questions to our sessions. This drove the point home that we clinicians need to be much more informed and comfortable in *going there* when our clients ask that of us.

This book has been a collaborative labor of love, birthed by many midwives/midspouses.

Although I belong to certain marginalized or historically oppressed groups (bisexual/omnisexual, cisgender woman/femme appearing, neurodiverse), I must acknowledge that my White, educational, and professional privilege has allowed me to pursue this project with relative ease. Lastly, I respectfully acknowledge my places of home and work, where much of this manuscript was created, are within the ancestral, unceded homelands of the Pocumtuck and Nonotuck peoples.

Resources

CLINICIAN RESOURCES

- **Worksheets, handouts, surveys, and articles** are available for download.

INSTRUCTOR RESOURCES

SPRINGER PUBLISHING CONNECT™ | A robust set of instructor resources designed to supplement this text is located at **http://connect.springerpub.com/content/book/978-0-8261-0041-2**. Qualifying instructors may request access by emailing **textbook@springerpub.com**.

- **LMS Common Cartridge With All Instructor Resources**
- **Instructor's Manual**:
  - Learning Objectives
  - Chapter Outlines
  - Chapter Summaries
  - Discussion Questions with sample answers
- **Instructor Test Bank**: 195 multiple-choice questions with detailed rationales
- **Instructor Chapter PowerPoints** summarizing chapter content

I

Foundations for Sexual Health

CHAPTER 1

Sexual Health Frameworks

Stephanie Baird

LEARNING OBJECTIVES

- Gain an introductory understanding of modern sexual health.
- Learn about the importance of approaching sexuality from a sex- and pleasure-positive framework (Global Declaration of Sexual Rights and Pleasure) versus erotophobia.
- Learn about several positive sexual health models (OWL, Planned Parenthood, 4-D Wheel, CREATE).
- Learn about the PLISSIT (Permission, Limited Information, Specific Suggestions, Intensive Therapy) model of sexual health communication.
- Learn about the importance of our ever-evolving and more explicit guidelines for sexual consent.
- Learn about factors interfering with discussing sexuality and increase comfort addressing sexual health.
- Explore one's sexological worldview and how it impacts the ability to help clients.

INTRODUCTION TO SEXUAL HEALTH

Congratulations on taking this educational step to empower yourself and your current or future clients toward full healthy sexual functioning. If you are like us, and most U.S. psychotherapists, clinicians, social workers, and other mental health and medical students and professionals, your education and background included very little information about sexual health. Most of us received zero to just 6 hours of basic sex education in public school, and depending on the decade and geographic region of your school, your education may have only mentioned menstruation and abstinence. Perhaps you can now take the single offered human sexuality class in college or graduate school (the course this textbook has been selected for), or perhaps you are lucky enough to choose from two or more sexuality classes. If you are this lucky, we urge you to take all the classes, as even one class is inadequate for the job of fully understanding the nuance, breadth, and depth of something as ordinary and extraordinary as human sexuality.

In other words, pursuing advanced specialization and/or certification in most therapies or mental health degree programs does not bring automatic access to basic, never mind sex-positive, resources and information.

An often-cited study indicated that 91% of the clients at a community mental health clinic reported being exposed to at least one or more traumatic events in their lifetime (Cusack et al., 2004). Most of our caseloads will overwhelmingly be composed of sexual trauma survivors who have had little to no access to positive and helpful sexual health information. It is estimated that sexual problems affect 40% to 45% of cisgender women (cisgender means the person identifies with the sex/gender assigned at birth) and 20% to 30% of cisgender men (Lewis et al., 2010), with a noticeable correlation between trauma and adult sexual issues (Yehuda et al., 2015), such as lower sexual interest, arousal, orgasms, and sexual satisfaction (Neumann et al., 1996). I find this statistic plays out in my own private practice again and again.

Additionally, the statistics regarding sexual assault trauma are sobering. More than 50% of cisgender women, nearly 33% of cisgender men, and two out of three transgender individuals experience sexual trauma involving physical contact (abuse, molestation, assault, etc.) in their lifetimes, much of it by the age of 18 (Centers for Disease Control and Prevention, 2024). These high statistics informed my drive to become a sexual trauma-focused EMDR consultant (certified in eye movement desensitization reprocessing [EMDR] therapy, which addresses the gamut of trauma). These statistics also inform my drive to integrate and share positive sexual health information, resources, and healing in our work with clients, many of whom are sexual trauma survivors. This chapter provides that foundation of sexual health, introducing several uplifting paradigms.

WHAT IS "SEXUAL HEALTH"?

The World Health Organization (WHO) defines sexual health as:

> a state of physical, emotional, mental, and social well-being related to sexuality; it is not merely the absence of disease, dysfunction, or infirmity. Sexual health requires a positive and respectful approach to sexuality and sexual relationships, as well as the possibility of having pleasurable and safe sexual experiences, free of coercion, discrimination, and violence. For sexual health to be attained and maintained, the sexual rights of all persons must be respected, protected, and fulfilled. (n.d., Overview)

The Office of the Surgeon General and Office of Population Affairs defines sexual health similarly as:

> inextricably bound to both physical and mental health. Just as physical and mental health problems can contribute to sexual dysfunction and disease, those dysfunctions and diseases can contribute to physical and mental health problems. Sexual health is not limited to the absence of disease or dysfunction, nor is its importance confined to just the reproductive years .... It includes freedom from sexual abuse and discrimination and the ability of individuals to integrate their sexuality into their lives, derive pleasure from it, and to reproduce if they so choose. (2001, p. 1)

WORKING DEFINITIONS OF SEX AND SEXUAL ACTIVITY

For the purposes of this book, sex and sexual activity may refer to any behavior that involves any amount of sexual interest/desire and/or arousal among any configuration of consenting individuals and genders, or with oneself. This nonexhaustive list of behaviors includes kissing, deep kissing, making out, outercourse (any nonpenetrative activity), touching sensitive and/or erogenous areas like breasts and genitals, erotic/sensual massage, solo or mutual masturbation, giving and/or receiving oral sex, penis-vagina intercourse, anal sex, manual stimulation, consenting adult kink/bondage and discipline, dominance and submission, sadism, masochism (BDSM) activities, and/or use of sex toys with any consenting gender and/or genitalia configuration.

WHAT IT MEANS TO BE SEX- AND PLEASURE-POSITIVE

Educators, activists, and researchers have increasingly moved from frameworks of intervention, disease, and disorder to frameworks prioritizing disease/disorder prevention along with sexual pleasure and well-being promotion. Many activists and educators such as Nagoski (2015), adrienne marie brown (2019), Tallon-Hicks (2022), and Dodson (1996) purposely center sexual pleasure in much of their writing. In agreement with the primacy of sex positivity, this textbook begins with elaborating some positive frameworks, in hopes of laying down a pleasure-based foundation from which to examine sexuality. And while individuals and organizations have been studying sex, sexuality, and sexual health for decades, in my work with clients I often come back to Peggy Kleinplatz's direct and arresting research question, "[W]hat kind(s) of sex would be worth wanting[?]" (Kleinplatz et al., 2009, p. 2).

DECLARATION OF SEXUAL RIGHTS AND PLEASURE

Since 1978, the World Association for Sexual Health (WAS) has worked toward sexual health and rights. Thousands of members attend global biennial congresses and in recent years have made declarations for sexual rights.

Declaration of Sexual Rights

According to the WAS, sexual rights may pertain to an individual's sexuality, but they are essentially fundamental human rights. Some of these rights are noted in the list that follows (WAS, 2014):

1. The right to equality and freedom of sexual expression
2. The right to make decisions about one's body in regard to sexuality
3. The right to be safe from all forms of sexual violence and coercion, and be free from inhumane treatment or punishment because of one's sexual or gender expression
4. The right to accurate scientific information and education about sexuality and sexual health
5. The right to freely create and dissolve marital and other similar relationships
6. The right to family planning resources
7. The right to organize freely to promote sexual rights and health
8. The right to privacy regarding sexual matters
9. The right to judicious laws and remedies regarding sexual rights
10. The right to the highest attainable standard of sexual health, including sexual safe and pleasurable sexual experiences

Declaration on Sexual Pleasure

At WAS's congress in Mexico City (October 2019), they improved their previous declaration by adding a separate declaration on sexual pleasure adapted from a definition from the Global Advisory Board for Sexual Health and Wellbeing (GAB):

> Sexual pleasure is the physical and/or psychological satisfaction and enjoyment derived from shared or solitary erotic experiences, including thoughts, dreams and autoeroticism. Self-determination, consent, safety, privacy, confidence and the ability to communicate and negotiate sexual relations are key … factors for pleasure to contribute to sexual health and wellbeing. Sexual pleasure should be exercised within the context of sexual rights [including] equality and non-discrimination, autonomy and bodily integrity, and the right to the highest … standard of health and freedom of expression. The experiences of human sexual pleasure are diverse and sexual rights ensure that pleasure is a positive experience for all concerned and not obtained by violating … human rights and wellbeing. (GAB, 2016)

Some of WAS's (2019) declaration includes:

- Sexual pleasure is a fundamental part of sexual and human rights and includes the possibility of diverse sexual experiences.
- Access to appropriate sources of sexual pleasure is part of human well-being.
- Sexual health and well-being include pleasurable and safe sexual experiences free of discrimination, coercion, and violence.
- Sexual pleasure shall be globally integrated into education, health services, research, and advocacy, and contributes to global health.

General Impact of Trauma and Erotophobia on Positive Sexual Health

Despite most of us walking by magazine covers at the grocery store touting advice like "Fifty Ways to Spice Up Your Sex Life" or "Achieve Your Most Powerful Orgasm Yet," our culture as a whole remains erotophobic, shaming, and "puritanical" when it comes to embracing sexual pleasure and health. *Erotophobia* is a term used by sex educators Dischavio (2016) and Klein (2010), among others, to refer to our society's (and a person's) fear of sexuality and sexual content. This can include anything from anxiety and fear preventing someone from examining their own genitals (and refusing Pap smears) to the avoidance of all sexual discussion or activity.

We have now had several decades of sex-positive activism, ramping up in the 1960s with the sexual revolution and burgeoning forms of birth control, continuing through the second wave liberation-oriented feminism of the seventies, surfacing again in the nineties with third wave feminism (partially in response to right-wing Christian/Reaganomic backlash in the eighties and the rise and stigmatization of HIV/AIDS). The nineties' third wave feminism increased public awareness of sexual assault and emphasized intersectionality of race, culture, class, gender, sexual orientation, and so forth. The nineties also brought an army of sex-positive feminist activists like Susie Bright (sex-positive essayist and author of *Sexual State of the Union* [1997]), Carol Queen (popular sex educator, adult toy store co-owner, and author of *Real Live Nude Girl* [2002]), and Tristan Taormino (writer, activist, and filmmaker), along with the mainstreaming of feminist sex toy stores like Good Vibrations in California and other states. Safer sex discussions also increased in response to the HIV/AIDS crisis. Much of the mainstream can thank Dr. Ruth Westheimer et al. (2012) for all of her trailblazing work candidly and openly tackling any sexual matter thrown her way, from the 1980s to the present.

Increasingly available internet pornography burst onto the scene in the late 1990s and early 2000s, single-handedly misinforming millions of individuals about average sizes of body parts and once again locking folks into stereotypes of masculine individuals actively seeking and receiving sex, and feminine individuals "happy to oblige" others' desires, passively neglecting their own sexuality and pleasure. However, the widespread availability of e-readers plus steamy erotic fan-fiction (e.g., the problematic *Fifty Shades of Grey* published in 2011) allowed feminine individuals to catch up with masculine individuals in viewing and engaging with erotic material.

The #metoo movement is one of our most recent cultural sexual history developments. Initially beginning in 2006 when Black, Indigenous, and People of Color (BIPOC) sexual assault survivor and activist Tarana Burke developed the phrase, it erupted in 2017 when actress Ashley Judd accused Harvey Weinstein of sexually assaulting her. This accusation soon unleashed a torrent of disclosures from other famous and nonfamous ciswomen (and some cismen) against (mostly) cismen in power. The #metoo movement has also brought with it much needed discussion of consent, which will be discussed in more detail shortly.

However, despite this ever-widening spiral of positive sexual health awareness, our puritanical and shaming culture is not going out without a cultural and political fight. This means that despite the availability of more sex-positive media content such as the television shows *Sex Education* (Netflix), *Bridgerton* (Netflix), *Mrs. Fletcher* (HBO), *Heartstopper* (Netflix), and *Welcome to Chippendales* (Hulu), legislation continues to be enacted that severely restricts individuals' autonomous expression of sexuality. These erotophobic laws include antiabortion actions such as the recent overturning of *Roe v. Wade* (2022) as well as the many transphobic laws that exist and get added in the majority of states. In fact, as of this writing (February 2025), 528 such bills exist across 46 states, with six having passed (Trans Legislation Tracker, n.d.). Even progressive Massachusetts has a bill on the docket that, if passed, would prohibit classroom "[i]nstruction by school personnel or third parties on sexual orientation or gender identity [in] Kindergarten through Grade 3" (MA H551 § 32B[c]).

Research (Calzo & Blashill, 2018) and other published accounts reflect that some LGBTQ adults knew they were not heterosexual as young as age 9 or 10, with some transgender folks knowing they did not feel comfortable in their assigned gender as early as elementary school. This is just one example of how our current erotophobic culture works against humans developing knowledge and comfort around the various aspects of their sexual identity.

I have included various sexual guidelines and declarations to emphasize the importance of including sexual health as a vital and essential piece of our clients' healing and lives. Van der Hart et al. (2006) often describe healing from trauma as a three-phase comprehensive approach. Phase One involves stabilization (resourcing, grounding, etc.). Phase Two includes the nitty-gritty of treatment (including EMDR therapy and trauma-focused cognitive behavioral therapy [CBT]). Phase Three of overall trauma treatment includes improving intimacy, sexual health, and self-actualization.

If we all had been lucky enough to receive sex education reflecting WAS values (as well as the OWL [Our Whole Lives] and Planned Parenthood values mentioned later in this chapter) from early childhood, with an emphasis on pleasure and consent, I believe the sexual trauma statistics would be greatly reduced and all of us would happily exist in "Phase Three" of overall treatment: empowered and fulfilling sexual health and intimacy.

POSITIVE MODELS OF SEXUAL HEALTH

Since being on this journey of integrating positive sexual health into my own clinical practice, I have discovered many wonderful models of sexual health. Some of the most well-known and helpful models are described in this section. Keeping these basic models in mind will help inform all your subsequent learning and exploration of human sexuality from the nuts and bolts of sexual and reproductive anatomy to treating diagnosable sexual disorders to promoting the enhancement of pleasure for everybody.

SEXUAL HEALTH MODEL

The *sexual health model* (Robinson et al., 2002) derives from a sexological approach to education, and defines 10 key components posited to be essential aspects of healthy human sexuality: communicating about sex, culture and sexual identity, sexual anatomy and functioning, sexual healthcare and safer sex, challenges to sexual health, body image, masturbation and fantasy, positive sexuality, intimacy and relationships, and spirituality. This model, holistically developed from several sexuality education sources (including sexual attitude reassessment workshops), as well as research, supported long-term HIV prevention through encouraging organizations to provide comprehensive, culturally and environmentally specific sexuality education.

PERMISSION, LIMITED INFORMATION, SPECIFIC SUGGESTIONS, AND INTENSIVE THERAPY MODEL

One of the first concepts I learned in my foray into sexual health involves the *PLISSIT* (**P**ermission, **L**imited **I**nformation, **S**pecific **S**uggestions, and **I**ntensive **T**herapy) model developed by Annon in 1976.

Permission is considered a first level intervention in which the clinician provides permission for the client to discuss/talk/ask questions and/or disclose their feelings and concerns related to specific sexual health issues. "By encouraging clients to share their thoughts, questions, etc., you validate the issue as a legitimate health matter" (Luchterhand, 2014, p. 1). This may be the most important step and help we can provide to certain clients who have been searching for answers or validation for years. You can explicitly provide permission by asking clients verbally or in your intake paperwork if they have any sexuality-related concerns. You can also make mention of your experience and comfort with sexual health on your website or listings. By having sex-positive posters, books, or pamphlets displayed in your waiting room and office, you can provide an environment that says, "We can talk about sex here."

Limited Information is a second level intervention that goes beyond the permission obtained in the first step and provides basic information about the topic. During this step, you might provide handouts, dispel myths and preconceptions, and refer clients to books and websites. This textbook references many educational tools and resources you can add to your library of knowledge.

Specific Suggestions comprise the third level and involve advanced levels of knowledge or specific expertise. If you are not comfortable or able to provide these, and the client continues to report sexual difficulty (even after processing and discussing sexuality-related aspects), you may need to refer your client to a specialized or certified sex therapist, pelvic floor physical therapist, midwife or sex-positive ob/gyn, or other sexual health specialist.

The fourth level intervention of *Intensive Therapy* (if needed) is typically provided by an outside specialist (e.g., sex therapist or pelvic floor physical therapist) for a particular issue, such as continued pelvic pain or erectile dysfunction.

OUR WHOLE LIVES SEXUALITY EDUCATION CURRICULUM

I fell in love with OWL in 2018 after my local Unitarian Universalist (UU) congregation asked me if I wanted to become trained to teach the seventh through twelfth grade curriculum, with the intent of volunteering to teach the 9-month-long curriculum to our congregational youth. I jumped at this lifelong chance to proactively prevent sexual trauma by inoculating youth (and later, adults) with as much factual, educational, and sex-positive information as the curriculum could provide.

The concepts and guidelines that inform this curriculum grew from the research of the Sexuality Education Task Force in the early nineties and from the work of many educators, as well as UU and United Church of Christ (UCC) congregations, who saw a lack of evidence and fact-based sexuality education for youth when developing curriculum for the life span. You do not have to be a UU or UCC member to receive training to teach the various OWL curricula (broken into these age ranges: kindergarten through first grade, fourth through sixth grade, seventh through ninth grade, tenth through twelfth grade, young adult, adult, and now older adult). Like taking a Sexual Attitude Reassessment (SAR) workshop, becoming OWL trained is a good way to open up one's mind and sexological (further elaborated in the text that follows) worldview.

Our Whole Lives Program Values

Keeping in mind these OWL program values, assumptions, and circles of sexuality makes excellent guidelines for sex-positive clinical health and therapy practice.

> *Self-Worth:* Every person is entitled to dignity and self-worth, and to their own attitudes and beliefs about sexuality.
>
> *Sexual Health:* Knowledge about human sexuality is helpful, not harmful. Every individual has the right to accurate information … . Healthy sexual relationships are consensual, nonexploitative, mutually pleasurable, safe [(low or no risk of sexually transmitted infections [STIs], emotional pain, unintended pregnancy)], developmentally appropriate …, based on mutual expectations and caring, [and] respectful. [Any type of] sexual intercourse is only one of the many valid ways of expressing sexual feelings.
>
> *Responsibility:* We enrich our lives by expressing sexuality in ways that enhance human wholeness and fulfillment [with potential to] express love and pleasure. All persons have the right and obligation to make responsible sexual choices.
>
> *Justice and Inclusivity:* We need to avoid double standards [and stereotypes]. People of all ages, [sexual identities,] races/ethnicities, genders, income levels, abilities, and sexual orientations must have equal value and rights. Sexual relationships should never be coercive or exploitative. Being romantically and sexually attracted to one's own gender (homosexual), another gender (heterosexual), one or more genders as well as one's own (bisexual), all genders (pansexual), or no one (asexual) is natural in the range of human sexual experience. (Tino et al., 2008/2023, pp. xii–xiii)

Our Whole Lives Assumptions

It can be helpful to hold these OWL assumptions in mind (Tino et al., 2023, p. xii):

- All humans are potentially sexual beings from before birth until death.
- "It is natural to express sexual feelings in a variety of ways."
- "Sexuality is a good part of the human experience [and] includes much more than sexual behavior."
- "People engage in healthy sexual behavior for a variety of reasons, including to express caring and love, to experience intimacy and connection with another, to share pleasure, to bring new life into the world, and [have] fun and [relax]."
- "Sexuality in our society is damaged by violence, exploitation, alienation, dishonesty, abuse of power, and the treatment of persons as objects."
- It is healthier for young teens to postpone forms of intercourse.

OWL has further clarified that while:

> all persons are sexual, this does not mean that all people are sexually interested or sexually active; rather, it means that we all have bodies to care for, decisions to make about sex and relationships, and an understanding of our gender or agender identity; and we are all affected by societal messages about sexuality. (Tino et al., 2008/2023, pg. xii)

Our Whole Lives Circles of Sexuality

This diagram, adapted by OWL, depicts the overlapping and intersecting circles of sexuality, which permeate human experience, according to OWL (see **Figure 1.1**). Dennis Dailey originally developed this for a youth education curriculum in 1995. It remains a solid framework from which to explore sexuality.

Sexuality encompasses nearly every aspect of our being, from attitudes and values to feelings and experiences. It is influenced by the individual, family, culture, religion/spirituality, laws, professions, institutions, science, and politics.

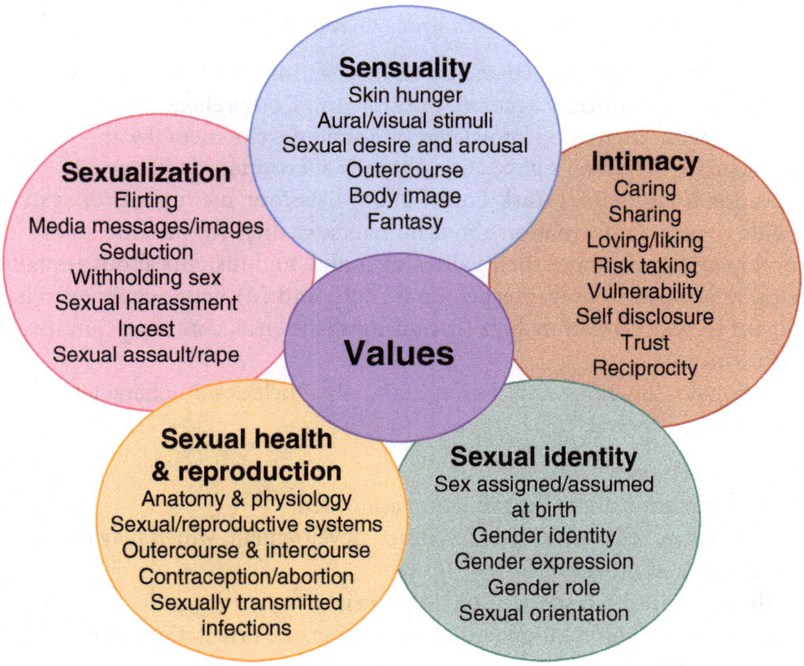

Sensuality involves our level of awareness, acceptance, and enjoyment of your own or others' bodies.

Intimacy is the experience of mutual closeness with another person.

Sexual identity is how we perceive ourselves as sexual beings.

Sexual health and reproduction focuses on attitudes and behaviors related to the sexual and reproductive systems, including health and hygiene, the health consequences of sexual behaviors, and the biology of producing children.

Sexualization involves the use of sexuality to influence, control, and/or manipulate others.

FIGURE 1.1. Circles of Sexuality

Source: Adapted from Life Planning Education. (1995). *Advocates for youth*. Washington, DC, Advocatesforyouth.org, based on the original work of Dennis Dailey, Professor Emeritus, University of Kansas.

PLANNED PARENTHOOD MODEL OF SEXUAL HEALTH

Planned Parenthood sex educators base their curriculum on material developed by ETR (Education, Training and Research), whose goal is to advance to health equity. ETR's textbook, *Sexuality Education: Theory and Practice* (Bruess & Schroeder, 2018), provides a wealth of history and information regarding sexuality education and lists several major guidelines for comprehensive sexuality education, such as the United Nations Educational, Scientific and Cultural Organization's (UNESCO) and the Sexuality Information and Education Council of the United States' (SIECUS) guidelines, as helpful psychoeducation. We can share these guidelines with our clients, pointing out that most of us never received any sex education at all, let alone comprehensive sex education adhering to these fairly extensive guidelines. Acknowledging the global and pervasive lack of helpful sex education can reduce our clients' sense of shame or inadequacy around any sexual health gaps they may possess.

UNESCO's sexuality education goals are:

> to equip children and young people with knowledge, skills, attitudes and values that will empower them to: realize their health, well-being and dignity; develop respectful social and sexual relationships; consider how their choices affect their own well-being and that of others; and, understand and ensure the protection of their rights throughout their lives. (2018, p. 16)

UNESCO advocates for both formal and nonformal settings, both in-school and out-of-school settings, and includes scientifically accurate information. Comprehensive sexuality education is incremental (building on increasing knowledge), age and developmentally appropriate, based on a curriculum, inclusive of human rights, and culturally appropriate and relevant.

SIECUS (National Guidelines Task Force, 2004) lists four main goals of sexuality education: (a) provide accurate information about human sexuality; (b) provide an opportunity for people to develop and understand their values, attitudes, and insights about sexuality; (c) help people develop relationships and interpersonal skills; and (d) help people exercise responsibility with regard to sexual relationships (including abstinence, contraception use, and coping with sexual pressure).

SIECUS (National Guidelines Task Force, 2004) also includes 30 characteristics of sexually healthy adults. Here are several:

- Appreciate one's own body.
- Seek further information about reproduction as needed.
- Affirm that human development includes sexual development, which may or may not include reproductive or sexual experience.
- Interact with all genders in respectful and appropriate ways.
- Affirm one's own sexual orientation and respect the sexual orientations of others.
- Affirm one's own gender identities and respect the gender identities of others.
- Reject sexual stereotypes and promote acceptance of diverse sexualities
- Express love and intimacy in appropriate ways.
- Avoid exploitative or manipulative relationships
- Develop and maintain meaningful relationships.
- Make informed choices about family options and relationships.
- Exhibit skills that enhance personal relationships.
- Identify and live according to one's own values.
- Take responsibility for one's own behavior.
- Practice effective decision-making.
- Develop critical-thinking skills.
- Communicate effectively with family, peers, and romantic partners.
- Enjoy and express one's sexuality throughout life.
- Express one's sexuality in ways that are congruent with one's values.
- Enjoy sexual feelings without necessarily acting on them.

GINA OGDEN'S 4-DIMENSIONAL WHEEL OF SEXUAL EXPERIENCE

Gina Ogden has developed a wonderfully comprehensive and holistic approach to sexual health, which is worth learning about briefly here and more on your own. Ogden's 4-Dimensional Wheel of Sexual Experience consists of four quadrants: physical, mental, emotional, and spiritual. These are similar to various psychotherapy frameworks (such as EMDR therapy) that include the three-prong approach of body, mind, and emotions (see **Figure 1.2**).

The physical quadrant involves the person's range of sensory experience (smell, touch, taste, sight, hearing), movement and stillness, comfort and safety, arousal, orgasm, and other physical pleasures/sensations. This quadrant can be characterized by heightened senses. The "shadow side" can contain pain, disgust, numbness, and dysfunction (Ogden, 2016a).

The emotional quadrant contains the person's range of feelings (love, passion, yearning, anger, hatred, and fear), empathy, self-compassion (defined by Kristen Neff [n.d.] as including the components of mindful awareness, self-kindness, and common humanity—we all suffer at some point), trust (the ability to let go of control), open-heartedness, and heightened feelings. The shadow side can include disappointment, anxiety, depression, restriction, anger, boredom, shame, and guardedness (Ogden, 2016a).

The mental quadrant includes beliefs and messages about sexuality and spirituality, including religious messages. Ogden also includes imagination, intuition, memory, dreams, waking dreams, and fantasies, along with wishes, intentions, anticipations, and expectations. This quadrant can involve a curious open mind, problem-solving, increased understanding, and expanded beliefs. The shadow side, however, may contain negative messages and rigid attitudes about what sex should be like (Ogden, 2016a)

The spiritual quadrant involves a deep sense of connection with one's self, partner(s), and/or "higher power." It can include inner visions, communication with divine forces, and experiencing oneself as part of all that is sacred. It can be characterized by ecstasy, increased energy, lasting satisfaction, connection, and transcendence. However, the shadow side can include a profound sense of isolation, depression, and paralysis (Ogden, 2016a).

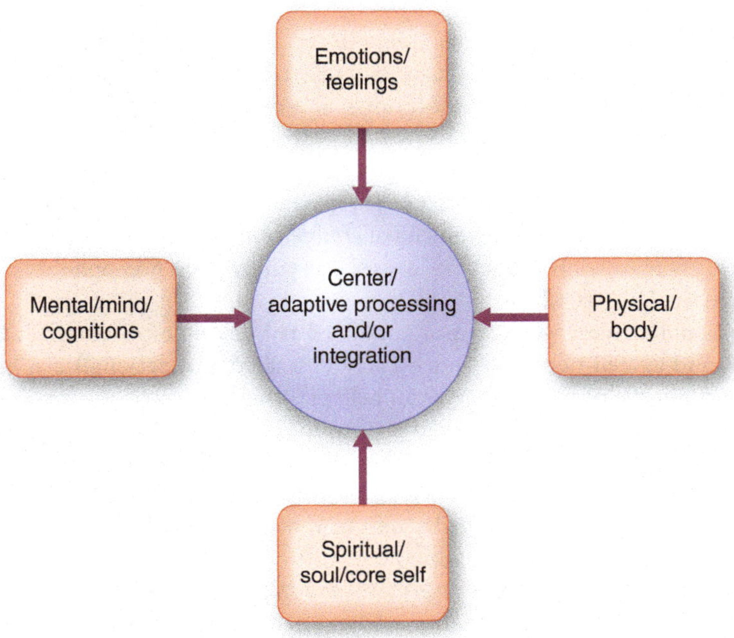

FIGURE 1.2. The Dimensions of Sexual Experience

Source: Adapted from Ogden, G. (2018). *Expanding the practice of sex therapy: The Neuro-update edition – An integrative approach for exploring desire and intimacy* (2nd ed.). Routledge.

The center of these four quadrants converging positively varies by individual. Some folks may report that visiting this center feels like a "high-definition Oz." The center "may feel like a place of mystery and paradox where opposites merge in an uncanny way" (Ogden, 2016b, p. 2). The person "may experience ... one-ness and, integration, shape-shifting, ... timelessness, light, and[/or] lightness of being" (2016b, p. 2). They may report communing "profoundly" with self and/or partner. The center may feel like "a place of clarity and vision, ... vastness, [and] unconditional love" (2016b, p. 2). As with the four quadrants, the center has a shadow side: hopelessness and despair (Ogden, 2016a).

You can have your client explore and address an issue using the four dimensions of the wheel. Create a sense of safety in the office, perhaps in one specific area (or one specific area in their home for teletherapy). Invite your client to try a movement to address the issue. Help your client develop a ritual. If possible, you may want to apply slow bilateral stimulation (BLS), such a butterfly hug tapping, to strengthen any positive responses. Concretize abstract concepts with tangible objects (feathers, rocks, shields, pillows, etc.) and have the client hold them while receiving the BLS and holding positive cognitions related to the concept.

Please refer to Ogden's 2018 book *Expanding the Practice of Sex Therapy* for full instruction on incorporating her 4-D Wheel into your client work. Consider completing the 4-D training and joining the 4-D network.

CREATE: SEX EDUCATION WITH ADULTS

Roz Dischiavo (2016) developed a holistic model for providing sex education to adults.

The CREATE acronym stands for:

- **C**reate community in the class.
- **R**educe erotophobia and disrupt systems of oppression.
- **E**stablish safety/"brave space."
- **A**cknowledge risks and encourage personal reflection.
- **T**each the information holistically.
- **E**valuate.

There are multiple ways to *create community* in the classroom from boundary and communication exercises to creating group collages or images. "Creating community requires an understanding of intersectionality, historical trauma, and oppressive systems that create divergent experiences in the room depending on race, ability, gender identity, orientation and other factors" (Dischiavo, 2023, p. 12).

Humor, factual information, open discussion, and "appropriate self-disclosure" can all help *reduce* the individual and cultural phenomena of *erotophobia* ("powerful, irrational fears about ... sexuality," [Ince, 2005, p. 7]). Erotophobia "causes everything from homophobia to laws against" abortion (Dischiavo, 2023, p. 12).

Offering optional activities and menus, graduated risk-taking of disclosure and interaction, trust exercises, and agreed-upon safe touch (fully described and optional) can help *establish* a sense of *safety* within the participants. We can help prevent and/or address "harm through community norms and ... plan for responding to racism, ableism, transphobia, ageism and homophobia" (Dischiavo, 2023, p. 13).

Personal reflection helps adults continue to consciously examine their own values and choices. This can also help students to acknowledge and take reasonable risks in the classroom such as sharing more deeply.

Teaching holistically involves utilizing many modalities of instruction, such as instruction that is experiential, involves practice, utilizes artistic expression, is based on accurate information, "demonstrate[s] an understanding of oppressive systems and use[s] approaches that create awareness of intersectional oppressions, [has] sexual proficiency as its goal, [is] embodied, and ... include[s] fun" (Dischiavo, 2023, p. 13).

Ideally, any learning is *evaluated* on four levels: reactions, actual learning, transfer of knowledge and skills, and results (such as an increased use of condoms or even pleasure-promoting devices such as adult sex toys). Both the content and the process should be evaluated (Dischiavo, 2023).

CONSENT

The concept of consent is relevant in all ways as we continue our journey toward integrating sexual health. Hopefully you are enthusiastically consenting to reading and integrating the information in this book. As we work with clients, particularly if we are helping them process potentially erotophobic environments, influences, and/or sexual trauma, we should constantly ask for and obtain consent. The #metoo movement has helped generate increased and essential discussion around sexual consent.

As someone who came of age in the eighties and nineties, not much was discussed or even known at that time about active negotiation of sex-related activities. During my work in the late nineties, primarily working with sexual assault survivors, consent concepts emerged in clinical work as well as in rape crisis educational campaigns. However, most of these campaigns centered around the "no means no" concept. This, of course, is paramount. Humans being able to say no to unwanted activities is the foundation from which we can later say yes to wanted activities.

Much of the 20th century stereotypical masculine and feminine gender expression involved the idea that a cisgender man should always want and try for sex, and that a "good" cisgender woman should be a "gatekeeper," saying no often, but eventually "giving in." One obvious and well-known example comes from Gone with the Wind, when Rhett Butler forcibly drags Scarlett O'Hara, kicking and fighting him, upstairs for sex. The very next scene shows her, apparently after sex, looking content. It wasn't okay for a woman to outright want and ask for sexual activity—that desire somehow put the woman in a "slut" category. Luckily, our wonderful 21st century has brought increased activism with folks naming "slut-shaming" as a bad thing, along with the creation of the problematic term *man-slut* (which I dislike), in an attempt to equalize notions of sexual desire.

Now that we are one-quarter into the 21st century, with #metoo solidly in place, humans thankfully continue to expand the conversation around consent. At a minimum, for a person to legally consent to any sexual activity (physical, verbal, or otherwise), the person needs to be of age (16 is the youngest age for any type of intercourse in Massachusetts; this varies state by state).

FRIES

Consent has further evolved into the excellent and helpful acronym FRIES. According to Planned Parenthood (n.d., What Is Consent), modern full consent is:

1. **F**reely given. "Consenting is a choice you make without pressure, manipulation, or under influence of drugs or alcohol."
2. **R**eversible. "Anyone can change their mind about what they feel like doing, anytime. Even if you've done it before" and you are preparing to do it again.
3. **I**nformed. "You can only consent if you have the full story. For example, if someone says they'll use a condom, but don't, then there isn't full consent."
4. **E**nthusiastic. "When it comes to sex, you should only do things you WANT to do, not things you are expected to do."
5. **S**pecific. "Saying yes to one thing (like going to the bedroom to make out) doesn't mean you've said yes to other" things (like intercourse).

I personally love the addition of enthusiasm, as this concept finally equalizes desire within all the genders. No longer does sex have to reflect the Western stereotype of a cisman being socialized all his life to seize any opportunity of sex (a concept resented by many cismen and others). Now ciswomen and other genders can seize the permission, and the imperative, to enthusiastically ask for what they want.

WHEEL OF CONSENT

Dr. Betty Martin developed the wheel of consent over the past few decades, resulting in her 2021 book publication on this topic (Martin & Dalzen, 2021). As a four-decade-plus bodyworker, she noticed the lack of attunement and awareness that many people experienced around what touch they were comfortable receiving and the difficulty they had noticing, advocating, and articulating their boundaries. She especially noticed that many people "endured unwanted and unsatisfying touch" over and over, tracing this pattern back to childhood socialization of unquestioned compliance with many kinds of boundary crossing edicts (i.e., hug your grandparents even if you don't feel like it). This socialization teaches people that their autonomy, choices, and "feelings do not matter." From these observations she developed her wheel of consent, consisting of these four quadrants—*serve, take, accept,* and *allow*—as a way to help people gain confidence in noticing and acting upon comfort and discomfort.

The *serve* quadrant involves "actions to benefit others" and is often called "giving." The *take* quadrant involves actions that benefit oneself. In both of these quadrants "you are doing" the action to someone else. The *allow* quadrant allows others to "act as they want" and the *accept* quadrant, also called "receiving," is where one "benefits from the actions of others." For these two quadrants the other person is the one doing or acting.

On the side of *serving* and *allowing*, actions by one person are "giving gifts" and are for the other person. On the side of the *take* and *accept* quadrants, someone is "receiving a gift" by the actions of another person.

At the center of the circle is where full consent exists, with actions of serving and receiving, taking and allowing fully articulated and agreed upon. Outside of the circle are the "shadow sides" of each quadrant: "do-gooder"/martyr (serve), perpetrator/thief/abuser/assailant (take), freeloader/entitled person (accept), and tolerating/enduring/victim/pushover (allow).

While the wheel is a bit more complicated to share with clients and students than the FRIES consent model, it may prove revelatory to many. Dr. Betty Martin encourages interested learners to review all of the information on her website and consider taking a workshop to gain true familiarity and facility in articulating these concepts to others (www.bettymartin.org).

FACTORS THAT PREVENT ADDRESSING SEXUAL HEALTH

Several factors can interfere with clinicians (even therapists who regularly discuss sexual trauma content) addressing positive sexual health with clients. Some of these factors include ongoing cultural erotophobia, clinicians' own discomfort in discussing sexuality, clinicians' own unexplored/unresolved issues regarding sexuality, and/or clinicians' own traumatic histories or propensity for vicarious traumatization (Saakvitne et al., 1996).

Even if we feel comfortable and confident discussing sexual health, we may harbor uncertainty about our clients' own comfort levels and interest, worrying that introducing sexual health material might make our clients uncomfortable. Other concerns for us may include perceived boundary issues, potential lawsuits, potential attraction/arousal, our own appropriate versus inappropriate curiosity, misspeaking a term, or introducing a topic on which we have less expertise.

However, according to Gallagher (2014), overall research shows that many clients want to bring up and discuss sexual concerns, yet most prefer their providers inquire first. Gallagher noted that, in fact, most clients rarely ever bring up their concern at all, likely due to concerns about whether they are "normal." In 2010, Klein noted that a typical view of "normal" sexuality includes: "sex when tired, too high or too low expectations, and awkwardness and self-consciousness," versus a joyful, fulfilling, and positive part of life.

Bringing sexual health into our intakes and conversations with our clients not only gives them much-needed permission to mention sexual concerns, but it also likely combats erotophobia in our society at large. In turn, our clients will be able to embrace a personal vision of their sexuality that goes beyond "normal," "typical," or "average" into the joyful and pleasurable extraordinary.

Finally, while perusing the *Psychology Today* therapist directory listings in 2020, sex therapy was not available as a psychotherapy focus/topic. As of May 2021, I am happy to report sex therapy is now an option.

THERAPIST'S SEXOLOGICAL WORLDVIEW

A sexological worldview is the "result of the socialization process that is comprised of values, beliefs, opinions, attitudes, and concepts specific to sexuality, including any and all sexual behavior and identities" (Sitron & Dyson, 2009 as cited in Sitron & Dyson, 2012, p. 2). This socialization comes from television, films, books, schools, the news, media, social media, pornography, religion, peers, family, and so on. As therapists, it is crucial that we continuously examine our own worldviews, remain aware that clients may not inhabit our worldview, and set aside our own biases in order to best help our clients.

Our goals for ourselves, and ultimately our clients, include moving away from a rigid right or wrong dualistic way of thinking, and instead move toward a more relativistic evolution of a changing, progressing world with room for greater sexual diversity and acceptance of others' realities. This larger worldview helps provide the foundation for a culturally competent sexual health practice.

Additionally, embracing the concept of polysemicity can help us attain this greater worldview. Polysemicity essentially means that someone else's experiences may not be what ours would be, even if we do the exact same thing (Klein, 2010). For example, two lesbian ciswomen can report very different experiences regarding the exact same sexual activity.

INCREASING COMFORT WITH ADDRESSING SEXUAL HEALTH

Two of the best ways to increase one's comfort level with addressing sexuality involve self-reflection (examining one's own biases and stereotypes) and continuously seeking information and education. Keeping a daily or weekly journal of your own experiences of sexuality and erotophobia helps increase self-reflection.

If reading this book is your first foray into accurate and empowering sexual health, it is a great step toward education. This book mentions many more resources that will hopefully find their way onto your office bookshelf or be bookmarked on your web browser. Stephanie Buehler's indispensable primer, *What Every Mental Health Professional Needs to Know About Sex*, Third Edition (2022), recommends topics for the professional to journal about at the end of each chapter, which is another wonderful step toward self-reflection and sexual health acclimation.

There are many organizations and individuals that offer specific training and workshops on sexual health. The national organization that addresses sex education and counseling is the American Association of Sexuality Educators, Counselors and Therapists (AASECT). For anyone wishing to pursue further sexuality certification, taking a 3-day SAR workshop is required. SARs are designed to "inundate participants with sexual material in order to bring awareness to areas of discomfort or bias, and through exploration and discussion, ease the participants into a place of greater comfort and confidence in approaching this work" (South Shore Sexual Health Center, n.d., What Is a S.A.R.?). I highly recommend signing up for a SAR workshop if you wish to expand your comfort with sexuality-related concerns. Not only will you learn about every imaginable sexual topic, often through videos, guest speakers/panels, interactive learning, and relevant readings, but you will meet a group of open-minded folks also willing to explore the outer limits of current societal norms. Completing a SAR will tackle both the self-reflection and educational piece, as well.

Another very effective strategy, one that I greatly benefited from in prior years, includes receiving regular consultation or supervision regarding your sexuality-related cases. I was fortunate to gather monthly with a small group of clinicians meeting at a sex therapy practice. These meetings provided education, validation, and space for reflection on bias and discomfort, as well as internalizing and integrating many of the concepts you will be reading further about in this book.

Case Study 1.1: Lily: Sexual Trauma, EMDR Therapy, Sexual Health, Sexual Rights and Values, PLISSIT, Consent, 4-D Wheel

The following case composite example draws from many clients for the purpose of illustrating the aforementioned sexual health frameworks, demonstrating how these additional lenses can help a clinician search for sexual health–related elements. Mostly sexual frameworks are touched upon in this example. The following chapters explore the intersection of therapy and sexual health in greater detail. This particular example showcases sexual health in relation to EMDR therapy.

Lily sought EMDR therapy to process and treat preteen sexual trauma by teenage neighbors, an early college sexual assault, and current sexual dissatisfaction. Lily has a full-time job in human resources, is a lesbian-identified ciswoman in her late thirties, is bicultural (Puerto Rican and Irish heritage), is a practicing Catholic, and is in a committed long-term monogamous relationship with another ciswoman. She also reported an abortion related to the college sexual assault.

Placing her life experience within the circles of sexuality, she experienced sexualization (unwanted sexual activity), reproductive concerns (she continues to harbor shame and guilt about the abortion), intimacy concerns (difficulty trusting her partner), and sensuality concerns (current lack of pleasure with touch, infrequent orgasms, poor body image, and lack of sexual fantasy). She reports comfort with her sexual identity as an out lesbian and ciswoman.

Lily met the criteria for posttraumatic stress disorder (PTSD) due to flashbacks, nightmares, avoidance of sexual interaction, irritability, and negative beliefs about herself. She also met the criteria for hypoactive sexual desire disorder due to a persistent reported lack of sexual interest. Due to the tendency of trauma and lack of sexual desire to substantially overlap, we decided to treat the trauma first.

We processed all the obvious substantial trauma ("large T" Trauma, i.e. trauma reported by Lily as severely disturbing) EMDR therapy processed the preteen sexual abuse and the college sexual assault to the point where those events no longer bothered her (and she was free of the prior reported PTSD symptoms).

We next determined that there were many small trauma ("small t," i.e., trauma reported by Lily as mildly to moderately disturbing) targets. These targets related to the negative messaging of sexuality she experienced within her family culture as well as from the religious Catholic culture within which she was raised.

Indeed, as we further explored, we found numerous EMDR therapy targets that rated three or higher on the subjective units of distress scale (SUDs) of 0 to 10 (0 is neutral, 10 is the most disturbing), such as nuns at her Catholic school shaming Lily's makeup, her mother's disapproval of her clothing choice (calling her "a slutty dresser"), and the neighborhood boys catcalling her (she had developed breasts and other puberty changes slightly earlier than her cisfemale peers).

Lily had never received any accurate sex education other than "don't have sex." No one in her family instructed her about menarche; menstrual pads simply showed up in her bathroom drawer one day.

Broadly speaking, she had not been provided with any healthy or accurate sexual education or framework. She had no idea, even through her late twenties, that she was entitled to a "positive and respectful approach to sexuality" (WHO, n.d.), a life free from sexual abuse, nor was she aware of the basic tenets of consent.

Throughout the therapy, permission (from the PLISSIT) was often given for Lily to discuss her trauma and sexuality concerns and questions. Often limited information was provided in the form of sexuality-related self-help resources such as books on women's sexuality. As she had reported some numbing in her genital region, she was referred to a local respected sex-positive ob/gyn to rule out any medical condition.

Many sessions were spent on normalizing sexual health and sexuality, including the right to engage in sexual behavior simply for pleasure and connection. Keeping in mind SIECUS's 30 characteristics of sexually healthy adults, the positive thought/cognitions of "I am normal and can enjoy my body," "I have the right to enjoy and express my sexuality," and "I can identify and ask for what I want" were identified and frequently used. Lily's initial negative cognitions were: "Something is wrong with me," "I can't be vulnerable," and "I don't have choice or voice."

Once all these "small t" EMDR targets were addressed, we then used Ogden's 4-D Wheel to identify any lingering difficulties or challenges. Physically, Lily continued to report some difficulty identifying arousal and other pleasurable signs. Emotionally, she noticed continued fear and shame. Mentally, she continued to harbor lingering messages of guilt around sexual enjoyment from her Catholic background, particularly in light of the homophobia she went through in her coming out process. These generated even more "small t" appearing targets, which ended up rating higher on the SUDs upon further activation, pushing them into more "big T" trauma territory. Spiritually, she reported a lack of deep connection to her body and her partner.

We were able to find more recent and current EMDR targets based on the 4-D Wheel categories. For example, Lily noted that when her partner approached her from behind to hug her, she froze and went numb, essentially shutting down. Once we processed these more current/present targets, we developed and processed several EMDR future templates (a form of future rehearsal) to navigate through any lingering negative experiences of her sexuality.

Additionally, Lily and her partner had joined an Episcopalian "welcoming" congregation a couple of years ago (specifically welcoming to LGBTQ+ folks). She was now able to parse out her own spiritual identity, retain similar pieces to her Catholic upbringing that continued to feel meaningful and positive (her relationship to Jesus and Mary), and enjoy a new comfort during church services knowing that she was "normal," loved, and enthusiastically accepted as herself.

Lily also chose to strengthen more positive resources via EMDR therapy into a vision of self-acceptance. This resource included envisioning her cherished Celtic cross given to her by a nurturing and warm Irish grandmother (representing unconditional love and spiritual connection), shells found in Puerto Rico (representing openness and sensual connection), and her engagement ring from her supportive partner (representing trust, healthy risk-taking, mutual sharing, and pleasure). Lily reported consistently being able to identify and ask for what she wanted, not only sexually, but in her profession, family of origin, and friendships.

At this point, criteria were no longer met for hypoactive sexual desire disorder. Lily noted consistent sensation perception throughout her body, including her genitals, more orgasms, and a greater interest and ability to receive and enjoy sexual connection with her partner. Her frequency of interest now more closely matched her partner's reported frequency. Lily also more easily accessed the "center" of her 4-D Wheel, experiencing timelessness, unconditional love, and integration of mental, physical, emotional, and spiritual quadrants during some of her sexual experiences. At the mutual decision of client and therapist, Lily discharged from therapy with many sex-positive resources, messages, sources of encouragement, and additional support to pursue pleasure and connection with herself and her fiancé.

SUMMARY

The WHO and the Office of the Surgeon General and Office of Population Affairs both have helpful definitions of sexual health. A working definition of sexual activity is provided, and the uplifting and affirming WAS's Declaration of Sexual Rights and Pleasure is shared.

The PLISSIT model is a consent-based and comprehensive model for sexual health communication and intervention.

The OWL and the Planned Parenthood curricula embrace many sex-positive values (e.g., dignity and self-worth, knowledge, choice, equal rights and value), which we can keep in mind in our work with clients. Gina Ogden's 4-D Wheel of Sexuality (mental, physical, emotional, spiritual, and center dimensions) also offers a helpful and holistic clinical framework. The CREATE model offers holistic guidance for sex education with adults. The concept of consent (particularly FRIES) is extremely important, not only regarding clients' experiences with sexual activity, but for ourselves as therapists as we inquire about our clients' sexual health.

Many individual and cultural factors (e.g., erotophobia) impact therapists' potential comfort and discomfort in addressing sexual health with their clients. Therapists also bring their own sexological worldview into the session; therefore, gaining knowledge and familiarity with sexual health is critical. There are many ways therapists can increase their comfort with sexual material, including training such as a SAR workshop.

DISCUSSION QUESTIONS

- How does a lack of standardized, fact-based, and comprehensive sex education contribute to an increased risk of sexual trauma?
- How has an ongoing lack of standardized and comprehensive sex education perpetuated erotophobia?
- How might increasing access to basic sexual health information regarding consent, as well as sexual rights and pleasure, result in decreased STIs, unplanned pregnancies, and reduced instances of sexual trauma/abuse?
- What would you choose to feature in a public service announcement (PSA) regarding your top 10 most important elements of positive sexual health (drawing from characteristics of sexually healthy adults, sexual rights and pleasure, and OWL values)?

LEARNING ACTIVITIES

CourseConnect

To access self-assessment questions and interactive, competency-based learning activities for this chapter, visit www.springerpub.com/courseconnect. See inside front cover and tear-out card for CourseConnect details.

ADDITIONAL RESOURCES

Additional resources are online and available at www.springerpub.com/courseconnect.

REFERENCES

Annon, J. S. (1976). The PLISSIT model: A proposed conceptual scheme for the behavioral treatment of sexual problems. *Journal of Sex Education and Therapy, 2*(1), 1–15. https://doi.org/10.1080/01614576.1976.11074483

Bright, S. (1997). *Sexual state of the union*. Touchstone.

brown, a. m. (2019). *Pleasure activism: The politics of feeling good*. AK Press.

Bruess, C., & Schroeder, E. (2018). *Sexuality education: Theory and practice* (7th ed.). ETR.

Buehler, S. (2022). *What every mental health professional needs to know about sex* (3rd ed.). Springer Publishing Company.

Calzo, J. P., & Blashill, A. J. (2018). Child sexual orientation and gender identity in the adolescent brain cognitive development cohort study. *JAMA Pediatrics, 172*(11), 1090–1092. https://doi.org/10.1001/jamapediatrics.2018.2496

Centers for Disease Control and Prevention. (2024, January 23). *Sexual violence prevention: About sexual violence.* https://www.cdc.gov/sexual-violence/about/#cdc_behavioral_basics_quick-quick-facts-and-stats

Cusack, K. J., Frueh, B. C., & Brady, K. T. (2004). Trauma history screening in a community mental health clinic. *Psychiatric Services, 55*(2), 157–162. https://doi.org/10.1176/appi.ps.55.2.157

Dailey, D. (1995). *Circles of sexuality as depicted in life planning education: A youth development program.* University of Kansas.

Dischavio, R. (2016). *The deep yes: The lost art of true receiving.* Spanda Press.

Dischiavo, R. (2023). *The exceptional educator: Sex education theory & methods.* Institute for Sex Education & Enlightenment.

Dodson, B. (1996). *Sex for one: The joy of self-loving.* Three River Press.

Gallagher, K. (2014, October). *Pandora's box: Sex from A to Z in clinical work* [Presentation]. Brattleboro Retreat.

Global Advisory Board for Sexual Health and Wellbeing. (2016). *Working definition of sexual pleasure.* https://www.gab-shw.org/our-work/working-definition-of-sexual-pleasure

Ince, J. (2005). *The politics of lust.* Prometheus Books.

Klein, M. (2010, April). *When sex gets complicated: Pornography, kink, cybersex, and other clinical challenges* [Workshop]. American Society of Sex Educators, Counselors and Therapists Northeast Region Meet and Greet, Florence, Massachusetts.

Kleinplatz, P. J., Menard, A. D., Paquet, M.-P., Paradis, N., Campbell, M., Zuccarino, D., & Mehak, L. (2009). The components of optimal sexuality: A portrait of "great" sex. *The Canadian Journal of Human Sexuality, 18*(1–2), 1–13. https://juliacolwell.com/wp-content/uploads/2017/05/The-components-of-optimal-sexuality-Kleinplatz-et-al.-2009.pdf

Lewis, R. W., Fugl-Meyer, K. S., Corona, G., Hayes, R. D., Laumann, E. O., Moreira, E. D., Jr., Rellini, A. H., & Segraves, T. (2010). Definitions/epidemiology/risk factors for sexual dysfunction. *The Journal of Sexual Medicine, 7*(4), 1598–1607. https://doi.org/10.1111/j.1743-6109.2010.01778.x

Luchterhand, C. (2014). *Whole health: Change the conversation: Advancing skills in the delivery of personalized, proactive, patient-driven care: The PLISSIT model clinical tool.* University of Wisconsin-Madison School of Medicine and Public Health.

Martin, B., & Dalzen, R. (2021). *The art of receiving and giving: The wheel of consent.* Luminaire Press.

Massachusetts General Court. (2025). *An Act relative to parental rights in education, H.551.* https://malegislature.gov/Bills/194/H551

Nagoski, E. (2015). *Come as you are.* Simon & Schuster.

National Guidelines Task Force. (2004). *Guidelines for comprehensive sexuality education: Kindergarten through 12th grade* (3rd ed.). Sexuality Information and Education Council of the United States. https://siecus.org/wp-content/uploads/2024/05/Guidelines_3ed.pdf

Neff, K. (n.d.). *What is self-compassion?* https://self-compassion.org/what-is-self-compassion

Neumann, D. A., Houskamp, B. M., Pollock, V. E., & Briere, J. (1996). The long-term sequelae of childhood sexual abuse in women: A meta-analytic review. *Child Maltreatment, 1*(1), 6–16. https://doi.org/10.1177/1077559596001001002

Office of the Surgeon General and Office of Population Affairs. (2001, July 9). *The Surgeon General's call to action to promote sexual health and responsible sexual behavior.* Office of the Surgeon General. https://www.ncbi.nlm.nih.gov/books/NBK44216

Ogden, G. (2016a, May). *Exploring the 4-D Wheel of Sexual Health.* Workshop presented at the AASECT Northeast Region Meet and Greet, Florence, MA.

Ogden, G. (2016b). *The four-dimensional wheel of sexual experience (4-D wheel): An organizing principle for exploring sexual stories—past, present, & future* [Handout]. AASECT Northeast Region Meet and Greet, Florence, MA.

Ogden, G. (2018). *Expanding the practice of sex therapy: The Neuro-update edition—An integrative approach for exploring desire and intimacy* (2nd ed.). Routledge.

Planned Parenthood. (n.d.). *Sexual consent.* Retrieved January 17, 2025, from https://www.plannedparenthood.org/learn/relationships/sexual-consent

Queen, C. (2002). *Real-live nude girl: Chronicles of sex-positive culture.* Cleis Press.

Robinson, B. E., Bockting, W. O., Rosser, B. R. S., Miner, M., & Coleman, E. (2002). The sexual health model: Application of a sexological approach to HIV prevention. *Health Education Research, 17*(1), 43–57. https://doi.org/10.1093/her/17.1.43

Saakvitne, K. W., Pearlman, L. A., & Staff. (1996). *Transforming the pain: A workbook on vicarious traumatization.* W. W. Norton & Company.

Sitron, J. A., & Dyson, D. A. (2009). Sexuality attitudes reassessment (SAR): Historical and new considerations for measuring its effectiveness. *American Journal of Sexuality Education, 4,* 158–177. https://doi.org/10.1080/15546120903001407

Sitron, J. A., & Dyson, D. A. (2012, March 13). Validation of sexological worldview: A construct for the use in the training of sexologists in sexual diversity. *SAGE Open, 2*(1). https://doi.org/10.1177/2158244012439072

South Shore Sexual Health Center. (n.d.). *Home page.* Retrieved January 29, 2025, from https://www.southshoresexualhealthcenter.com/getcertified

Tallon-Hicks, Y. (2022). *Hot and unbothered: How to think about, talk about, and have the sex you really want.* HarperCollins.

Tino, M. J., Millspaugh, S. G., & Haave, L. A. (2023). *Our Whole Lives: Sexuality education for young adults, ages 18–35.* Unitarian Universalist Association. (Original work published 2008)

Trans Legislation Tracker. (n.d.). *2025 anti-trans bills tracker.* Retrieved February 18, 2025, from https://translegislation.com

United Nations Educational, Scientific and Cultural Organization. (2018). *International technical guidance on sexuality education: An evidence-informed approach* (2nd rev. ed.). https://unesdoc.unesco.org/ark:/48223/pf0000260770/PDF/260770eng.pdf.multi

van der Hart, O., Nijenhuis, E. R. S., & Steele, K. (2006). *The haunted self: Structural dissociation and the treatment of chronic traumatization.* W. W. Norton and Company.

Westheimer, R., Grunebaum, A., & Lehu, P. (2012). *Sexually speaking: What every woman needs to know about sexual health.* John Wiley and Sons.

Wilson, P. (2014). *Our Whole Lives: Sexual education for grades 7–9* (2nd ed.). Unitarian Universalist Association.

World Association for Sexual Health. (2014, March). *Declaration of sexual rights.* https://www.worldsexualhealth.net/_files/ugd/793f03_779f193815894895b9d1480bde676c37.pdf

World Association for Sexual Health. (2019). *Declaration on sexual pleasure.* https://www.worldsexualhealth.net/was-declaration-on-sexual-pleasure

World Health Organization. (n.d.). *Sexual and reproductive health and rights.* Retrieved January 17, 2025, from https://www.who.int/health-topics/sexual-and-reproductive-health-and-rights

Yehuda, R., Lehrner, A., & Rosenbaum, T. Y. (2015). PTSD and sexual dysfunction in men and women. *The Journal of Sexual Medicine, 12*(5), 1107–1119. https://doi.org/10.1111/jsm.12856

SUPPLEMENTAL MATERIALS FOR CLINICIANS AND CLIENTS

For PDF versions of this material, access the "Downloads" feature on Course Connect (www.springerpub.com/courseconnect).

DECLARATION OF SEXUAL RIGHTS, PLEASURE, AND CONSENT HANDOUT

Since 1978, the World Association for Sexual Health (WAS) has worked toward sexual health and rights. Thousands of members attend global biennial congresses and in recent years have made declarations for sexual rights.

DECLARATION OF SEXUAL RIGHTS

1. The right to equality and freedom of sexual expression
2. The right to make decisions about one's body in regard to sexuality
3. The right to be safe from all forms of sexual violence and coercion, and be free from inhumane treatment or punishment because of one's sexual or gender expression
4. The right to accurate scientific information and education about sexuality and sexual health
5. The right to freely create and dissolve marital and other similar relationships
6. The right to family planning resources
7. The right to organize freely to promote sexual rights and health
8. The right to privacy regarding sexual matters
9. The right to judicious laws and remedies regarding sexual rights
10. The right to the highest attainable standard of sexual health, including sexual safe and pleasurable sexual experiences

Source: Adapted from the World Association for Sexual Health. (2014, March). *Declaration of sexual rights*. https://www.worldsexualhealth.net/_files/ugd/793f03_779f193815894895b9d1480bde676c37.pdf

DECLARATION ON SEXUAL PLEASURE

> Sexual pleasure is the physical and/or psychological satisfaction and enjoyment derived from shared or solitary erotic experiences, including thoughts, dreams and autoeroticism. Self-determination, consent, safety, privacy, confidence and the ability to communicate and negotiate sexual relations are key ... factors for pleasure to contribute to sexual health and wellbeing. Sexual pleasure should be exercised within the context of sexual rights [including] equality and non-discrimination, autonomy and bodily integrity, and the right to the highest ... standard of health and freedom of expression. The experiences of human sexual pleasure are diverse and sexual rights ensure that pleasure is a positive experience for all concerned and not obtained by violating ... human rights and wellbeing. (GAB, 2016)

Some of WAS's Declaration of Sexual Rights include:

- Sexual pleasure is a fundamental part of sexual and human rights and includes the possibility of diverse sexual experiences.
- Access to appropriate sources of sexual pleasure is part of human well-being.
- Sexual health and well-being include pleasurable and safe sexual experiences free of discrimination, coercion, and violence.
- Sexual pleasure shall be globally integrated into education, health services, research, and advocacy and contributes to global health.

CONSENT

According to Planned Parenthood (n.d., What Is Consent), modern full FRIES consent is:

1. Freely given. "Consenting is a choice you make without pressure, manipulation, or under influence of drugs or alcohol."

2. Reversible. "Anyone can change their mind about what they feel like doing, anytime. Even if you've done it before," and you are preparing to do it again.
3. Informed. "You can only consent if you have the full story. For example, if someone says they'll use a condom, but don't, then there isn't full consent."
4. Enthusiastic. "When it comes to sex, you should only do things you WANT to do, not things you are expected to do."
5. Specific. "Saying yes to one thing (like going to the bedroom to make out) doesn't mean you've said yes to other" things (like intercourse).

CHAPTER 2

Sexual and Reproductive Anatomy and Health

Stephanie Baird

LEARNING OBJECTIVES

- Learn elementary internal and external generative and erectile sexual anatomy and development.
- Learn about the complex interplay of chromosomes, hormones, and anatomy that can result in a variety of biological expression, demonstrating the spectrum (versus binary) nature of sex and gender (including intersex).
- Learn basic sexual health information regarding fertility and pregnancy.
- Learn essential sexual health information (sexually transmitted infections [STIs], HIV, pregnancy prevention, abortion, safer sex).

INTRODUCTION

If this is your first book and/or class addressing sexual health, this chapter provides some basic medical and scientific reference information, including explanations of reproductive/sexual systems. Other books that go into much greater biological detail include *What Every Mental Health Professional Needs to Know About Sex*, Third Edition (Buehler, 2022); *Our Bodies, Ourselves* (Boston Women's Health Book Collective, 2011), and the more lay-person friendly *The Guide to Getting It On* (Joannides, 2017).

IN UTERO SEXUAL/REPRODUCTIVE ANATOMY DEVELOPMENT AND DIFFERENTIATION

In a college level Women's Studies class in conservative Texas in the early 1990s, I learned that all human embryos start out with undifferentiated potential reproductive organ morphology. If there were no Y chromosome and/or low testosterone, the initially ambiguous gonadal material usually defaulted into commonly grouped organs designated "female," such as ovaries, vulva, and clitoris. My mind was blown. The professor explained that as the embryo grows, around week eight, the specific chromosomes indicate which sex hormones will begin releasing. I had always suspected that we humans had a lot more in common with each other, versus differences. And here was proof that we all start out with similar formats!

Biology has continued to evolve a much more complex picture of embryonic development (Toulson & Landon, 2021). More specifically, initial "primordial structures include egg shaped organs" and tissues. These structures later differentiate into "generative and erectile organs" including gametes where androgens (hormones) such as testosterone, estrogen, and progesterone will be produced (Toulson & Landon, 2022). Additionally, "two pairs of ducts … will differentiate into the tubes that gametes travel through when they leave the gonads along with other urinary and reproductive structures" (Toulson & Landon, 2022, p. 1). Sex chromosomes alone do not dictate which structures develop. Hormones, cellular receptors, *and* the environment (particularly industrial and pharmaceutical chemicals, which can act as androgen or antiandrogen mimics) *also greatly* influence reproductive and tissue differentiation (Toulson & Landon, 2022).

If the chromosomes are XX, with appropriate androgen levels and cellular receptors, the gonadal material develops into the default labia and vulva (versus scrotum) and clitoris (versus penis). For an XY chromosomal presence, the ambiguous gonadal genitalia generally will morph into testosterone-producing testes (along with a penis), as long as specific levels of androgens and cellular receptors enable the cells to respond to these hormonal signals (Toulson & Landon, 2022).

Folks born with intersex or ambiguous genitalia or organs may have chromosomal variations (XXY, XO, XXX, XYY, etc.) or have experienced different hormonal influences while in the womb. This can result in less typically combined *intersex* external and/or internal sex organs, as explained later in this chapter.

ESTROGEN-DOMINANT ANATOMY AND DEVELOPMENT

EXTERNAL SEXUAL ANATOMY: CLITORIS, VULVA, LABIA, PERINEUM

Someone who experiences an estrogen-dominant body and puberty develops external genitalia that generally include "the *mons pubis* (or fatty pad below the abdomen); the *vulva* that consists of the *labia majora* (larger "lips") and *labia minora* (smaller lips); the *clitoris*; and the entrance to the vagina, called the *introitus*. The *perineum* is the strip of skin between the vagina and anus [and can be sensitive to touch. The *external urethral orifice* (exit for urine)] is located between the clitoris and vagina" (Buehler, 2022, p. 20; see **Figure 2.1**).

An article in *The Guardian* reported research by El-Hamamsy and colleagues (2021) that half of nearly 200 British patients in hospital waiting rooms surveyed could not identify the urethra,

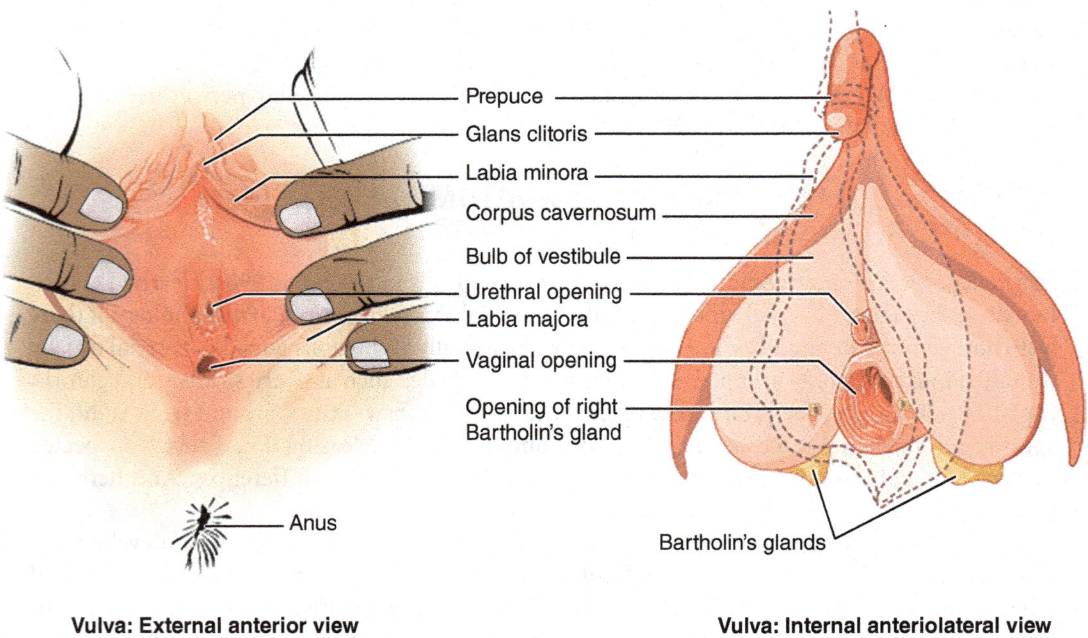

FIGURE 2.1. Vulva, External Anterior View and Internal Anteriolateral View

Source: Betts, J. G., Young, K. A., Wise, J. A., Johnson, E., Poe, B., Kruse, D. H., Korol, O., Johnson, J. E., Womble, M., & DeSaix, P. (2013, April 25). *Anatomy and physiology* (2nd ed., Fig. 27.10). OpenStax. https://openstax.org/books/anatomy-and-physiology/pages/27-2-anatomy-and-physiology-of-the-female-reproductive-system. Licensed under CC BY 4.0 (https://creativecommons.org/licenses/by/4.0).

while 37% mislabeled the clitoris—regardless of their gender (Geddes, 2021). Only 46% of this sample correctly identified that people with vaginas have three "holes" (vagina, urethra, and anus). Additionally, the respondents were given diagrams of external and internal sexual and reproductive anatomy to label. Only half even attempted to label the diagram, and of those who did, just 9% labeled the requested structures correctly. Many respondents confused the urethra with the clitoris, and vice versa. Based on my own clinical practice with clients over the years, I have little reason to think that folks on this side of the pond would do much better with these diagrams. Such a poor understanding of sexual anatomy does not bode well for self-advocacy, informed consent, or even basic health seeking (El-Hamamsy et al., 2021).

Erectile Organs and Tissues

Clitoral Complex (Erectile Organ)

The clitoral complex, an incredibly sensitive organ with thousands of nerve endings, is the only organ in any body that appears to have an exclusive pleasure function and not play double duty. Due to this high concentration of nerve endings (the highest in any organ), the clitoris (an external **AND** internal glans) is covered by a "hood" of skin that can retract when aroused. The clitoris was only recently discovered to be much larger than believed, having two leg-like extensions that are contained internally within the pelvis (Pauls, 2015) and connected to the vulva. Therefore, it is more of a dual organ, configured both externally and internally. Internally, this system possesses a "root, crura, and bulbs."

The overall average size from external visible glans to internal legs comprises a 4-inch range. The dorsal nerve of the clitoris, part of the pudendal nerve, is responsible for "clitoral somatic innervation" (Pauls, 2015) and are the primary source of sensation. Just recently, Uloko et al. (2023, Results) confirmed that the "mean number of myelinated nerve fibers innervating the human clitoris was 10,281," far higher than the previously assumed and frequently cited 8,000 nerve endings.

Most aroused clitorises will experience vasocongestion and swelling (both in the external glans and in the internal "legs") from blood accumulation due to sexual stimulation (physical and/or mental stimulation). The clitoral glans may eventually pull back inside the clitoral hood, perhaps due to increased sensitivity, with high arousal.

Some clients may report a lack of sensitivity in their clitoral area. If possible, refer your client for a full genital evaluation by a respected and preferably feminist-oriented skilled sex-positive midwife or ob/gyn in your area. [Be careful with your referrals as many clients may disclose uncomfortable past experiences at gynecologist offices.] If medical causes are ruled out, this numbness may be related to overall body numbness from dissociative symptoms related to prior (most likely sexual) traumatic experiences. With the PLISSIT (**P**ermission, **L**imited **I**nformation, **S**pecific **S**uggestions, and **I**ntensive **T**herapy) model in place (giving clients permission to feel and explore their anatomy, plus psychoeducation about the clitoris and orgasm), sensitivity may return to the clitoris. Often, once traumatic, erotophobic, and/or disturbing material is processed and worked through (possibly via eye movement desensitization and reprocessing [EMDR] therapy), a sense of comfort or safety can be established within the client's own physical environment, body, and mind, allowing them to more easily notice and interact with physical sensation.

Psychological Clitorectomy

The notable journalist Peggy Orenstein, in interviewing 70 teen girls for her book on *Girls and Sex* (2016), coined the term *psychological clitorectomy*. This refers to the lack of instruction to females about the existence and role of the clitoris in sexual pleasure, leaving essentially a blank space in their sexual functioning. This omission deemphasizes and decenters female sexual pleasure, placing the emphasis on male sexual pleasure. Of note, it was either in the aforementioned Women's Studies college class, or in another Human Sexuality college-level class (circa 1993), when I first heard the word *clitoris* uttered out loud. Although I was 20 years old at the time, I knew very little about my own anatomy. Much of modern medical research has mostly been conducted on cismale-gendered bodies. Only in the recent decade have scientists even begun to research pregnancy! Paul Joannides (2017) corroborates that even recently, in the late 2010s, when he asked large college audiences how many of them learned about the clitoris from a parent, very few students raised their hands.

In the *Science Vs* podcast episode "The G-Spot" (Zuckerman, 2016), Wendy Zuckerman discusses how researcher Helen O'Connell suggests using the term "clitoral complex" to indicate the vastness and complex relationship of clitoral elements to the nearby urethra, vulva, and vagina, especially during arousal and engorgement. O'Connell et al. (2005) noted that throughout history, going back to the year 1561 when anatomist Fallopia described the clitoris, information about the clitoris has alternated between accessible and available to hidden and disappeared. Historical information documenting its existence appeared again around 1700, and again in 1900, when it was labeled in the 1901 edition of *Gray's Anatomy*. However, in the 1946 edition, there was no mention or depiction of the clitoris.

Case Study 2.1: Richita, Genital Numbness

This brief EMDR and sexual health case example illustrates the return of genital sensation.

Richita, a ciswoman restaurant chef, sought EMDR therapy for adolescence sexual abuse targets. She reported being raised by "overprotective, rigid," and noncommunicative Southeast Asian professional immigrant parents in a suburb of Boston. She also reported abuse by an older male cousin, which was never disclosed until now. As a result of this perceived parentally oppressive environment, plus the sexual abuse, she reported "acting out" sexually in her late teens and early twenties, yet deriving no sexual sensation, pleasure, nor satisfaction. She also began engaging in substance use during this time, to help "numb" out.

Now in her early thirties, Richita reported success with obtaining and maintaining sobriety from substances. At this point in her recovery she wanted to heal from the sexual trauma and get in touch with her sexual body. As we worked through the EMDR targets relating to the sexual abuse, her parents' oppressive parenting behaviors, and many of her negative experiences with addiction and sexuality, she reported beginning to notice sensation in her genitals. Sensation had largely been absent for many years. She was referred to Betty Dodson's book on learning how to have orgasms, called *Sex for One: The Joy of Self-Loving* (1996).

Between EMDR therapy and sexual health psychoeducation, she noted a gradual increase of sensation, eventually reporting pleasurable masturbation accompanied by orgasms. She also realized that it was easier to focus on pleasure and experiencing orgasms by playing music to help drown out outside noise. Additionally, she became more comfortable with explaining her sexual needs to current partners, thereby increasing her presence, sensual enjoyment, and positive genital experience with said partners.

Labia (Appears to Swell, Due to Erectile Clitoral Bulbs of Vestibule)

Labia have sensitive nerve endings and can appear to engorge and deepen in color with stimulation. Due to the rise of easily available pornography, some people have become self-conscious about their labia color or size and have fallen prey to surgical procedures such as "labiaplasty" (to change the shape and/or size of the labia) or even "vaginoplasty" (to supposedly tighten a loosened vagina). These costly procedures are neither medically necessary nor recommended, as genitals come in all shapes and sizes, and surgery may cause lasting scarring and interfere with sexual function and pleasure (American College of Obstetricians and Gynecologists [ACOG], 2020). If your clients report any dissatisfaction with the appearance of their genitalia, these dissatisfactions may be good topics to explore with a sex therapist or other well-boundaried practitioner comfortable with helping the client attain acceptance and celebration of their unique genitals.

Nipples (Erectile)

For many bodies (of any gender), breasts/chests and nipples may show sensitivity and harden when stimulated. Some breasts may visibly increase in size when aroused, and the skin tone/color may flush or change in color. Some folks may feel self-conscious of their nipple color or the size of the areolas (the dark area around the nipples), as well as breast/chest size (clients may consider this area too big, too small, too "unusually" shaped, or too saggy), or presence or absence of hair in the nipple area. Once again, any unease or discomfort related to appearance can be explored during therapy, with the goal of acceptance and celebration.

Orgasm

Pleasurable physical stimulation and positive mental sexual context generally must occur in order to facilitate an orgasm (or multiple orgasms). An orgasm is often experienced as release of sexual tension through rhythmic contractions of the uterus and vagina, for people with vulvas and clitorises. People with clitorises are more likely to have longer orgasms and to be able to orgasm again quickly after the first orgasm. For people with penises, it is often experienced as a release of tension of the prostate gland and seminiferous tubules (during orgasm, semen is often ejaculated from the penis, though not always).

During orgasm, heart rate, respiration, and blood pressure are at their peak. People may also notice myotonia, which is the tightening of muscles, aka muscle tension. Orgasms may last from a few seconds to a couple minutes, depending on anatomy and other factors. People with clitorises are more likely to have longer orgasms and to be able to orgasm again very quickly after the first orgasm.

For all brains and bodies experiencing orgasm, various brain euphoria and craving-related regions and neurotransmitters (dopamine and oxytocin) are associated with orgasm. Orgasm results from a convergence of activity between these neurotransmitters and areas in the hypothalamus, cerebellum, amygdala, and hippocampus, among other brain regions (Komisaruk & Rodriguez Del Cerro, 2021). So, yes, the brain can be considered the most important pleasure organ.

Clitoral Stimulation Orgasm

Unfortunately, despite all the consciousness-raising groups in the 1970s where ciswomen examined their genitalia with hand mirrors, very few ciswomen have ever visually inspected their genitals once, let alone regularly. People with penises have frequent opportunities (typically during urination or masturbation) to observe their genitals. I, and many other authors of sexual health books, recommend that folks with clitorises, vulvas, and labias consider bringing a mirror to this region regularly for general health inspection and awareness of appearance and condition, similar to occasional breast self-examination. For bonus self-appreciation, folks can articulate positive affirmations and intentions to this area (e.g., "My clitoris is an important source of pleasure, which I treasure" or "I take care of my vulva, labia, clitoris, and vagina by bringing it love and pleasure"). Clients can add slow bilateral stimulation (BLS, such as butterfly hug tapping) or listen to audio BLS to intensify positive feelings.

Additionally, despite the prevalence of those *Cosmopolitan* magazine covers claiming "Top 10 Tricks for Stronger Orgasms," many ciswomen continue to report lack of orgasm during sexual activity, even with the progress in deemphasizing so-called "vaginal-based orgasms." I have found that a small but persistent number of my own cisfemale-identified clients have never or rarely masturbated to orgasm. Those who have masturbated have yet to share their preferred technique or strategies with a partner, out of embarrassment, fear of hurting their partner's feelings, or placing a greater value on their partner's needs.

I highly recommend Dodson's book *Sex for One: The Joy of Self-Loving* (1996), a classic for assisting those with a clitoris, vulva, and vagina to learn how to have orgasms and share that information more easily with others. Betty Dodson also has a guest appearance on Gwenyth Paltrow's Netflix Series, *The Goop Lab*, in the episode "The Pleasure Is Ours" (2020), where she essentially schools the audience in correct anatomical terminology (vulva vs. vagina) and encourages participants to truly see and embrace their vulva.

INTERNAL SEXUAL AND REPRODUCTIVE ANATOMY: VAGINA, G-SPOT, PELVIC FLOOR, AND SO FORTH

Internal parts that often develop together in an estrogen-dominant body and environment include the *introitus* (vagina's entrance), *vagina, Grafenberg* or *G-spot area, cervix, uterus, fallopian tubes*, and *ovaries* (see **Figure 2.2**). Ovaries are the gonads that produce and release eggs during the menstrual cycle and also produce sex hormones. A released egg travels the approximately 4-inch-long fallopian tube (oviducts) to the uterus, where, if fertilized by sperm, it can implant and become an embryo. The cervix is tissue at the mouth of the uterus and protrudes into the uppermost part of the vagina, connecting the uterus to the vagina. The uterus, a pear-shaped and -sized muscular organ, sheds its lining during menstruation and houses a fetus during pregnancy. The *urethra* (tube from which the body releases urine) and *urethral opening*, in this anatomical configuration, is usually located between the clitoris and the vagina. The *Bartholin glands* are two small, round glands on either side of the vaginal opening that secrete fluid during sexual arousal (Goldfarb & Casparian, 2000).

The *hymen* is a very thin piece of tissue that in many bodies nearly covers the vagina until it is worn away from exercise, injury, or, infrequently, intercourse (Buehler, 2022). At different eras throughout history, intact hymens have been associated with "virginity" and weaponized

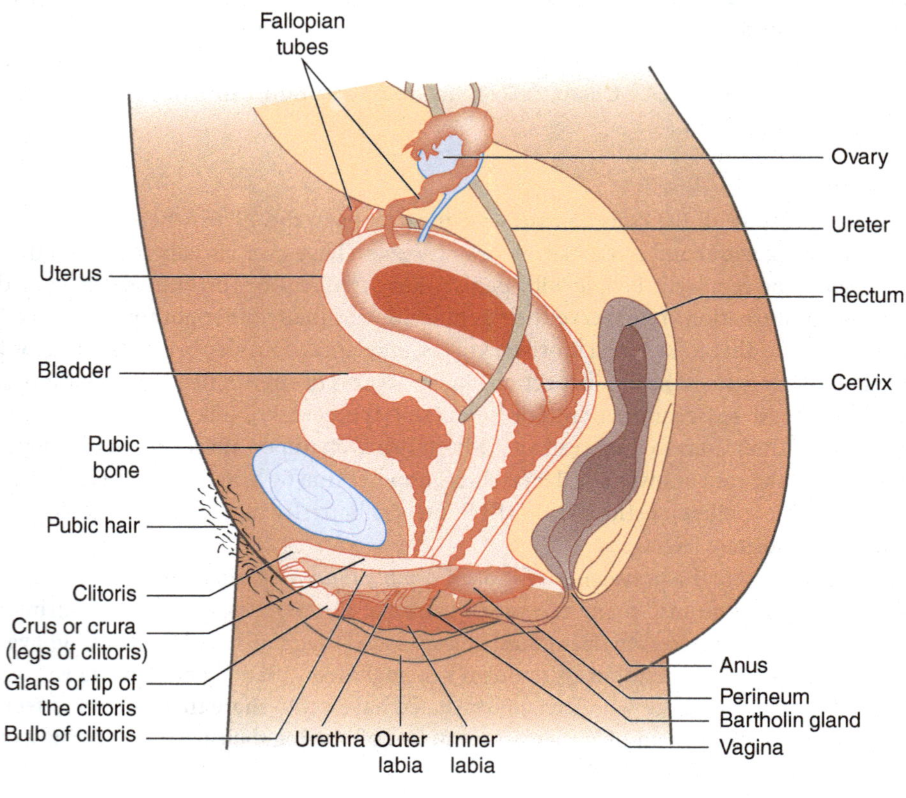

FIGURE 2.2. Vulva, Anterolateral View

to accuse individuals of being impure if a hymen appeared to be absent before marriage. On the other hand, some individuals may possess a very thick hymen that may require surgery to allow comfortable penetration.

Vagina (Generative Organ)

The vagina (the canal through which menstruation blood, birth, and/or semen can travel) automatically strives to maintain a certain pH-level for daily health and functioning, as well as for comfortable intercourse. Mental and/or physical sexual stimulation can result in lubrication of the vagina lining via pores (and can occur in 30 seconds or less). However, vaginas may not produce and discharge lubrication at any given moment due to a variety of reasons such as hormonal interference (i.e., birth control), dehydration, or even something like cold and flu medicine, despite adequate and/or pleasurable mental or physical sexual stimulation. This presence or lack of lubrication can create difficulties for bodies with vaginas, particularly if the lubrication (or lack of) is in opposition to a desired activity. Becoming familiar with water-based lubrication can resolve many of these situations. The vagina is not known to be very sensitive to touch or pressure and contains much fewer nerve endings than the clitoris or labia.

Physically aroused vaginas generally expand, with the uterus pulling upward, creating more comfort for penetration.

Aging clients may report dissatisfaction with the tightness (or looseness) of the vaginal wall. Nonsurgical "vaginal rejuvenation" uses radiofrequency to increase tightness, which may help with urinary incontinence as well. Clients should obtain second opinions from sex-positive medical practitioners before proceeding with any altering procedure, and could potentially benefit from in-depth exploration in therapy regarding acceptance and celebration, or empowerment to pursue any pleasure- and health-affirming helpful interventions.

G-Spot Area (Erectile Area)

The G-spot area, once viewed with complete skepticism, is reported to be about 2 inches inside the vagina on the anterior side (toward the upward front of the body), and may be part of the clitoral system. Anatomists remain divided about the shape, purpose, exact location, and area size. Biology professor Toulson (personal communication, June 11, 2021) believes it is analogous with the prostate. Stimulation of this area, whether via penis, fingers, or sex toy, can result in female ejaculation and/or orgasmic sensation for some bodies. This "vaginal" orgasm may in actuality be related to the clitoral structure. Other bodies may find this stimulation painful or related to feeling the need to urinate (Buehler, 2022). Every body is different and normal, and should not be pathologized.

Pelvic Floor

Pelvic floor muscles hold up the uterus and other organs in the abdomen, and are responsible for *continence* (the ability to retain or evacuate urine and feces; Buehler, 2022).

The pelvic floor is an area that has begun to receive more attention in the medical establishment within the last couple of decades. The pelvic floor muscles act like a basket holding in and up the internal organs. They form a diagonal path supporting the clitoris, urethra, vagina, and anus. "For optimal sexual health, the pelvic floor muscles must be in good tone. Muscles that are too tight, or *hypertonic*, can contribute to a variety of medical problems, including painful intercourse" (Buehler, 2022, p. 22). Muscles that are loose, or *hypotonic*, can make it difficult for someone to experience appropriate stimulation, potentially leading to weak or no orgasms.

Thankfully, some physical therapists have specialized in pelvic floor physical therapy for decades and have been busy helping folks regain sexual health and functioning, as well as improve continence. Bodies that have given birth often suffer for years, involuntarily urinating while sneezing and coughing, believing that nothing can resolve their incontinence. Directing such a client to a well-informed pelvic physical therapist can not only reduce or eliminate the incontinence, but the exercises learned and practiced may also result in regaining orgasmic strength.

Also, many of our sexually traumatized clients hold tremendous physical and emotional pain in their pelvis, particularly in the form of constant (usually unconsciously) tensing of these muscles. Pelvic physical therapy can help these clients retrain their muscles to a more balanced tension, ultimately allowing for fuller and enhanced sexual health. For some clients, this *intensive therapy* (from PLISSIT) referral may be the best thing that can come out of psychotherapy.

Many folks have heard of learning and practicing Kegel exercises to improve continence and decrease postchildbirth vaginal wall slackness. Clients should make sure they have accurate information and instructions. I myself suffered from reduced continence, 7 years after giving birth vaginally. My own physical therapist, Stacy Troy, MS, PT, noted that most people learn and perform Kegels inaccurately, and emphasized the importance of learning and practicing Kegel exercises correctly. The proper exercise involves pulling up and squeezing the pelvic floor muscles for both short and longer periods. It does *not* involve practicing stopping urine midstream (although that can be helpful to *initially* identify these muscles) nor does it involve squeezing your abdomen or buttocks together. The Mayo Clinic has a very helpful and accurate guide to performing Kegel exercises on their website (www.mayoclinic.org/healthy-lifestyle/womens-health/in-depth/kegel-exercises/art-20045283).

REPRODUCTIVE DEVELOPMENT: PUBERTY THROUGH MENOPAUSE

Menstruation

The average age of menarche and puberty for estrogen-dominant people with ovaries in the United States is around 12.4 years of age (with children as young as age 8 and as old as 16 having their first period). In menstruation, around every 28 to 29 days the body releases an egg from the ovary into the fallopian tubes where it eventually lands in the uterus that has been prepared with extra lining. The menstrual cycle has four phases: the menstruation (shedding of the uterine lining), follicular (follicles are produced on the ovary's surface, uterine lining begins to thicken), ovulation (ovary releases a mature egg into the fallopian tube), and luteal (progesterone and estrogen release, thickening the uterus lining) phases. Should fertilization occur by a sperm, a pregnancy may develop. If there is no fertilization, then the lining will be released as menstrual blood.

Many menstruating folks may experience any of the following difficulties with their cycles: premenstrual syndrome (e.g., headaches, fatigue, irritability, cramps), dysmenorrhea (painful periods), heavy bleeding, and/or amenorrhea (absence of periods), among other syndromes or disorders.

People with ovaries are born with a wide average range of 35,000 to 2.5 million ovarian follicles (potential eggs).

Puberty Developments and Concerns

Breasts are also beginning to develop during puberty, along with other secondary sex characteristics such as increased body hair, body odor (due to more active sweat glands), and widening of the hips. Skin may develop acne. Significant height and foot growth spurts likely occur. Fat may redistribute around the body. The clitoris and labia also generally grow and mature, possibly increasing a bit in size. Mood swings may be reported by any body going through puberty.

Inquiring as to your clients' experiences with development, menstruation and pregnancy may also reveal potential explorable issues, as some clients may have had very little information about menstruation prior to menarche, may report embarrassing memories about their development (having their first period while wearing white shorts, being teased for having small or large breasts, etc.), or may have had difficult pregnancies or deliveries that still elicit disturbance of mind and body in their recollections.

Conversely, some clients may appreciate elements of their physical appearance, including their visible sexual and reproductive organs. This esteem, appreciation, and pride may be utilized as a strength amid other treatment concerns.

Menopause and Beyond

Menopause on average occurs around the age of 51 to 53 in the United States. However, clients may enter perimenopause as early as 35. Either way, clients undergoing menopause may experience decreased estrogen, hot flashes, night sweats, vaginal dryness or changes, and sometimes a lower sex interest. Testosterone also declines, possibly contributing to lower sexual interest and less sensation in erogenous zones such as nipples and clitoris. Between 40% and 60% of postmenopausal clients experience atrophic vaginal symptoms (Resh, 2018). Resh (2018) has also observed symptoms such as labial fusion, or even the "labia minora completely vanish."

Many clients do not report these changes and may not schedule gynecology appointments as often as they did earlier in life, missing opportunities to bring up such changes to health professionals. Not all perimenopausal, menopausal, or postmenopausal clients report lower sex interest. Some older clients, especially ciswomen, may finally feel free enough to explore their sexuality at this stage in life. It can be good practice to inquire with permission and curiosity about your clients' experiences with hormones, aging, and so forth, versus making assumptions or stereotypes based on generalities. Chapter 12 on aging has more information regarding aging vaginal and vulvar health.

A Note on Lubrication

Vaginal lubrication differs greatly, and every moment for every vagina is different, depending on the time of day, month, age of person, hormones present or not, where they are in the menstrual cycle, whether peri- or menopausal, daily stress toll, use of alcohol or cigarettes, and generally how hydrated they are that day (the more hydrated, the better). Remember, there is no patented direct correlation between lubrication, arousal, and interest in sexual activity at any given moment. Some people may report copious lubrication at all sorts of times, yet not be interested in sexual activity in those particular moments (or at all). Others may be as aroused as they have ever experienced themselves, yet not secrete a drop of lubrication. There may be noticeable lubrication that occurs during unwanted sexual activity—possibly the vagina's way of reducing or preventing injury and tears.

There has also been a slight perceived prejudice of "naturally" well-lubricated vaginas over vaginas that benefit from added lubrication. Even a person who every day of their adult life notes regular secretions and fluids may have an off day for any of the preceding reasons.

The simplest solution to any lubrication concern is to keep quality water-based lubrication on hand. Additionally, it is useful to know a little bit about lubrication as clients may report difficulty finding one that does not irritate, therefore leading to uncomfortable intercourse experiences. It can be helpful to provide some basic consumer education.

There are many different lubrications available, from organic to paraben-free to plant oil-based to water-based to items one can find around the kitchen. Sex educators generally favor water-based lubrications over oil-based as these are least likely to cause allergic reactions, infections, or to dehydrate. Also, they are safe to use with latex condoms and sex toys, keeping the latex and toy material intact.

The badvibes.org website has a wonderfully educational and informative section on lubrication. Osmolality refers to how concentrated the dissolved particles are per unit of water in a solution or serum. Osmolality is important because the "body's natural mucus is constantly trying to maintain homeostasis" (badvibes.org, n.d., Osmolality). Osmolality is measured in milliosmoles per kilogram of solvent (mOsm/kg). Ideally, vaginas prefer an isosmotic lubricant around 285 to 295 mOsm/kg, which is equal osmotic pressure as the body's hydration level. Badvibes.org notes that Good Clean Love and Sliquid Organics lubricants both fall within that "genital-friendly" ideal range.

pH levels are also helpful to consider when selecting lubrication, especially for the vagina. Vaginal pH ranges from 3.8 to 4.6 (and higher if postmenopausal). Individuals should look for lubrications in their general range so as not to disturb the environment more than necessary. Good Clean Love and Astroglide fall right in that sweet spot (although Astroglide has very high osmolality, somewhat canceling out the pH benefit). Slippery Stuff Liquid and Sliquid Organics at 6.8 might be more ideal for the postmenopausal vagina.

Humectants are another ingredient often added to lubricants as preservatives and to increase viscosity. Natural and/or organic humectant alternatives that many may find nonirritating can include honey, shea butter, and jojoba oil. Many manufactured lubricants may contain petrochemicals such as "propylene glycol, … benzene, benzoic acid" (badvibes.org, n.d., Petrochemicals). These can "dehydrate mucus and cause skin irritation, leaving mucous membrane more vulnerable to bacterial vaginosis or STIs [sexually transmitted infections]" (badvibes.org, n.d., Petrochemicals). Most medical practitioners recommend avoiding lubrications that contain parabens, petroleum, glycerin, and sugars.

Some manufactured lubricants may contain microbicides to kill or reduce the infectivity of viruses or bacteria added as spermicides. While obviously helpful to kill unwanted sperm, frequent use may also irritate the incredibly self-regulating vaginal environment. (Sperm themselves are chemically not welcome by the vagina, which is why seminal fluid contains a solution of immunosuppressants to neutralize the vagina's environment and help sneak the sperm through.)

Some clients may prefer using naturally occurring products from their cupboards. Sweet almond oil (also helpful for oral and anal sex), virgin coconut oil (con: it can stain sheets), olive oil (con: it can clog pores, so wash off when done), and avocado oil (not as long-lasting as the aforementioned) can be used. Remember that any oil-based lubes should NOT be used if one is using a condom to prevent STIs and/or pregnancy.

Aloe vera is a water-based substance that can be used with condoms and may feel very soothing as well. Less known household lubes include Ghee butter (great for moisturizing, but bad for condoms and must be washed off right away to avoid going rancid) and Nagaimo (a type of slippery yam that is very popular in China, Japan, and Vietnam). Lastly, room-temperature egg whites can be applied with a liquid dropper.

Clients should avoid these household items at all costs: baby oil, petroleum jelly, and any kind of vegetable, canola, or other similarly refined oil. These may have unpleasant chemicals, may increase risk of infections, may stain sheets, and may degrade condoms or sex toys.

As for anal penetration, lubrication must be used. The anus does not produce any natural lubrication, so to avoid tears, pain, infections, and so on, one must employ a lubrication. Smittenkittenonline.com has a great collection of lubricants recommended for anal play, most made by Sliquid (including an organic option). They also sell "Backdoor balm–anal aftercare" southern butter that contains healing nutrients such as calendula, plantain, chickweed, yarrow, and vitamin E.

TESTOSTERONE-DOMINANT ANATOMY AND DEVELOPMENT

EXTERNAL SEXUAL ANATOMY: PENIS, SCROTUM, PERINEUM

Testosterone-dominantly developed external genitals usually include the penis, scrotum, and perineum.

Penis (Erectile and Generative Organ)

The penis is comprised of three main parts: the *root* (contained internally), the *shaft* (the main part that extends from the body), and the *glans penis* (the top or "head" of the penis; Buehler, 2022). Penises naturally come with a *prepuce* (foreskin) at birth, yet, as circumcision is the most common surgery worldwide, many penises no longer have foreskins (see **Figure 2.3**).

The *urethra* (internal tube that carries urine and/or semen) opening appears at the glans penis's tip. "On the underside of the nonerect or flaccid penis, the *corona* (which means "crown" in Spanish) appears as a ridge. The *frenulum* is a cordlike structure also on the underside of the penis that connects the corona to the shaft. The entire glans penis is the most sensitive part of the penis, filled with nerve endings that help with arousal and orgasm" (Buehler, 2022, p. 24).

When sexually aroused, the penis becomes erect due to vasocongestion (accumulation and swelling of blood in the vesicles), the scrotal skin smooths out, and the testicles are drawn into the body.

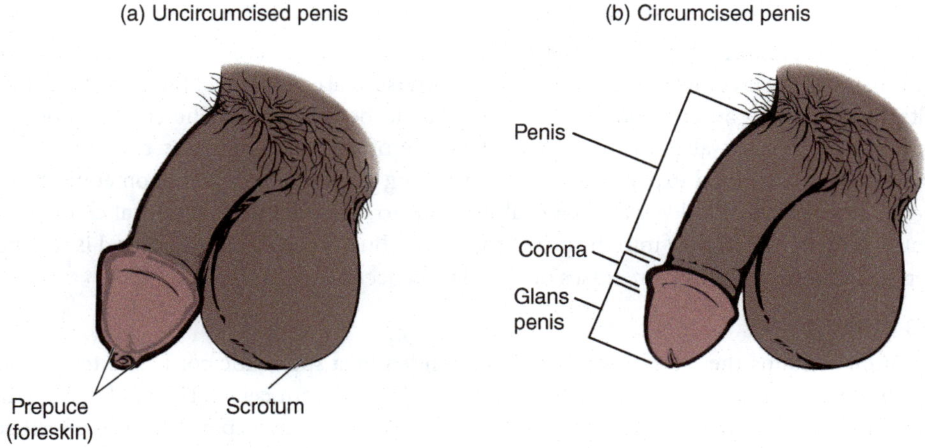

FIGURE 2.3. External Sexual Anatomy: Penis and Scrotum

Source: Modified from Betts, J. G., Young, K. A., Wise, J. A., Johnson, E., Poe, B., Kruse, D. H., Korol, O., Johnson, J. E., Womble, M., & DeSaix, P. (2013, April 25). *Anatomy and physiology* (2nd ed., Fig. 27.10). OpenStax. https://openstax.org/books/anatomy-and-physiology/pages/27-1-anatomy-and-physiology-of-the-male-reproductive-system. Modified by adding color/skin tones. Licensed under CC BY 4.0 (https://creativecommons.org/licenses/by/4.0).

Some clients may struggle with questions about their penis size and specific memories of feeling belittled or shamed. It is important to validate that penises come in a range of sizes (with the average size reported to be around 5 inches, smaller than what people expect it to be) and circumferences, and offer psychotherapeutic help with any size-related concerns, doubt, or shame. It may also be important to provide psychoeducation for heterosexual cismen about clitoral sexual anatomy, expanding their sexual repertoire to understand the importance of the clitoris in sexual pleasure. This can help reduce the pressure they may have placed on themselves about penis size and performance.

Scrotum and Perineum (Sensitive)

The "sack-like" external *scrotum* contains the *testes*, the organs that produce sperm and sex hormones. When cold, "the scrotum pulls close to the body to keep the testicles warm, and when … warm, the scrotum hangs away from the body. The *perineum* is the strip of skin that is visible from behind the scrotum to the anus" (Buehler, 2022, p. 24). Most scrotums and perineums enjoy stimulation. Scrotums also typically pull up close to the body just prior to ejaculation, enhancing the orgasm experience.

Medical Trauma or Injuries

Some clients report medical trauma regarding penises or scrotums, perhaps relating to injury, early surgeries, badly performed circumcisions (especially if the child receives a circumcision after the age of 1 year), or adult medical problems (e.g., Peyronie disease can result in scarring of penis tissue). If the client reports these events as currently disturbing, then psychotherapy (particularly EMDR therapy) may help to reduce the emotional/mental disturbance associated with the difficulty.

INTERNAL SEXUAL ANATOMY: CHAMBERS, TESTICLES, SEMINAL VESICLES, PROSTATE

The *Cowper glands* (or *bulbourethral glands*) are the two pea-sized glands that secrete preejaculate, assisting in neutralizing the acidic environment of the urethra (Goldfarb & Casparian, 2000).

Penis Chambers (Erectile and Generative)

The penis includes three interior chambers: two *corpus cavernosum* (very erectile) and one *corpus spongiosum* (slightly erectile). The two "corpus cavernosum are … parallel tubes in the penis that fill with blood during an erection, causing the penis to become rigid. The corpus spongiosum [(mostly generative, but also erectile)] is a "structure of spongy tissue that runs the length of the front of the penis [and expands] with blood during an erection. When [someone] becomes aroused, nerves cause blood vessels in a healthy penis to expand. Other chemical changes occur that cause more blood to flow into the penis, than out" (Buehler, 2022, p. 24). Blood is retained in the penis until either stimulation ceases or ejaculation occurs.

Testes (Generative)

The *scrotum* contains the *testicles* (or *testes*), suspended by a spermatic cord. The testes contain (long) *seminiferous tubules* (where sperm is generated from germ cells). The *epididymis* (tightly coiled tube that stores maturing sperm) and "the *vas deferens* carry sperm from the testicles to the *urethra*." The urethra is "the tube that carries sperm or urine from [inside] the body to its exit [through] the tip of the penis" (Buehler, 2022, p. 25; see **Figure 2.4**).

Seminal Vesicles and Prostate (Generative and Sensitive Glands)

The *seminal vesicles* are located at the back of the bladder and create about 60% to 80% of the ejaculated semen (Buehler, 2022; Joannides, 2017). The *prostate* (meaning "guard of the bladder") produces the remaining 20% to 40% of fluid (Buehler, 2022; Joannides, 2017). Stimulating the prostate with either anal play or anal penetration can be very pleasurable for gay, straight, and/or bisexual individuals with prostates. Unfortunately, the prostate can acquire diseases like cancer or prostatitis (Buehler, 2022). Some individuals may report shame related to desires of receiving anal penetration or prostate stimulation. Psychoeducation and psychotherapy can address and eliminate this shame.

INTERSEX

The original Intersex Society of North America website explains the category and definition of *intersex* succinctly. Intersex is a general term used for a variety of conditions in which a person is born with reproductive and/or sexual anatomy that do not seem to fit the "typical"

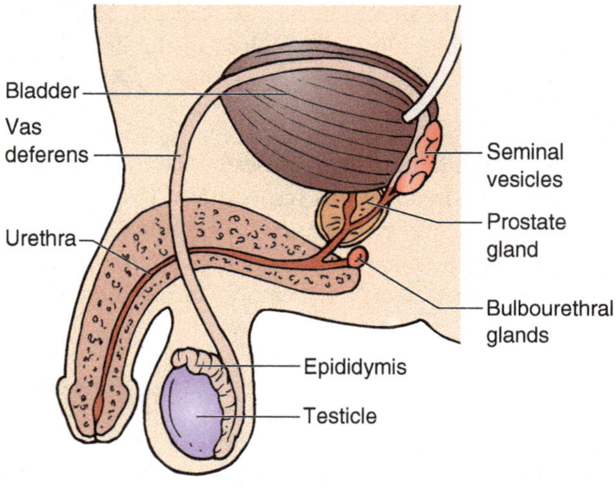

FIGURE 2.4. Gross Internal Sexual Anatomy of Penis, Scrotum, Prostate, and So Forth

Source: Reprinted from Tkacs, N., Herrmann, L., & Johnson, R. (2020). *Advanced physiology and pathophysiology* (1st ed.). Springer Publishing Company.

definitions of "female" or "male." They note that it is humans who have defined sex in binary norms, and that in reality, perhaps penises, testes, clitorises, and vulvas come in a variety of shapes and sizes.

STATISTICS

Statistically, it seems that about 1.7 infants in every 100 births may be intersex in some way, and are as common as redheads. Some researchers estimate this number to be higher than 2%.

CHROMOSOMAL VARIATIONS

Humans can have many chromosomal combinations other than XX (generally related to an estrogen-dominant person with vulva, ovaries, etc.) or XY (generally related to a testosterone-dominant individual with penis, testes, and related organs). Some examples are XO (Turner syndrome), XXX, XXY (Klinefelter syndrome), or XYY, or some cells that are XY and some that are XX, and so on. Many of these individuals have no medical problems related to the chromosomal variations, although some may have fertility difficulties or inabilities.

HORMONAL AND ANATOMICAL VARIATIONS

Intersex individuals can possess internal structures (e.g., ovaries) that do not seem to match external structures (e.g., penis), which is often not discovered until puberty, they try to conceive, or they receive an autopsy.

Examples of hormonal and/or anatomical variations include XX salt-wasting congenital adrenal hyperplasia (SWCAH), androgen insensitivity syndrome (AIS), XY complete gonadal dysgenesis (Swyer syndrome), and XY partial gonadal dysgenesis.

INTERSEX ACTIVISM AND ADVOCACY

InterAct is an activist organization fighting to outlaw any surgeries that could potentially be performed on ambiguous or atypical genitals while the child is still a minor. Many states and organizations now recognize that it is best to perform as little surgery as possible (only allowing for life-saving surgeries such as creating a way for urine to exit the body). However, such surgeries have not been outlawed entirely and the medical establishment may still pressure parents to give permission for unnecessary hypospadias repair (the urethra not exiting the glans penis in the expected place), vaginoplasty (removing penis, testicles, and scrotum to create a vagina), clitoroplasty (creation of or reduction in size of clitoris), or gonadectomy (removing testes or ovaries). All these procedures meant to conform organs to the historical gender binary can have a life-long deleterious impact on physical and mental health. Recent standards of care include assigning a gender at birth that makes sense, but being open and honest with the child about what is known about their sexual and reproductive organs, supporting the child in their gender journey, and leaving any surgical options up to them for when they are of consenting age.

I mention intersex concerns as there may be the occasional client who has an experience with this possibility, whether due to childhood surgery or due to a recent discovery via an infertility clinic of different internal organs than had been assumed. Affirming and validating their experiences with psychoeducation and supportive psychotherapy may be of invaluable help.

SEX HORMONES: ESTROGEN, PROGESTERONE, AND TESTOSTERONE

All healthy bodies produce various levels of estrogen, progesterone, and testosterone at different ages, based on chromosomal and gonadal makeup.

TESTOSTERONE

Relatively large amounts of testosterone are produced in adult testicles. "Normal" levels of testicle-produced testosterone contribute to good muscle mass, overall energy, and healthy erections. Once a testosterone-dominant individual with a penis and testes turns 35, levels slowly decline over the years and estrogen increases. For individuals with ovaries and vulvas, healthy testosterone contributes to positive mood, energy, and bone and muscle heath, as well as specific sexual health elements such as sexual interest, pleasure, arousal, and orgasm. Some individuals may experience "abnormally low levels of testosterone, which can result in low sex drive, loss of muscle mass, weight gain, fatigue, and difficulty attaining and maintaining an erection" (Buehler, 2022, p. 25). As these symptoms can overlap with depression, it is recommended to refer these clients for a physical with testosterone and hormone testing.

ESTROGEN

Estrogen assists with the growth of breasts, pubic hair, body hair, and menstruation. In all bodies, estrogen helps regulate brain function, bone health, skin health, lipid metabolism, erectile function, and sexual desire. Lower or higher estrogen in folks with ovaries may contribute to a range of problems: hot flashes, trouble sleeping, vaginal dryness, difficulty with menstruation, fibroids, mood swings, fatigue, and decreased sexual interest, among others. High estrogen in people with penises and testes may result in enlarged breasts, infertility, difficulty with erections, dry skin, and loss of sexual interest.

Estrogen-dominant clients with vaginas and ovaries may seek therapy complaining of lower energy and interest in sex. They may benefit from a physical as well, although many other factors can also be responsible. Some clients with estrogen-producing ovaries experience a decline in estrogen and testosterone as they age, resulting in vaginal dryness and thinning of the vaginal and vulvar tissue, potentially leading to painful intercourse (Buehler, 2022). Thankfully, there are many potential solutions such as topical estrogen, vitamin E cream, dehydroepiandrosterone (DHEA) cream, barium rings, and water-based lubricants (Resh, 2018). Chapter 12, "Aging Sexual Health," has more information.

PROGESTERONE

Progesterone is the reproductive hormone most associated with pregnancy and helps maintain a healthy pregnancy. It helps prepare the breasts for producing milk, helps balance other hormones, and can help prevent bone loss and heart disease. It can also help with sleep as well as general calming. Excessive cortisol and prolactin, polycystic ovary syndrome (PCOS), thyroid conditions, and menopause can result in low progesterone. Depressed mood, fatigue, and ovarian cysts and some cancers may correlate with higher progesterone levels.

FERTILITY, PREGNANCY, BIRTH, PREGNANCY LOSS

FERTILITY

Clients may seek therapy due to anxiety, stress, concerns, or prior disturbing events related to childbirth and fertility. Some clients who want to have children may have gone through years of fertility treatment, arriving at your office discouraged, in despair, and perhaps holding medical trauma related to prior fertility procedures, miscarriages, or stillborn births.

Other clients may report harrowing childbirth experiences that continue to haunt them physically and/or emotionally, impacting their desire to engage in penis–vagina intercourse, or in any sexual activity, for that matter. It can be a good idea to gently inquire about any difficulties with getting pregnant, the pregnancy, and/or birth in your clinical assessment.

INFERTILITY

For reproductive-aged individuals in the United States, about 9% of people with testes, and about 11% of people with ovaries, have experienced *fertility* problems. In one third of infertile couples, the difficulty is with the testes and/or related organs. In one third of infertile couples, the difficulty is with the ovaries and related organs. In the remaining third, the difficulty cannot be identified, or is with both people (Chandra et al., 2013). Overall, people are more and more delaying giving birth to their first child. A *Forbes* article noted that the worldwide average age of an individual giving their first birth has moved back to 31; in the United States, the age has moved from 21 to 26 (Stahl, 2020).

CONCEPTION

For a new human to be conceived, a viable *egg* (or *ovum*, a sex cell developed in the ovaries) and *sperm* (sex cell developed in the testes) must meet and join. This can be done in a variety of ways. Vagina/penis intercourse, where sperm is ejaculated in or near the vagina, is the most common way for conception to occur. According to Planned Parenthood and the Centers for Disease Control and Prevention (CDC), unprotected adult penis/vagina intercourse will lead to a 75% to 85% chance of pregnancy over the course of a year. For those with limited fertility options, medical technology may offer assistance. *Artificial insemination* (aka *intrauterine insemination* [IUI]) is when sperm is pushed through a catheter or other device through the vagina and cervix, into the uterus. For *in vitro fertilization* (IVF), eggs are removed from ovary follicle sacs. An egg is fertilized by injecting a single sperm into the egg or mixing the egg with sperm in a petri dish. The fertilized egg, called an embryo, is then transferred into the uterus. In a *surrogate* pregnancy, someone with a uterus carries and gives birth to a baby for a person who is not able to have children. In this scenario, eggs from the person who will carry the baby, or from an egg donor, are fertilized with sperm to make an embryo.

PREGNANCY

Healthy pregnancies involve a fetus growing inside a uterus for about 40 weeks, divided into three trimesters.

The first trimester (weeks 1–12) is the most important one for predicting the health and viability of the fetus (and is when most miscarriages occur). The fetus's major organs and brain begin to form and develop. Gonadal differentiation begins to occur around week eight. The embryo starts out with undifferentiated potential reproductive organ morphology, which includes primordial structures such as "egg-shaped organs" and tissues. These primordial structures later differentiate into "generative and erectile organs" (i.e. clitoris or penis), based on the presence and absence of specific chromosomes, hormones, cellular receptors, and environmental factors (as discussed earlier in the "In Utero" section). The brain, spine, neural tube, cardiac tissue, kidneys, pancreas, arm and leg buds, and cartilage for fingers and toes begin to form.

Pregnant people in the first trimester often experience strong fatigue, morning sickness or nausea, breast tenderness, mood swings, food cravings and/or aversions, menstruation cessation (though some spotting may happen), more frequent urination, constipation, heartburn, bloating, and gas.

In the second trimester (weeks 13–27), pregnant people may experience ankle and feet swelling, leg cramps, constipation, itchy skin, stretch marks, darker areolas, hemorrhoids, varicose veins, and so on. The fetus is undergoing important brain development; they can open their eyes, hear sounds, move arms and legs, and taste different foods through the amniotic fluid. Kicking can be felt, digestion is working, and they may be able to suck their thumb.

In the third trimester (weeks 28–40), the pregnant person may experience shortness of breath, frequent urination, constipation, heartburn, indigestion, breasts leaking colostrum (pre-milk), vivid dreams, and Braxton Hicks "practice" contractions. The fetus's lungs and kidneys finish maturing and the brain continues developing at a fast rate. Bones harden, the circulatory and musculoskeletal systems are ready, and more fat forms under the skin.

Difficulties can arise at any point, creating or increasing stress for the parent(s). First-time parents may have increased anxiety due to having yet to experience pregnancy, childbirth, and child-rearing. Therapy, along with supportive and experienced midwives/obstetricians, can help allay many of these concerns.

BIRTH

Most babies are born between 38 and 41 weeks of pregnancy, via vaginal delivery, without any complications. However, in 2023 about a third of babies in the United States were born via cesarean (C-section), often due to maternal health variables like gestational diabetes, hypertensive disorders, environmental influences, and possibly higher reimbursement for doctors (and reduced worry of lawsuit).

Up until around 2006, episiotomies were routinely performed (surgical incision in the perineum to widen the vaginal opening for childbirth). These were thought to minimize complications from vaginal birth tearing and maintain or enhance a smaller closure for intercourse. However, this has since been disproven; the ACOG now recommends against routine episiotomies. The rate is now less than 12%, with a target rate of less than 5%. In addition to simply repairing the tears or lacerations from vaginal delivery, some doctors added a "husband stitch," often without the person's consent, designed to tighten the vaginal opening a bit more, to enhance the pleasure of the person with the penis. This practice is not considered an approved medical procedure or accepted practice.

The 12 weeks following the birth of the baby is sometimes referred to as "the fourth trimester." It is a time of great physical and emotional change as the baby adjusts to being outside the womb, and parents adjust to this new role. It is suggested that one should try to recreate, for another 3 months, the kind of environment the baby had in the uterus with the use of swaddling and swaying and skin-to-skin contact, especially during feeding and bath time.

PREGNANCY LOSS

Miscarriages and pregnancy loss affect many people. "About 10% to 20% of known pregnancies result in miscarriage" (Mayo Clinic Staff, n.d., para. 1). About one in 100 pregnancies are stillborn (babies lost at 20 weeks of pregnancy or later; MacDorman & Gregory, 2015). Any or all of these losses can result in ongoing grief and PTSD symptoms for the people involved. Supportive, grief, and/or trauma-informed therapy can assist in targeting and working through the emotional aftershock.

IMPACT ON SEXUAL FUNCTIONING

Any of the previously noted aspects of pregnancy and birth can impact someone's sexual functioning both positively and/or negatively.

Some pregnant people report increased sexual interest, vitality, and freedom, perhaps related to a possible vibrancy and health experienced during pregnancy (as well as the knowledge that another pregnancy is not possible, while already pregnant). Partners of pregnant people may find them especially glowing and attractive.

The stress of trying to conceive may hinder sexual interest and functioning in all involved. Both vulvas and penises may have difficulties with arousal and orgasm due to the pressure to engage in intercourse for procreation. Negative or traumatic prior pregnancy and birth-related events may loom over sexual activity, impeding pleasure and ease. Any lingering physical problems from birthing (e.g., episiotomies, scar tissue) may reduce pleasure, or even result in pain during intercourse.

ESSENTIAL SAFER SEX INFORMATION: SEXUALLY TRANSMITTED INFECTIONS AND PREGNANCY PREVENTION

SEXUALLY TRANSMITTED INFECTIONS

For the most updated information, refer to websites such as Planned Parenthood or your local STI clinics. However, since some of our clients may mention concerns about STIs or unwanted pregnancy, it is helpful to have a basic understanding of common STIs and protection.

Possible STIs include chlamydia, genital warts, herpes, gonorrhea, human papillomavirus (HPV), pubic lice, scabies, syphilis, trichomoniasis, hepatitis B, and HIV/AIDS. Most of these are very treatable if caught early, so it is recommended that sexually active individuals get tested regularly, regardless if they always use barriers and feel symptom free. Even some skin-to-skin contact that does not include any penetration can spread an STI such as HPV, herpes, pubic lice, or scabies.

Using condoms or dental dams can reduce the likelihood of spreading an STI as well as prevent pregnancy, if penile–vaginal penetration is involved. For anal sex, it is important to use water-based lubrication with a condom, thereby increasing the protection a condom provides. To prevent the spread of HIV, using condoms or dental dams is a must. However, if your client is HIV-positive, there are now treatments (antiretroviral or ART) that allow an individual to live a long, healthy life, as well as greatly reduce the risk of giving HIV to anyone else. Individuals at risk of HIV exposure can also take preexposure prophylaxis (PrEP), which effectively prevents acquiring HIV.

Unfortunately, despite the fact that millions of people contract an STI sometime in their lives, a great deal of shame continues to accompany these diagnoses. Anywhere you find shame, you find potential psychotherapeutic content to process, whether it is the moment of diagnosis, when your client told their partner(s) about the STI, or their impending fear about mentioning the STI to a new partner.

PREGNANCY PREVENTION AND ABORTION ACCESS

Again, consult Planned Parenthood or local family planning clinics for the most updated information. Currently there are many methods available to prevent sperm and eggs from meeting. These methods range from barriers such as condoms and internal condoms to hormonal disruption of the sperm or egg's journey (e.g., emergency contraception such as Plan B, monthly or quarterly birth control pills or injections, some intrauterine devices (IUDs), implants, birth control patches, vaginal rings) or other methods like diaphragms, birth control sponges, cervical caps, and spermicide. They all have varying degrees of success. Only abstinence from penis–vagina intercourse has a 100% success rate of preventing pregnancy. If a client is most focused on preventing pregnancy, then helping them broaden their view of sex to include outercourse (kissing, massage, dry humping/grinding), oral sex, manual sex, and mutual masturbation (and other kinds of sex play that does not involve sperm potentially meeting eggs) may reduce pregnancy anxiety and enhance overall sexual pleasure.

Abortion involves the termination of the fetus and can happen via a medical abortion (taking the abortion pill within 11 weeks of the pregnancy) or a surgical outpatient abortion, which uses suction and/or medical tools to remove the pregnancy from the uterus, up to 16 weeks after the pregnancy.

Some clients may have experiences related to pregnancy scares, abortions, or partners not using condoms when they were asked to use them. Abortion-related issues may increase due to the antiabortion legislation and climate in the United States since the overturning of *Roe v. Wade* in June 2022. As of March 2024, 14 states have a total ban on abortion and 27 states have bans based on gestational duration. In 2023, more than 166,000 people had to travel to other states to obtain abortions. These people may be encountering shaming antiabortion sentiments and judgment in their home states. Also worth noting is that over 55% of people seeking abortions have already had one live birth. Abortion access and care also disproportionately and negatively impact people of color (Guttmacher Institute, 2024). It may be important to inquire about these potential experiences as you assess your client's sexual health and functioning.

Client reports of shame or embarrassment regarding access of abortion or contraceptive health care may help to identify clinical material for processing. It is critical, as a mental health provider, that no matter one's personal views or opinions on abortion, to respond compassionately and nonjudgmentally, with warmth and care, and create a safe space where clients can disclose, discuss, and process their experiences regarding abortion.

SUMMARY

Human sexual and reproductive anatomy is not as simple and binary as was once thought. Chromosomes, hormones, cell receptors, and environmental factors together influence which groups of organs tend to develop together. An estrogen-dominant androgen system, along with XX chromosomes, tends to result in the development of the clitoris, labia, vagina, ovaries, fallopian tubes, cervix, uterus, and so forth. A testosterone-dominant androgen system, along with XY chromosomes, tends to result in the development of the penis, scrotum, testes, prostate, and so on. About 2% of the population has combinations of chromosomes, hormones, and gonads falling into the *intersex* category. Most healthy bodies have various levels of estrogen, progesterone, and testosterone, as well as a perineum, urethra, anus, and nipples. Some individuals may report discomfort with body parts; this discomfort can alert us to potential clinical material for processing.

Unprotected sexual activity can result in STIs and pregnancy. STI prevention, pregnancy prevention, and abortion options and availability remain concerns for many sexually active individuals. Experiences with STIs and unwanted pregnancies can lead to shame; this shame can unearth possible clinical material to process. Clients may also bring fertility concerns to their therapy sessions.

DISCUSSION QUESTIONS

- With what similar structures do all embryos start?
- What are some examples of the biological sex spectrum beyond the historically discussed female and male binary?
- What organ is most responsible for pleasure for estrogen-dominant, vulva-possessing individuals, and why are researchers only just recently discovering and expanding the known medical information?
- What are some areas that experience pleasure (upon stimulation), other than the penis, for bodies with penises?
- What is the most full-proof way to prevent an unwanted pregnancy? To prevent an STI transmission? What are some ways to greatly reduce the risk of both unwanted pregnancy and STI transmission?

LEARNING ACTIVITIES

CourseConnect

To access self-assessment questions and interactive, competency-based learning activities for this chapter, visit www.springerpub.com/courseconnect. See inside front cover and tear-out card for CourseConnect details.

ADDITIONAL RESOURCES

Additional resources are online and available at www.springerpub.com/courseconnect.

REFERENCES

American College of Obstetricians and Gynecologists. (2020, January). *Elective female genital cosmetic surgery* (Committee Opinion No. 795). https://www.acog.org/clinical/clinical-guidance/committee-opinion/articles/2020/01/elective-female-genital-cosmetic-surgery

badvibes.org. (n.d.). *The science of lubricants: Science behind body lubricants and their role in humans sexual life*. Retrieved January 29, 2025, from https://badvibes.org/the-science-of-lubricants

Boston Women's Health Book Collective. (2001). *Our bodies, ourselves*. Simon & Schuster.

Buehler, S. (2022). *What every mental health professional needs to know about sex* (3rd ed.). Springer Publishing Company.

Chandra, A., Copen, C. E., & Stephen, E. H. (2013). Infertility and impaired fecundity in the United States, 1982–2010: Data from the national survey of family growth. *National Health Statistics Reports, 67*, 1–19. https://www.cdc.gov/nchs/data/nhsr/nhsr067.pdf

Dodson, B. (1996). *Sex for one: The joy of self-loving*. Three River Press.

El-Hamamsy, D., Parmar, C., Shoop-Worrall, S., & Reid, F. M. (2021). Public understanding of female genital anatomy and pelvic organ prolapse (POP); a questionnaire-based pilot study. *International Urogynecology Journal, 33*(2), 309–318. https://doi.org/10.1007/s00192-021-04727-9

The pleasure is ours (Season 1, Episode 3) [TV series episode]. (2020, January 24). In A. Fried, D. Lillegard, E. Loehnen, S. Minoprio, & G. Paltrow (Executive Directors). *The Goop Lab.* Boardwalk Pictures.

Geddes, L. (2021, May). Most Britons cannot name all parts of the vulva, survey reveals. *The Guardian*. https://www.theguardian.com/lifeandstyle/2021/may/30/most-britons-cannot-name-parts-vulva-survey

Goldfarb, E., & Casparian, E. (2000). *Our Whole Lives, sexuality education for grades* 10–12. Unitarian Universalist Association.

Guttmacher Institute. (2024, June). *Abortion in the United States* [Fact Sheet]. https://www.guttmacher.org/fact-sheet/induced-abortion-united-states

Joannides, P. (2017). *Guide to getting it on, unzipped V.9.0.* Goofy Foot Press.

Komisaruk, B. R., & Rodriguez Del Cerro, M. C. (2021). How does our brain generate sexual pleasure? *International Journal of Sexual Health, 33*(4), 602–611. https://doi.org/10.1080/19317611.2021.1989534

MacDorman, M. F., & Gregory, E. C. W. (2015, July 23). *Fetal and perinatal mortality: United States, 2013* [National Vital Statistics Report, Vol. 64, no. 8]. U.S. Department of Health and Human Services, Centers for Disease Control and Prevention, National Center for Health Statistics. https://www.cdc.gov/nchs/data/nvsr/nvsr64/nvsr64_08.pdf

Mayo Clinic Staff. (n.d.). *Miscarriage*. Retrieved September 17, 2021, from https://www.mayoclinic.org/diseases-conditions/pregnancy-loss-miscarriage/symptoms-causes/syc-20354298

O'Connell, H. E., Sanjeevan, K. V., & Hutson, J. M. (2005). Anatomy of the clitoris. *The Journal of Urology, 174*(4 Pt 1), 1189–1195. https://doi.org/10.1097/01.ju.0000173639.38898.cd

Orenstein, P. (2016). *Girls and sex: Navigating the complicated new landscape*. Harper Collins Publisher.

Pauls, R. N. (2015). Anatomy of the clitoris and female sexual response. *Clinical Anatomy, 28*(3), 376–384. https://doi.org/10.1002/ca.22524

Resh, E. (2018). *Hormones, health, and love* [Presentation]. Brattleboro Retreat.

Stahl, A. (2020, May). New study: Millennial women are delaying having children due to their careers. *Forbes*. https://www.forbes.com/sites/ashleystahl/2020/05/01/new-study-millennial-women-are-delaying-having-children-due-to-their-careers/?sh=18f10a0d276a

Toulson, A., & Landon, A. (2021, May). *Gender, sex, and sexuality inclusion in anatomy & physiology education* [Conference workshop]. Human Anatomy and Physiological Society.

Toulson, A., & Landon, A. (2022, March). *Bio 218 Most important points: Anatomy of sex and reproductive organs* [Class handout]. Department of Biology, Holyoke Community College.

Uloko, M., Isabey, E. P., & Peters, B. R. (2023). How many nerve fibers innervate the human glans clitoris: A histomorphometric evaluation of the dorsal nerve of the clitoris. *The Journal of Sexual Medicine, 20*(3), 247–252. https://doi.org/10.1093/jsxmed/qdac027

Zuckerman, W. (Host). (2016, September 1). The G-spot [Audio podcast episode]. In *Science Vs*. Spotify Studios. https://open.spotify.com/episode/3NCf6DAWtiWOShQr6MNqNY

CHAPTER 3

Sexology History, Desire and Arousal Models, and Sexual Compatibility

Stephanie Baird, Katherine Hertlein, and Wendy Stock

LEARNING OBJECTIVES

- Learn about sexology and 20th-century sexual research on desire and arousal (Kinsey, Masters and Johnson, Basson's nonlinear model).
- Learn about the 21st century broadly applicable *dual control model* of sexual response.
- Learn about spontaneous and responsive desire and arousal concordance and nonconcordance.
- Learn about sexual compatibility (including sexual personality styles) and how to administer the accompanying sexual personality style questionnaire.
- Learn about *erotic templates* and how they may relate to client presenting concerns.

HISTORY OF SEXOLOGY

DEFINING SEXOLOGY

Sexology is the interdisciplinary study of human sexuality. It draws upon biology, psychology, sociology, anthropology, medicine, and history, among other disciplines, to investigate human sexuality topics such as sexual development and health, behaviors, reproduction, sexual orientation, gender identity, sexual dysfunction, and societal norms and attitudes. Sexology researchers and practitioners may work to understand the diversity of human sexual behaviors and experiences across histories and cultures, advance knowledge, promote sexual health and well-being, and contribute to policies and practices that support sexual rights and equality.

SEXOLOGY RESEARCH

In the 1940s and 1950s, pioneering and groundbreaking early sex researcher Alfred Kinsey demonstrated that most sexual problems were related to ignorance about sexual functioning and the many variations from what was considered "the norm" (Kinsey et al., 1948, 1953). Kinsey and his researchers collected data from over 10,000 women and men (cisgender subjects) through interviews, questionnaires, and direct observation of sexual behavior in laboratory settings. This early research revealed the diversity of sexual activity and behavior among adults, particularly spotlighting a broad and far-reaching spectrum of sexual orientation beyond heterosexual. His research, in fact, resulted in the 1948 development of the Kinsey scale (measuring sexual orientation and/or preference). The scale goes from 0 (exclusively heterosexual) to 7 (exclusively homosexual), with data showing that most of his subjects fell somewhere in the 1 to 6 range.

SEX RESEARCH/MODELS OF SEXUAL DESIRE AND AROUSAL

MASTERS AND JOHNSON

From the 1950s to the 1970s, Masters and Johnson (1966) studied sexual pleasure through observations and measurements of human subjects in laboratory settings. From their data and measurements they concluded that healthy sexual functioning involves the following physiological sequence: *excitement* (i.e., flushing of skin, muscle tension, erections of clitoris and penis, faster breathing), *plateau* (continued genital arousal and preparation for orgasm), *orgasm* (rhythmic contractions of genital muscles at the height of arousal and pleasure), followed by *resolution* (post-sexual restful state, return to regular heart rate, etc.). Their important research continued to help destigmatize and normalize human sexual behaviors and functioning (debunking many misconceptions), and they also recognized the importance of communication and emotional intimacy in sexual interactions and relationships.

HELEN SINGER KAPLAN

Helen Singer Kaplan expanded Masters and Johnson's research, recognizing the cismale focus of their model and adapting it into a triphasic model of *desire*, *arousal* (excitement and plateau), and *orgasm*. *Desire* finally became a critical component, with the understanding that our brains account for a great deal of our sexual response abilities (Kaplan, 1977). She described her triphasic model as nonlinear, noting that more than one stage or part can co-occur. She also noted the importance of psychological factors such as motivation, emotional connection, and expectation in sexual response, for both the individual and the couple involved. She wrote extensively about understanding sexuality and dysfunction through a comprehensive and integrative lens of psychological, biological/physiological, medical, and interpersonal factors.

ZILBERGELD AND ELLISON

Zilbergeld and Ellison (1980) also made contributions to understanding sexual response and arousal by advocating for both cognitive and affective factors impacting arousal. At the time, this was a substantial shift in trying to move the field past solely considering the physiology of sexual response; these researchers also incorporated other elements not observable to the naked eye. Their approach covered five phases: desire, the experience of arousal cognitively and/or affectively by sexual interaction, the ability to have a physiological arousal response, the experience of an orgasm, and an appraisal as to whether that interaction was satisfactory.

SHERE HITE

Shere Hite was a prominent sex researcher in the 1970s and 1980s. Hite coordinated her questions and efforts with National Organization for Women (NOW) resources, resulting in the development and initial distribution in 1972 of her first open-ended questionnaires for the "feminist sexuality project." This questionnaire included many questions about how, why, and how often (cis) women masturbate, and how many orgasms they find sexually fulfilling, among many other very personal and specific questions. Many thousands of questionnaires were sent all over the United States, and a bit over 3,000 were returned.

The major finding of the resulting *Hite Report* on female sexuality (Hite, 1976/2011) was that around 70% of female respondents easily had orgasms via clitoral stimulation through masturbation, but rarely had orgasms from penis-vagina intercourse alone.

Hite and her data were questioned during press conferences, articles, and television interviews. Geraldo Rivera raised the "fear that masturbation will become the ultimate sex act and men will become irrelevant" (Rivera & Morris, 1977, 27:00). A defender at a NOW press conference gave the analogy, "What if men were expected to only orgasm by stimulation of the testicles, not the penis?" Men were staggered to learn that clitoral stimulation was much more important than vaginal penetration. However, early sex research by Masters and Johnson had confirmed the greater likelihood of orgasms occurring via clitoral stimulation versus vaginal penetration (and even then, Masters and Johnson noted that the orgasms were due to indirect clitoral stimulation), yet somehow this had been forgotten by the time Hite conducted her research.

After years of gathering questionnaires answered by men, Hite then published *The Hite Report on Male Sexuality* (1981) based on over 7,000 respondents. Some of the radical conclusions in the study included how the majority of respondants felt "pressured" to perform sexually. In a documentary on the study, one of the original male editors said, "[W]hen [the men] started answering the questions about their emotional life, I haven't had many sadder experiences as an editor in my life" (Newnham, 2023, 1:04:47). Many of the respondents mentioned the lack of acceptance and denigration of showing sadness, and a lack of connection with their own fathers. This book, by virtue of the answers, demonstrated a very early critique of toxic masculinity, in the voices of men.

Both *The Hite Report on Male Sexuality* and Hite's third book, *Women and Love: A Cultural Revolution in Progress* (1987), pointed out the rampant rates of affairs among both married women and men—both around 70% within the first 5 years of marriage—as well as emotional dissatisfaction present among most women (84%) and nearly universal reports of emotional and/or psychological harassment from men (95%). Again, despite another large sample size, these findings were questioned and scoffed at by the general media and academia.

Even with selling five million copies of her books, which were translated into 14 languages and banned in eight countries, and her original *Hite Report* named the 30th bestselling book of all time by *Newsweek*, Hite felt forced to flee the United States for Europe due to overt hatred and censorship, renouncing her citizenship in 1995 and passing away at the age of 77 in 2020.

I (S. Baird) have spent this time discussing Shere Hite's work to illustrate how easily groundbreaking sexology can be disparaged and disappear, particularly if it challenges stereotypes and misconceptions of "normal heterosexual" sexual functioning. I highly recommend the recent 2023 documentary, *The Disappearance of Shere Hite,* as an important overview of society's ongoing ambivalence and suppression regarding sex research, particularly research oriented toward vulvar pleasure.

THE WILLINGNESS MODEL

The willingness model, created by JoAnn Loulan, a lesbian sex therapist, provides a useful way to help couples with decreased frequency of sex or low desire. Loulan (1984), based on her observations of lesbian couples' sexuality, developed a model of sexual response that contained a new component—willingness. This model reflects the fact that for many ciswomen, desire does not always occur spontaneously. However, if individuals decide that they are willing and interested in engaging in sexual activity—despite lacking desire—they may find that desire occurs as they become physically aroused and experience pleasure.

True willingness requires consent; it is not an excuse for sexual coercion. The guidance to couples utilizing this technique is for the low desire partner to be willing to engage in physical affection and sexual touching to explore whether their desire can be "kindled." If the flames of arousal catch on, then the couple can proceed to have a sexual encounter, however this is defined. If no "kindling" occurs, the partners do not need to proceed. The higher desire partner must be willing to accept frustration if this happens.

The willingness model is helpful for people who know they enjoy having sex with a partner, but report feeling too tired, depressed, or stressed to want to initiate sex—they "want to want" sex.

It gives permission to say to one's partner, "I'm not really in the mood, but I might be if we start to fool around," and then see what happens. Sexual interest will then more likely develop if the initially uninterested person finds the interaction pleasurable and positive in some way. This is explained even further in the following discussion on responsive desire.

ROSEMARY BASSON

Rosemary Basson developed a nonlinear model of emotional intimacy, sexual stimuli, and relationship satisfaction that was initially focused on female sexuality and response (Basson, 2000). This model, often referred to as "the circular model of sexual response," includes the specific elements *spontaneous* desire (e.g., laying in a hammock on a warm sunny day that happens to light up erogenous zones), *sexual motivation* linked to emotional and physical satisfaction, and *responsive* desire.

Responsive desire is when partner A may not necessarily be thinking about sexual interaction, but partner B applies all of partner A's favorite courtship rituals and touches, resulting in partner A now developing interest and/or arousal to engage in sexual activity with partner B in that situation. To be clear, responsive desire is NOT about "giving in" (especially in this essential, long overdue #metoo zeitgeist of "enthusiastic and freely given consent"), but rather about being receptive to sexual activity in the context of what one considers to be erotic. Responsive desire involves external and internal stimuli (such as physical touch, emotional connection, or erotic thoughts) facilitating sexual desire and arousal. "Responsive desire emerges in *response* [emphasis added] to pleasure. Spontaneous desire emerges in *anticipation* [emphasis added] of pleasure. Both *are* [emphasis added] normal" (Nagoski, n.d., p. 16).

The Basson model (see **Figure 3.1**) also includes the presence, absence, or degree of willingness and receptivity to sexual activity. Basson notes that sexual interest and activity may begin and end anywhere in her model, emphasizing that sexual satisfaction and intimacy can reinforce desire in future sexual encounters, creating a circular pattern of sexual response.

WALEN AND ROTH

Walen and Roth (1987) offered a cognitive component to their sexual response model. They believed that at any given point of the journey to arousal, people evaluate their situation as something that is either positive or negative. If the situation receives a positive evaluation, then the

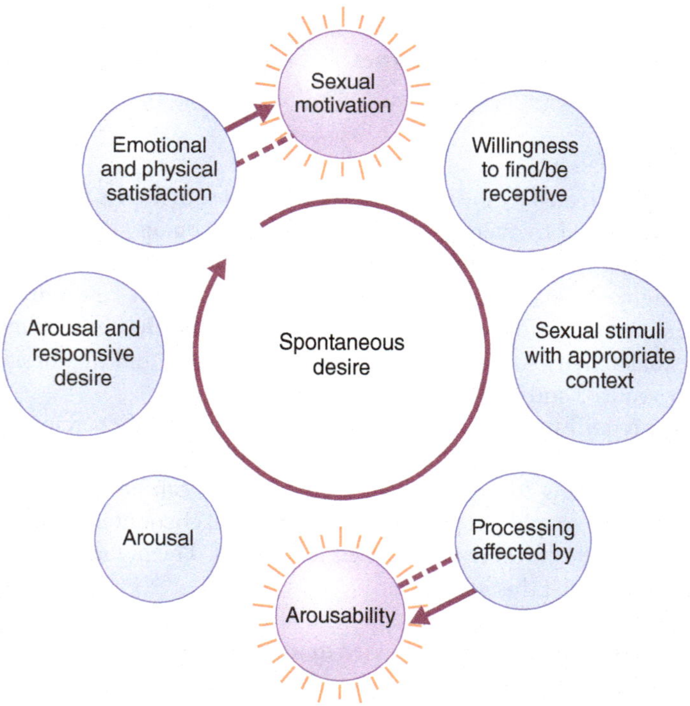

FIGURE 3.1. Basson Model of Sexual Motivation

Source: Basson, R. (2001). Female sexual response: The role of drugs in the management of sexual dysfunction. *Obstetrics & Gynecology, 98*(2), 350–353. https://doi.org/10.1016/s0029-7844(01)01452-1

journey to pleasure and orgasm continues. If the situation receives a negative evaluation or is appraised negatively, the situation moves toward the sexual arousal ending. At each point in the process, appraisal can be guided by a host of events including those that are from a biological basis, a cultural or contextual basis, and/or those from family origin, past relationships, prior trauma, and so on. This provides a holistic approach to understanding arousal and its various components.

DUAL CONTROL MODEL OF SEXUAL RESPONSE

In the late 1990s, Erick Janssen and John Bancroft of the Kinsey Institute (Bancroft & Janssen, 2000; Bancroft et al., 2009) developed the dual control model of sexual response. This model consists of two parts: the sexual excitation system (SES) and sexual inhibition system (SIS).

Emily Nagoski, a national sexpert and Smith College professor and researcher, has an entire chapter devoted to the dual control model in her sexual bible for people with clitorises and vaginas (and the people who love them): *Come as You Are* (2015). Essentially, Nagoski states that "your central nervous system (... brain and spinal cord) is made up of a series of partnership of accelerators and brakes—like the pairing of your sympathetic nervous system ('accelerator') and your parasympathetic nervous system ('brake')." Therefore, the "brain system that coordinates sex [has] a sexual accelerator and sexual brake" (2015, p. 48), called the SES and SIS.

The SIS has two brakes: an emergency brake that notices all the immediate dangers and turn-offs in the environment such as a child screaming in the next room or a grouchy text from one's supervisor. There is also a second brake that emits more of a "chronic, low-level 'No thank you' signal [possibly associated with a] 'fear of performance failure' like worrying about not having an orgasm" (Nagoski, 2015, p. 49). Humans do not necessarily need to know the specifics of a brake, just that we all have these two brakes, and we all have sexual accelerators. Some humans may have a sensitive SES and/or a sensitive SIS, independent of their environment. Because of how well this model is easily understood, I (S. Baird) talk almost exclusively with my clients about their sexual accelerator and brakes.

Talking to your clients about the dual control model, as well as the inclusion of elements such as emotional intimacy and sexual responsiveness, can help them figure out how to turn off their sexual brakes and turn on their sexual accelerators. We currently live in a very hectic world that can include multiple intersecting brakes such as juggling parenting and chauffeuring busy children along with work demands, household chores, hobbies, exercise routines, errands, managing finances, and so on.

Sometimes the best therapeutic intervention is giving clients permission to define better boundaries, stake out private time, or ask for something to change in the environment or their partner's behavior that is impacting their brakes. Therapy goals relating to the dual control model might include role-playing and rehearsal (including eye movement desensitization and reprocessing [EMDR] future templates) of saying no to that 100th task/favor, increasing comfort with resigning from a draining committee or job, asking for household help from a partner or child, and/or setting an important boundary with a relative. It can also be helpful for clients to identify potential sexual accelerators so that they may ask their partners for help in activating those accelerators.

Many clients seeking therapy often mention both a concurrence of a sexual trauma history and a current lack of sexual desire for any sexual activity (whether alone or partnered). In this case, we can hypothesize that their sexual brakes are fully engaged and need to be released by using trauma-informed therapy (i.e., EMDR therapy) to treat their sexual trauma. Once their trauma history has been fully processed, their interest in sex may return on its own (as their emergency and/or chronic brakes are no longer engaged).

Sometimes clients may still report lower interest in sex, yet no longer feel negatively triggered. In this case, they will need to work on identifying and releasing any other limiting brakes (e.g., lack of privacy, overwork, fatigue, medical problems), and then identify and engage with their sexual accelerators. This may be a long process for some trauma survivors who rarely have had the chance to freely engage with sexual context solely for themselves.

Emily Nagoski now has a companion workbook called *The Come as You Are Workbook: A Practical Guide to the Science of Sex* (2019) that can help folks investigate and expand their sexual accelerator contexts. If at this point the client continues to report low or no sexual interest (and is not distressed by this), then exploring the possibility of asexuality or greysexuality may be helpful.

SEXUAL TIPPING POINT

The sexual tipping point model offers a way to think about arousal from a biopsychosocial perspective (Perelman, 2018). In this approach, sexual turn-ons and turn-offs are weighed against each other as if in a ratio. If there are more turn-ons present, the individual will be aroused. If there are more turn-offs or the turn-offs have more weight or are more intense, the result will be the experience of impaired arousal. The model does not dictate what types of turn-ons and turn-offs might be involved. For example, someone might be engaging with an appealing erotic visual cue, but the cue may be paired with a medication they are taking that inhibits their sexual response. In this case, the braking (turn-off) influence of the medication will cancel out the potential accelerator (turn-on) of the visual stimuli.

AROUSAL CONCORDANCE AND NONCONCORDANCE

During sexual stimulation or fantasy, all genders may report or notice increased skin sweat, flushing of the skin, faster breathing, erect nipples, and pupil dilation, along with the genital-specific arousal of clitoral or penile erection, vulvar engorgement, vaginal lubrication, and so on. Unfortunately, many of these responses can occur during unwanted sexual contact, causing a great deal of confusion and distress for sexual trauma survivors who lack this information. Some survivors (regardless of gender identity or anatomical configuration) have reported orgasm during a sexual assault, creating intense confusion and shame.

A very important concept to explain to your clients (especially to clients who have reported erect penises, lubricated vaginas, and/or orgasms against their will) is *arousal concordance* and *nonconcordance*.

Arousal concordance is when a person feels aroused physically and reports a strong penile or clitoral erection *and/or* noticeable vaginal lubrication *and* also mentally desires to engage in the sexual activity. Arousal nonconcordance is when these two elements do not correspond (i.e., there is "sexually relevant" stimulation, but no sexual response or interest).

Cismen have about a 50% overlap of sexually relevant material and confirmed sexual interest, whereas ciswomen have only about a 10% overlap. In other words, in studies showing pornography to adults, cismen's erections correlated 50% of the time with their subjective reports of sexual arousal whereas ciswomen's subjective reports only correlated about 10% (Nagoski, 2015).

Use of typical pornography may introduce a confound that could cause a disjuncture between women's physical arousal and subjective desire. Although sexually explicit, the frequent decontextualized, nonrelational, and sometimes degrading aspects of standard pornography, could function as a brake to women's awareness of sexual desire.

Sexually relevant stimuli such as an erotic image, nipple stimulation, or kissing does not automatically equal sexually appealing stimuli, and vice versa. What is confusing is that if someone's body seems to be responding to sexual stimulation (because the body interprets the information as sexually relevant), they sometimes believe (or are told) that they want that stimulation. Assailants often tell targets things like, "Your nipples are hard" or "You are wet; therefore, you want this."

Conversely, established consensual partners can notice a lack of lubrication or other arousal signs and therefore question whether the partner really is "turned on." You may have clients who report either of these as disturbing or traumatic events. If so, it is critical to provide this psychoeducation and ample time for processing this information and any related shame your client may be holding, due to lack of knowledge of this biological concept.

Lubrication also varies greatly according to many factors—no one should feel ashamed or judged about their amount (or lack) of lubrication. A good analogy that helps clients understand is that most of us cry when we cut an onion, without having any correlating sadness, or that our mouths may salivate at the sight of a baguette that at first glance looks edible, only to discover upon picking it up that it is moldy or inedible.

SEXUAL COMPATIBILITY

DEFINITION

Sexual compatibility is often a misunderstood construct. While it is typically construed by couples to speak specifically to frequency of interest in sexual activity, it is instead a multifaceted construct that involves agreement in *emotions, cognitions,* and *behaviors* (Adeli et al., 2023; Mark et al., 2013; Offman & Matheson, 2005). Several studies have highlighted the value of sexual compatibility in a couple due to its association with sexual satisfaction (Mark et al., 2013) and sexual functioning (Offman & Matheson, 2005). Mark et al. (2013) distinguish between actual and perceived sexual compatibility. The former refers to the extent to which two partners have agreement about what activities constitute turn-on and turn-off responses; the latter refers to the more emotional elements of compatibility such as alignment between wants, needs, and the extent to which each person feels sexually satisfied.

COMPATIBILITY COMPONENTS

As previously mentioned, sexual compatibility is influenced by sexual function, which in turn is also influenced by sexual depression, sexual anxiety, and sexual satisfaction. The *emotional* component of perceived sexual compatibility involves the extent to which each partner understands the other. The *cognitive* component refers to the extent to which beliefs are shared. Finally, the *behavioral* component refers to the extent to which there is agreement and concordance of sexual practices and behaviors (Offman & Matheson, 2005).

For some ciswomen, sexual satisfaction (which can underwrite sexual compatibility) is in part explained by their perception of emotional closeness and involvement in the relationship and their partner. However, for some cismen a primary predictor of the perception of sexual compatibility is related to frequency of sexual interaction (Ahmadnia et al., 2023). At this time there is no data regarding sexual compatibility/satisfaction among transgender, gender nonconforming, intersex, and nonbinary individuals.

SEXUAL PERSONALITY STYLES

The concept of *sexual styles* was originally observed and posited by Donald Mosher (1980). Mosher proposed that orgasm quality is mediated by "effective sexual stimulation" that is experienced as "pleasurable sexual sensations" and feeling excited and joyful. Therefore, Mosher suggests that effective sexual engagement results from both pleasurable physical stimulation as well as "involvement" and interest in the activity. Mosher describes three categories of psychological involvement—*sexual trancer, partner engager,* and/or *role enactor*—and suggests that most of us gravitate toward one dominant style for ourselves.

Sexual trancers are a bit like the introverts of the Myers–Briggs personality test. They tend to like privacy and freedom from distractions. They enjoy a calm, relaxed, and serene mood. They like slow pacing and repetitive movements, and can be passive, sensual, and inwardly oriented. They prefer less frequent talking during sex so that they might be absorbed more easily into sensations. Their own fantasies may revolve around visual or sensory images.

Partner engagers enjoy being psychologically engaged with their partner, preferably involved in what they consider a "good" relationship. They relish a romantic and loving mood, lots of kissing, eye contact, and full body contact. Affectionate sharing, mutual pleasuring, romantic endearments, and love songs can be important parts of their repertoire. They expect their partners to act lovingly toward them, and enjoy a flowing, harmonious union with their partner. Their fantasies may include the face of their partner, memories of union with their partner, and other romantic images.

Role enactors are more like the extroverts of the Myers–Briggs and enjoy more interactive sex play. They may show a tendency toward dramatic, possibly even slightly exhibitionist, elements, bringing a very playful mood, pride in variety and skill of sexual techniques, active movements and sounds, and animated facial expressions. Lusty sex talk, dramatic orgasms, novel situations, role-plays, and interest in ecstasy also show up in this style.

Dr. Kathy McMahon later developed a helpful short sexual styles survey (personal communication, February 26, 2021) that you can provide to your clients to answer if they are interested in better understanding how they and their partners prefer and experience sexual activity. This survey is at the end of this chapter.

Many folks, just like in the Myers–Briggs personality classifications, can demonstrate flexibility in their sexual personality style. A client might mostly be a sexual trancer, but if they have a role enactor partner, that person brings out more playfulness and variety. Or perhaps a client's main style is partner engager, with a side of sexual trancer. This client needs to feel connected and mutual with their partner, allowing for the trance state for orgasm.

There is no right or wrong sexual style, just like being classified as an introvert in the Myers–Briggs classifications is as valid as being an extrovert. Where trouble can brew is when a sexual trancer client is matched up to a role enactor partner. Those are fairly different styles, which means they might have to work hard to make sure everyone's needs are met. For example, the role enactor may create an elaborate role-play scenario, bringing in sex toys, props, blindfolds, and so on. The sexual trancer then may be requested to engage in this active style for some time to fulfill the role enactor's emotional and sexual needs. Once fulfilled, the role enactor can more readily and easily provide a distraction-free, sensual focused zone for the sexual trancer's sensation absorption.

Also, just like in life, sexual opposites often attract. So, instead of clients thinking, "There is such a big river to cross," we can help them think about how fun it can be to build that sexual bridge with their sexual teammate. This is a great exercise in creative thinking and coming up with ways for differently sexually styled folks to feel satiated, together.

Lastly, long-term partners can notice a waning sex life over time and might jump to certain fatalistic conclusions about this, whereas it could be as simple as different sexual styles. In romantic beginnings, people easily cross all the bridges of differences, showing high flexibility in moving back and forth between sexual styles. However, as time goes on, and life gets in the way, folks tend to stratify back to their main style. A couple complaining of reduced sex life, or very different interests in sex frequency, might actually be grappling with very different styles. The role enactor may not be getting their curiosity piqued, and so they have given up on sex. The partner engager may not have felt emotionally connected to their partner in some time, so they turn to Netflix instead. Helping clients learn about their own preferred sexual style and asking for their needs to be met can help correct the ship's course.

Some of these incongruous style issues may be addressed through individual or couples therapy. For example, role-playing/rehearsal can help a client practice speaking up about asking for specific sexual needs, according to their dominant sexual style. If a role enactor client is paired up with a sexual trancer, then a possible rehearsal or EMDR future template might go like this:

Clinician: "Imagine yourself effectively asking for your partner to engage in role-play or use of props (or talking, etc.) during sex." (Client notes body sensation and bilateral stimulation is applied until negative sensation becomes neutral, or positive sensation is enhanced.)

Clinician: "Let's pair a positive thought with this event. How about, 'I am worthy and capable of asking for what I need.'" Continue the rehearsal or EMDR future template from there.

Case Study 3.1: Incongruous Sexual Personality Styles

Bianca and Viviana, cisgender lesbians, have been together for 3 years and have both noticed that their frequency of sexual activity has greatly decreased. Both are in their late twenties, and both work in human services at different corporations. Viviana has begun to explore the process of in vitro fertilization (IVF) pregnancy, as she is looking forward to having a family with Bianca. Bianca is also excited about eventually having a family, but is happy to wait a few more years as they continue to advance in their careers. They decided to seek couples counseling due to decreased intimacy and increased animated discussion around family planning and timing.

After completing a thorough intake process, including administering the sexual styles questionnaire, the therapist discovered that Bianca's answers reflected the *trancer* style, while Viviana's answers reflected the *role enactor* style. This also made sense as during the therapy sessions the therapist observed Viviana's frequent playfulness and sense of fun, whereas Bianca appeared more reserved and focused. When the therapist reported these observations and the results of the questionnaire to the couple, they both agreed the descriptions resonated.

Upon further exploration, Viviana reported how early in the relationship they engaged in frequent sexual role-play, as well as utilized many fun props such as blindfolds and handcuffs, alongside vibrators. While they continue to use vibrators, their blindfolds and handcuffs have remained buried deep in a closet drawer. Bianca noted that it can be hard to have an orgasm when she is engaged in more active sexual activity. A quiet, clean, dark room, and the ability to focus on the sensation, is most conducive to her being able to orgasm. Viviana added that for herself, that type of sex feels boring, and that she'd rather not have sex at all than feel bored. Viviana also noted that she anticipates the process of getting pregnant to be pedantic and "work-like"—making it even more unappealing to have similar "work-like" sex.

When asked why the role-plays and use of props diminished, Bianca noted that they had moved about a year ago, and never brought those toys back out. Not only that, but at that time she experienced some major changes at work, creating a period of intense stress. During those months, it was all she could do to make sure the vibrator was plugged in and clean for sex. Bianca also noted that she feels she has a more "responsive" style of sex, and therefore was often not an initiator of sex. Viviana took this to mean that perhaps Bianca was not as attracted to her anymore. For Viviana, having her partner woo and romance her were also important parts of the sexual interaction. The lack of this courtship behavior has felt deflating to Viviana's sense of sexual self.

The therapist worked with them to develop a bridge between their two different styles. First, they were asked to set aside weekly "context dates," with all available sex toys and props visible and accessible. They brainstormed a multitude of intimate and connecting activities they could do during those dates and came up with this list: listen to erotic audiobooks, tickling, flirting, cuddle in bed and reminisce about some earlier zestful sexual experiences with each other, give each other nonsexual massages, take a shower together, look at adult sex toy websites to see what new items were available, enjoy deep kissing, engage in manual and/or oral sex, share sexual fantasies, and/or utilize any of their sex toys. The therapist assured them that anything they ended up doing would be fine, as long as it felt pleasurable and connecting. The therapist also reiterated that if one of them no longer wanted to engage in the activity, they should stop it and switch to something else for the rest of that context date.

After a month of enjoying context dates focused on mostly kissing, Viviana massaging Bianca, and Viviana sharing some of her sexual fantasies and favorite prior sexual experiences with Bianca, on their own they set aside a longer Sunday afternoon to enact one of Viviana's recent fantasies. Bianca agreed to orchestrate most of the setting, prop, and behavioral details to activate Viviana's sexual accelerators. Viviana agreed that once she felt satiated, she would turn down the lights and create an environment where Bianca could more easily focus on having an orgasm. They agreed to keep the communication lines open so that either could speak up any time they were no longer feeling pleasure or excitement.

They arrived at the therapist's office on Tuesday with big smiles and described how they were able to arrange this magnificent sexual encounter, each meeting their partner's needs, getting their own needs met, and each finding renewed pleasure, excitement, and amazement at their partner's heightened sexual arousal during this encounter.

EROTIC TEMPLATE FORMATION

Jack Morin's innovative book *The Erotic Mind* (1995) introduced the concept of *core erotic themes* (CETs). He posits that these CETs develop during infancy and childhood from sexual or sensual triggers or events and lay the groundwork for our future sexual experiences. Specifically, these CETs form the bases of the specific types of feelings (not necessarily scenarios) we require for sexual engagement. Examples of feelings that one's CET might contain include a desire to be ravished, dominating, submissive, taboo, spiritually merged, and so on.

Patrick Carnes (2001) discusses the "sexual arousal template" which can include "thoughts, images, behaviors, sounds, smells, sights, fantasies, and objects" that sexually arouse an individual. While his take on "sex addiction" has been taken to task in recent years by more affirming and sex-positive therapists, there is some reality regarding the overexposure to internet pornography and how this easy access to what were once fringe and/or illegal images might be shaping clients' erotic templates into something they are ashamed or dismayed by, resulting in behaviors that feel "compulsive" or "out of control" to them. Additionally, it is worth noting that many individuals first stumble upon internet porn around the age of 9 or 10, endangering them toward developing unrealistic or negative associations with sexuality.

One short case vignette is "Travis," a senior cismale college student who sought EMDR therapy due to lingering feelings of disgust around seeing sexual images. As we developed our EMDR target list, several targets of early exposure (around age 8) and viewing of internet pornography were discovered. Working through these targets allowed him to have mental and emotional room to sort out for himself his own sexual likes and dislikes, without the accompanying disgust. He went on to have enjoyable sexual experiences with a new partner.

Another case vignette involves a young cisfemale child, "Mackenzie," around the age of 12. She had been exposed to pornographic images unwillingly at an earlier age (around age 6). Her presenting complaint was seeing unwanted flashes of the imagery in her mind and feeling anxious in general. After completing EMDR therapy on the identified targets and identifying difficult life circumstances relating to the early exposure (i.e., parents divorcing), she reported no longer experiencing the interfering thoughts and felt more "peaceful" and at ease.

Compassionately helping your adult clients explore their erotic templates (images, feelings, and themes) by using an open-minded, nonjudgmental, and curious stance can help them gain insight into their origins. If these CETs are truly distressing to the client or are illegal (such as looking at underage or violent pornography), processing of the specific themes and images can help to eliminate the shame, disturbance, and possibly the "positive charge" of those images. If necessary, we can help our clients find more positive, judgment-free ways to experience some of those formerly distressing erotic feelings (whether dominance, submission, rebellion, connection, etc.).

SUMMARY

Since the 1940s, there have been many scientists, biologists, sociologists, and psychologists researching human sexuality (e.g., Kinsey, Kaplan, Hite, Basson). Jannsen and Bancroft are recent researchers who formulated the dual control model of sexual response. According to this model, the brain system coordinates the SES and SIS. Interest and desire for sexual activity correlates with one's *sexual accelerator* being engaged. Active *sexual brakes* correlate with a disinterest and/or rejection of sexual activity. Many things can press on someone's sexual brakes, ranging from small things such as arguments or misunderstandings with partner(s), to large things like a history of trauma.

Spontaneous desire occurs when someone notices an interest in sexual activity arising that is unrelated to anything sexual in the mind or environment. *Responsive desire* can occur when one person, with full consent, engages their ambivalent partner with pleasurable sexually relevant or erotic stimulation, resulting in that ambivalent partner now becoming interested in sexual activity.

Arousal nonconcordance is when someone reports incongruous sexual arousal and interest. For instance, a trauma survivor may ashamedly report having had an erection, lubrication, and/or orgasm during unwanted sexual activity, and affirm they mentally and emotionally did not want the activity at all. Bodies often respond to sexually relevant stimuli regardless of actual interest or desire; therefore, sexual trauma victims should never be blamed or made to feel that "they wanted it." Any of these reported situations (unwanted arousal, lubrication shame) might benefit from supportive psychoeducation and therapy.

Sexual compatibility is a multifaceted construct that involves agreement in behaviors, emotions, and cognitions. High alignment of these agreements is often associated with positive sexual satisfaction and sexual functioning. Most folks can benefit from identifying a preferred sexual personality style (sexual trancer, partner engager, and/or role enactor) for themselves. Differences in sexual personality style may relate to some sexual incompatibilities.

Erotic and/or sexual arousal templates develop from birth to present. Helping our clients explore and understand these templates can lead to clinical material for exploration, particularly if shame or discomfort is reported.

DISCUSSION QUESTIONS

- What do you think was the most important discovery in sexology research in the 20th century (before the year 2000) and why?
- What are some common examples of "sexual brakes" reported by individuals? What might some examples of "sexual accelerators" be? How might someone turn off their reported "brakes" in order to access more "accelerators"?
- What can you tell a client who reports shame about having a penile or clitoral erection or vaginal lubrication during an unwanted sexual interaction?
- Do you think it is "better" to generally experience "spontaneous" desire or "responsive" desire? Why?
- What are some factors that might promote or enhance sexual compatibility within intimate partners?

LEARNING ACTIVITIES

CourseConnect

To access self-assessment questions and interactive, competency-based learning activities for this chapter, visit www.springerpub.com/courseconnect. See inside front cover and tear-out card for CourseConnect details.

ADDITIONAL RESOURCES

Additional resources are online and available at www.springerpub.com/courseconnect.

REFERENCES

Adeli, M., Moghaddam-Banaem, L., Shahali, S., & Soori, T. (2023). Genital warts and women's sexual challenges: Is sexual compatibility possible? A qualitative study. *BMC Women's Health, 23*(1), 610. https://doi.org/10.1186/s12905-023-02771-9

Ahmadnia, E., Ziaei, T., Yunesian, M., Haseli, A., Nazari, A. M., & Keramat, A. (2023). Sexual compatibility and its associated factors among heterosexual couples: A systemic review. *Sexual and Relationship Therapy, 38*(4), 603–621. https://doi.org/10.1080/14681994.2020.1849608

Bancroft, J., Graham, C. A., Janssen, E., & Sanders, S. A. (2009). The dual control model: Current status and future directions. *Journal of Sex Research, 46*(2–3), 121–142. https://doi.org/10.1080/00224490902747222

Bancroft, J., & Janssen, E. (2000). The dual control model of male sexual response: A theoretical approach to centrally mediated erectile dysfunction. *Neuroscience and Biobehavioral Reviews, 24*(5), 571–579. https://doi.org/10.1016/s0149-7634(00)00024-5

Basson, R. (2000). The female sexual response: A different model. *Journal of Sex & Marital Therapy, 26*(1), 51–65. https://doi.org/10.1080/009262300278641

Carnes, P. (2001). *Out of the shadows: Understanding sexual addiction* (3rd ed.). Hazelden.

Hite, S. (1981). *The Hite report on male sexuality.* Ballantine Books.

Hite, S. (1987). *Women and love: A cultural revolution in progress.* St. Martin's Press.

Hite, S. (2011). *The Hite report: A nationwide study of female sexuality.* Seven Stories Press (Originally published 1976).

Kaplan, H. S. (1977). Hypoactive sexual desire. *Journal of Sex & Marital Therapy, 3*(1), 3–9. https://doi.org/10.1080/00926237708405343

Kinsey, A. C., Pomeroy, W. B., & Martin, C. E. (1948). *Sexual behavior in the human male.* Indiana University Press.

Kinsey, A. C., Pomeroy, W. B., Martin, C. E., & Gebhard, P. H. (1953). *Sexual behavior in the human female.* Indiana University Press.

Loulan, J. (1984). *Lesbian sex.* Spinster's Ink.

Mark, K. P., Milhausen, R. R., & Maitland, S. B. (2013). The impact of sexual compatibility on sexual and relationship satisfaction in a sample of young adult heterosexual couples. *Sexual & Relationship Therapy, 28*(3), 201–214. https://doi.org/10.1080/14681994.2013.807336

Masters, W. H., & Johnson, V. E. (1966). *Human sexual response.* Little, Brown.

Morin, J. (1995). *The erotic mind: Unlocking the inner sources of sexual passion and fulfillment.* Harper Perennial.

Mosher, D. (1980). Three dimensions of depth of involvement in human sexual response. *Journal of Sex Research, 16*(1), 1–42. https://doi.org/10.1080/00224498009551060

Nagoski, E. (n.d.). *Ten tips for making the most of responsive desire.* Nagoski Booklet.

Nagoski, E. (2015). *Come as you are.* Simon & Schuster.

Nagoski, E. (2019). *The come as you are workbook: A practical guide to the science of sex.* Simon & Schuster.

Newnham, N. (Director). (2023). *The disappearance of Shere Hite* [Documentary]. NBC News Studios; Sony Pictures Television; TeaTime Pictures.

Offman, A., & Matheson, K. (2005). Sexual compatibility and sexual functioning in intimate relationships. *Canadian Journal of Human Sexuality, 14*(1-2), 31–39.

Perelman, M. A. (2018). Sex coaching for non-sexologist physicians: How to use the sexual tipping point model. *Journal of Sexual Medicine, 15*(12), 1667–1672. https://doi.org/10.1016/j.jsxm.2018.10.010

Rivera, G. (Writer), & Morris, M. (Director). (1977, March 3). The Hite report: A sexual survey (episode 28) [TV series episode]. In M. M. Berman (Producer) & J. Weintraub (Executive Producer), *Good Night America.* Maravilla; ABC Studios. https://www.geraldo.com/the-hite-report-a-sexual-survey

Walen, S. R., & Roth, D. (1987). A cognitive approach. In J. H. Geer & W. T. O'Donohue (Eds.), *Theories of human sexuality.* Plenum Press.

Zilbergeld, B., & Ellison, C. R. (1980). Desire discrepancies and arousal problems in sex therapy. In S. R. Leiblum & L. A. Pervin (Eds.), *Principles and practice of sex therapy* (pp. 65–101). Guilford Press.

SUPPLEMENTAL MATERIALS FOR CLINICIANS AND CLIENTS

For PDF versions of this material, access the "Downloads" feature on Course Connect (www.springerpub.com/courseconnect).

SEXUAL STYLES SURVEY

Dr. Kathy McMahon

Couples Therapy Inc., 125 Guest Street, Boston, Massachusetts

Following are characteristics that happen in sex. These can be thought of as preferred pathways of involvement. I want you to imagine your ideal sexual situation with your ideal sexual partner. Alternatively, imagine the kind of sex you'd like to have when you want sex to be "normal" or maximally satisfying for you. While many answers might fit, rank order them as (3) "most important," (2) "less important" or (1) "not important."

There are no right or wrong answers.

1. Setting: In the ideal setting, I'd like:

___ Privacy: Temperature, lighting, and freedom from distraction may all be important.
___ Psychological: A good relationship.
___ Freedom: Playful, inventive, fantasy, drama.

2. Mood: Ideally, I'd like to feel:

___ Calm: Relaxed and serene. Relaxing and getting in the mood can be a necessary preliminary to concentrate on sexual stimulation.
___ Romantic: Loving toward my partner.
___ Good about myself: High self-esteem, playful.

3. Sexual technique: What we do ideally should be:

___ Slow: Familiar, slow-paced, nothing sudden or unexpected. Gentle, rhythmic sensation without abrupt alterations in tempo or pressure leads to a familiar sense of enjoyed pleasure.
___ Tender: A lot of kissing, eye contact, and full body contact.
___ Innovative: Full of variety, skillful in love making in all areas of sexuality and the ability to be sexually responsive.

4. Sexual style: I'd like sex that is:

___ Sensation-focused: Good sex is all about connecting with the sensations, being receptive to one's partner, and being in touch with your inner self. Passive, receptive concentration and surrender, rather than the active pursuit of the novel thrill or novel self-expression, are preferred.
___ Mutual: Good sex is all about affectionate sharing, cuddling, and mutual pleasuring.
___ Active: Expressive in action, sound, and facial expression. I don't have to guess that they are enjoying themselves. Novelty adds spice.

5. Role expectations: In the ideal, my partner is:

___ In tune: They are sensitive to where I'm at, and aren't jarring in the way they interact with me.
___ Affectionate: They demonstrate their love for me in word and deed.
___ Complementary: Good sex happens with partners who are complementary and work well together to turn up the heat.

6. Sex talk:

___ "Shhh": Unless I'm hurting them or need to provide important feedback, I'd prefer to let our bodies do the talking. Mention pleasurable sensations or feelings ... that's okay.
___ Romantic endearments: I want to know how they feel about me. Intimate conversation may be a good seduction or may accompany the sex.
___ Arouse me: I like lusty or directive language, some might call it "dirty talk."

7. Fantasies:

___ Scriptless: My fantasies are often visual, sensory, or synesthetic. They don't have to have a plot, I can imagine a kiss, a touch, or an image and that's enough.
___ Romantic: I imagine my lover's face from precious moments, tender things we've done together, or the romance of our sex in my fantasies.

___ Novel: I like to imagine more innovative or daring fantasies, even if I wouldn't want to act them out in real life. "Let's pretend," is fun. Hey, it's just a fantasy, right?

8. Conception of sex:

___ An altered state: Great sex lets me escape the cares of my everyday life with the one I love. Or feeling ecstatically transported, floating on a sea of sensations.

___ Loving merger: Great sex for me reminds me of the love bond I feel. It is being deeply connected to my partner.

___ Ecstasy: Great sex is an adventure involving ecstatic expression and is "nonvolitional." It is so passionate that I'm swept away by it. Novel scripts or new props keeps things interesting.

9. Orgasm:

___ Absorbing: The best orgasms are intense sensations with a fading of my consciousness.

___ Flow: The best orgasms are like two people merging into one ... we lose our individuality and become one in union with each other.

___ Intense: The best orgasms are dramatic, expressive, and nonvolitional. They sweep me away without any effort on my part.

Use the following scale (1–5; 1 = *Not true for me* and 5 = *True for me*) to indicate "how true" the following statements are. Write your answer before each statement.

10. ___ The most important aspect of my mood when I get into sex is that I be relaxed and receptive.
11. ___ I believe that I would feel very excited having secret sex in a semipublic place.
12. ___ Ideally all sexual techniques begin and build from kissing the partner's face and lips.
13. ___ I like to have sex at a time when I am sure that there will be no distractions to interrupt or interfere with my enjoyment.
14. ___ When I'm feeling really good about myself, then I love to make love.
15. ___ The setting in which I have sex is less important than the present feelings existing between me and my partner.
16. ___ I like my partner to stay with a sexual activity that is feeling good rather than skipping around from here to there.
17. ___ I use my imagination to increase my absorption into the sensory experience of sex.
18. ___ When my heart is bursting with love, I know our sex will be bursting with pleasure.
19. ___ I pride myself in being quite accomplished in the techniques of oral sex.
20. ___ To increase my excitement, I often imagine during sex that I am with another partner or in a more exotic setting.
21. ___ Sometimes I imagine that my partner is pledging their love to me for life in the act of sexual intercourse.

SCORING

For questions 1 through 9, if the respondent most frequently ranks the first option (i.e., privacy, calm, etc.) as most important, then they likely fall under the "sexual trancer" category. If they most frequently rank the second option (i.e., psychologic, romantic, tender, etc.) as most important, then they likely fall under the "partner engager" style. If they most frequently rank the third option (i.e., freedom, innovative, active, etc.) as most important, then they likely fall under the "role enactor" style.

For questions 10 to 21, the following "highly true" categories apply to sexual trancer, partner engager, and role enactor, respectively.

Sexual trancer: 10, 13, 16, 17

Partner engager: 12, 15, 18, 21

Role enactor: 11, 14, 19, 20

CHAPTER 4

Human Sexual Development

Katherine Hertlein, Eterniti Claggett, and Desia Thrower

LEARNING OBJECTIVES

- Understand the models of sexual education.
- Describe the role of communication and sexual skill-building in sexual development.
- Describe how Erikson's psychosocial stages apply to sexual development.
- Describe the role of cultural and social factors in sexual development.

INTRODUCTION

Sexual development is an experience occurring throughout the life span, from childhood into old age. It reflects a complex interplay of hormones, genes, history, experiences, biology, and the environment. Healthy sexual development is often observed as having the following characteristics: (a) the use of accurate, age-appropriate terminology to describe anatomy and physiology; (b) healthy communication; (c) consent; (d) respect for bodily functions; (e) respect for erotic responses; (f) gender roles; (g) appropriate sexual boundaries, (h) ability to practically and affectionately touch and engage in physical interaction; (i) promoting healthy sexual decision-making; and (j) appropriate knowledge of sexual functioning. In other words, development that would be considered sexually healthy would include attention to one's physical development (including bodily changes) and emotional development (including attention to relationship development).

THE ROLE OF SKILL BUILDING AND COGNITION IN SEXUAL DEVELOPMENT

Cultivating healthy sexual development involves the application of different practices and skill-building activities to improve and expand one's knowledge, attitudes, and behaviors about sex (Boustani et al., 2017; Ghaffari & Feizollahe Vahid, 2020; Heard et al., 2015).

SEX EDUCATION

Providing education to enhance sexual development often includes details about one's body and bodily functioning, the influence of gender and sex roles, sexual behaviors, consent, and demonstration of affection. Education has been shown to have a positive influence on sexual development (McKay et al., 2022; Sell et al., 2023), especially for vulnerable groups such as men with mild intellectual disabilities in reducing their risk of victimization (Verbeek et al., 2023). At the same time, formal sex education programs are controversial in many cultures and societies. Formal sex education strategies refer to those models and programs taught in schools and other educational settings. In the United States, for example, three models of formal sexual education dominate the training: abstinence only until marriage (AOUM), abstinence-plus education (APE), and comprehensive sex education (CSE).

Abstinence-Only Programs

Abstinence-only programs teach that sex should only be experienced in the context of a legally married couple (Clark & Stitzlein, 2016). Such programming can negatively impact healthy sexual development if they omit critical information about sexual minorities, LGBTQ+ individuals, pregnant and/or parenting youth, and even survivors of sexual violence (Santelli et al., 2017) and shame people who have sex outside of the bounds of marriage (Lamb & Gilbert, 2019). In addition, many of the educational programs do not include information about the couple's relationship itself. Common examples include a lack of information on violence, communication, disease transition, and other related aspects of sexual relationships. Further, a general lack of education around sexuality tends to limit literacy in health matters generally.

Without appropriate education across the life span, young people may not receive medically accurate information about reproductive health, nor about how to approach relationships generally. At the same time, as young people become sexually active, the lack of medically relevant education leaves them at risk for medical and physical consequences such as sexually transmitted diseases and pregnancy, and also subject to problematic consequences of unhealthy relationships (Finkelhor et al., 2014; Kann et al., 2018). In fact, a significant number of young people report sexual assault, abuse, and an engagement in dating violence during their adolescent years, each of which would shape their view of sexuality, their self-confidence, sexual self-efficacy, and so on.

Comprehensive Sex Education

Programs that incorporate attention to pregnancy, disease prevention, dating violence, healthy relationships, healthy communication, gender roles, media management, and the role of parents in sexual communication reduce risky behavior and improve sexual health overall for young people (Coyne et al., 2019; Goldfarb & Lieberman, 2021; Scull et al., 2022). One such example is the "Our Whole Lives" (OWL) curricula. This program curricula is informed by comprehensive sexual education standards and includes information that is respectful of gender identity, ability status, and cultural background. It provides education through parents, peers, electronic media, and other formats and shapes the delivery to be appropriate for various target age groups.

Effective Communication

One such skill to be developed is effective communication as it supports healthy development through teaching people to understand how to express and receive messages of consent, how to communicate sexual wants and needs, and how to set boundaries (Widman et al., 2018). For example, Boustani et al. (2017) effectively implemented a program based in part on developing communication skills to reduce risky sexual behaviors in underrepresented youth. The same is true for older adults: partnerships with open sexual communication were rated as having greater satisfaction in sex than those partnerships without (Gillespie, 2017). The content of communication that fostered more satisfying sexual relationships for adults later in the life span included conversations about sexual synchronicity (that is, the opportunities for sexual interaction, how alike each preference was in desire and activities, and a reciprocal exchange of ideas and attitudes about sex; Gillespie, 2017).

SKILL-BUILDING

The timing of skill-building is important to one's sexual development. Just as one's sexual capacity changes over the life span, so does the need to be provided with updated and life-stage relevant information. For example, the communication skills that are taught to 4-year-olds about how to set boundaries around their body are different from the skills taught to adults. The conversation about consent is very different depending on the age and developmental level of the person. Martino et al. (2008), as cited by Aydoğdu et al. (2021), consider healthy sexual development in children to revolve around the child's values; some have created ways to frame it as a story, which is more consistent with youth development (Senior & Chenhall, 2016). Those with healthy sexual development in childhood value their personal health and body; express love and intimacy in ways consistent with their values, abilities, and preferences; and can interact with others appropriately.

COGNITIONS

Cognitions also influence one's level of sexual development. One category of cognition, *sexual-self-concept,* refers to all the cognitions and emotions one has related to their sexual relationships (Musavi et al., 2024). It also can include one's level of sexual self-awareness. Sexual self-concept, like general self-concept in other areas, can inform how one views themselves in certain situations. One's sexual self-concept is not necessarily a stable construct. It can be influenced by previous sexual experiences, trauma, bodily changes influenced by weight changes, childbirth, postpartum, hormonal changes, and perception of overall relationship well-being and satisfaction. It provides a broader view of one's thoughts and feelings about sex and sexuality and includes attention to concepts like arousal, anxiety, commitment, and self-exploration (Simsek et al., 2020).

With heightened sexual self-concept comes a second category of cognition, known as *sexual self-confidence*. As another important factor contributing to healthy sexual development, it is defined as "an individual's ability to experience their sexual desire and feelings comfortably and to have sexual awareness" (Musavi et al., 2024, p. 2). Individuals high in sexual self-confidence are less depressed, less anxious, and have an easier time in social relationships. They may experience other comorbidities as well, such as anxiety and harming behaviors (including homicidal and suicidal ideation; Simsek et al., 2020). These comorbidities alongside the lack of confidence can in general contribute to impairments in one's sex life and contribute to sexual problems more generally. This may potentially cause someone to avoid sexual situations and avoid sex altogether, thus fueling both the lack of confidence and the sexual impairments together (Simsek et al., 2020).

The third construct, *sexual self-efficacy*, refers to "one's perceived ability to engage in sexual activities and be desirable to their sexual partner" (Musavi et al., 2024, p. 3). Sexual self-efficacy is associated with sociodemographic factors, relationship factors, psychological factors, and sexual history factors.

The sociodemographic factors influencing sexual self-efficacy include social and parental support, socioeconomic status, religious requirements, the extent to which one can negotiate, and any other physical problems.

Some of the factors that affect sexual self-efficacy related to sexual history include one's sexual experience, the presence of childhood sexual abuse, whether the individual has any sexual difficulties, what their beliefs about sex are, and the extent to which they have had sex education and/or therapy training.

Relationship factors influencing sexual self-efficacy include satisfaction and quality of the relationship, how intimate the relationship is, and how long the relationship has lasted.

Finally, psychological factors include mental health disorders such as anxiety and depression, paranoia, psychosis, phobia, obsessions, aggression, and being a sensitive person (Assarzadeh et al., 2019; Atrian et al., 2019). While it is out of the scope of this chapter to report on body image and its connection to sexual self-efficacy, sexual self-efficacy reduces when one becomes more dissatisfied with their body image, which ultimately can have an impact on one's romantic relationship.

Besides the factors associated with sexual self-efficacy, this concept is important for healthcare practitioners as it is a window into understanding whether a sexual problem has a physical or psychological ideology. For example, people who have a high level of sexual self-efficacy tend to have sex more frequently. When they have sex more frequently, they report that they are more sexually compatible with their partner. On the other hand, people with low levels of sexual self-efficacy may have sex less frequently and potentially can engage in high-risk sexual behaviors. In addition, sexual self-efficacy is key to the development of healthy sexuality in youth (Byers et al., 2018).

Each of these cognitive concepts interacts with one another and contributes to one's psychological sexual development. For example, in cisgendered men, when sexual self-confidence drops, sexual self-efficacy drops as well because an individual who loses self-confidence begins to feel less desirable and may perceive themselves as being less effective in sexual situations (Batmaz & Çelik, 2021). The result is a recursive decline of confidence and satisfaction overall with one's sexual life (Yazdkhasti et al., 2023).

SEXUAL DEVELOPMENT ACROSS THE LIFE SPAN

IN UTERO

Human sexual development begins in utero (Aatscha et al., 2023; Arnold, 2017). A series of hormonal influences, chromosomal combinations, and gonadal development influence the structure of the developing human (Bramble et al., 2017). The differentiation of sex is a process by which (or if) gonads transition into testes at the initiation of certain styles of cells. Once the testes or ovaries have been formed, hormones are released that guide the continued development of structures. There are innumerable outcomes in how we differentiate from one other, and one's physical sexual development is no exception. Predictable outcomes of sexual development may result in an ability to distinguish one's sex and gender more easily, based on prior simplistic views of biology (i.e., binary classifications of "maleness" or "femaleness").

Intersex

If one's physical presentation does not follow in a predictable way, there are a vast number of combinations that result, contributing to a recent view of expansive biology and nonbinary gender. These natural variations in the differentiation process have historically (and harmfully) been referred to as *disorders of sexual development (DSD*; reinforcing previously pejorative and anxious attitudes), which can affect the way in which someone is identified by and self-identifies their sex and gender (Barseghyan et al., 2015, 2018). These physical, hormonal, and chromosomal variations are also known as *intersex*, seen in perhaps as much as 2% (or more) of the population, and highly varied in presentation. Intersex individuals in the past have been dangerously targeted and considered pathological because of the poor research base on this topic, and cultural fears of nonbinary presentations. The proportion of people who are intersexed experience challenge in obtaining advocacy and understanding what constitutes good care. Furthermore, managing these variations may be difficult, as they may co-occur with other conditions such as cancer or dysphoria, thus amplifying the effects of psychosocial issues.

ENVIRONMENTAL FACTORS

Environmental factors also impact sexual development in both physical and psychological ways. From a physical perspective, evidence suggests that sex determination can be impacted to some degree by environmental climate and temperature, along with the tendency for women to seek out partners who have the best potential to maximize offspring (Schwanz & Georges, 2021). Another example of this is the presence of evidence that environmental factors such as adolescent body mass index (BMI) and nutrition intake can influence the age of menstruation (Richardson et al., 2023). Early environmental stress, however, has been shown to be related to age of first sexual experience, but not with age of onset of menstruation (Richardson et al., 2023).

SEXUAL BEHAVIORS

Another consideration for healthy sexual development is evaluating the appropriateness of sexual behaviors in people across the life span. For example, as discussed earlier, we tend to view children as being innocent and not having any sexual desires, despite biological evidence to the contrary. Several studies have shown that infants and young children masturbate, though it is not believed to be intentional in infants. Hesapcioglu et al. (2017) discovered that individuals with higher scores on impulsivity and who score higher on the novelty-seeking scale are more likely to masturbate than others. Lamb and Gilbert (2018) dedicated a text to understanding what is considered appropriate across the life span for young people and is a helpful resource for helping parents and caregivers gain confidence in how to talk about sex to youth.

PUBERTY RITUALS AND YOUTH BEHAVIORS IN VARIOUS CULTURES

Puberty is a transitional life period marked by changes in body composition, size, and shape that vary distinctively across individuals. Typically it is an indication of health for an adolescent individual (Rogol et al., 2002), and marked by an event such as a growth spurt or first menstruation. Puberty also marks the entrance into adolescence, a transitional life stage that typically involves rituals, which can include ceremonies and celebrations; these vary across cultures.

Puberty rituals across cultures often function as rites of passage or a period of transition as outlined by Victor Turner in *The Ritual Process* (Turner, 1969, Ch. 3). This early text references *Les Rites de Passage* (van Gannep, 1909), which guides individuals through a three-phase journey: separation from childhood, a transformative liminal stage (may involve trials, tests, or symbolic death, reflecting this transitional state), and reintegration into society with a new adult status. An example of this could be the transition from undergraduate to graduate school. While the biological aspects of puberty are virtually the same across cultures, puberty rituals vary greatly all over the world. Much of the puberty rites in other cultures come from old text, and have likely evolved from that time. Turner's work makes reference to the circumcision of Ndembu males or the seclusion of females in Zambia, Southern Africa (1969).

Erik Erikson's Theory of Psychosocial Development

Erik Erikson's theory of psychosocial development offers a valuable framework for understanding the significance of these rituals. Erikson posits that individuals progress through eight stages throughout their life span, each presenting a psychosocial crisis that needs to be resolved for healthy development. During adolescence, individuals face the challenge of identity versus role confusion (E. H. Erikson, 1968). They grapple with questions like "Who am I?" and "What is my place in the world?" Puberty rituals, with their emphasis on separation from childhood and incorporation into adult roles, can be seen as supporting adolescents in navigating this crisis.

The Xhosa Imbali exemplifies this structure. Young men undergo a period of separation from their families and community (Turner, 1969). This physical and social detachment symbolizes a break from their childhood identity and aligns with Erik Erikson's (1968) concept of identity versus role confusion. During the liminal stage, the initiates face challenges and learn tribal lore, preparing them for their new roles as warriors (Mead, 1928). These challenges contribute to their development and foster a sense of identity as they approach adulthood. The Imbali culminates in a public ceremony (reintegration) where they are presented as warriors, gaining new rights and responsibilities within Xhosa society (Turner, 1967). This public recognition signifies their identity as adults within the community.

Even geographically distant cultures like those practicing the Hindu Upanayana and the Jewish bat mitzvah share similar themes. Both rituals mark religious adulthood and emphasize intellectual and spiritual growth, contributing to the development of a well-rounded identity. The Upanayana ceremony, for young boys, involves wearing a sacred thread symbolizing commitment to religious study (a form of separation; Bhandarkar, 1928). This act signifies their separation from childhood and their dedication to acquiring knowledge, thereby shaping their religious identity.

Another example of a female puberty ritual is a quinceañera. This celebration in Latinx families marks the transition of a girl into womanhood. It is a two-part celebration that includes both a religious element and a reception. The religious portion (typically a mass) includes a tradition of leaving flowers by a statue of the Virgin Mary to symbolize the purity of the 15-year old quince girl. Another portion of the ceremony is to give a porcelain doll to a younger sister to symbolize the transition.

These examples highlight the diverse expressions of puberty rituals across cultures, all serving to guide adolescents through the complexities of puberty and emerging adulthood. While the specific practices and symbols may vary, the underlying themes of separation, transformation, and reintegration often resonate with Erikson's psychosocial development theory, particularly the stage of identity versus role confusion. These rituals provide a structured and meaningful context for adolescents to navigate this critical stage, fostering a sense of identity, belonging, and social responsibility within their cultural framework. It is important to remember that these themes are not universally present and can vary significantly across cultures. Additionally, cultural norms and practices evolve, and contemporary versions of these rituals may differ considerably from their traditional forms.

Young Adult Sexual Behaviors

Emerging adulthood is a period marked by feelings of exploration, contemplation, and other factors, according to Erikson. The key features of emerging adulthood include the age of identity explorations, the age of instability, the self-focused age, the age of feeling in-between, and the age of possibilities.

For instance, there are distinct cognitive, emotional, and behavioral features that set young adulthood apart from younger and older individuals. Additionally, transitions to careers, marriage, and parenthood are occurring later, as postsecondary education has increased in need. The increased tolerance for premarital sex has also allowed marriage to be delayed. Finally, emerging adulthood has its own specific period, not to be associated with adolescence or older adulthood.

Erik Erikson's (1950, 1968) psychosocial theory of development posits that *young adulthood* (ages loosely defined between 19–40) is a period characterized by the navigation of the psychosocial crisis of *intimacy versus isolation* (Keniston, 1971, as cited in Arnett, 2000). This period is characterized by the search for meaningful and deep connections with others. In terms of sexual behaviors, individuals in this stage may explore and establish intimate relationships, seeking both physical and emotional closeness with their partners.

Having successfully grappled with identity formation in the intimacy versus isolation stage, young adults now focus outward, seeking to establish deep and meaningful connections with others (Orlofsky et al., 1973). Failure to achieve this developmental milestone can lead to feelings of isolation and a stunted sense of self.

The traditional conceptualization of young adulthood often overlaps with adolescence, leading scholars like Levinson (1978) to propose the "novice phase" (ages 17–33): a time for experimentation with careers and romantic relationships. Keniston (1971) termed this period "youth," highlighting the internal struggle between individual identity and societal expectations. Arnett (2000), however, recognized the limitations of such terms, as "youth" can also encompass childhood and adolescence. His concept of *emerging adulthood* (18–25) specifically addresses the unique psychosocial state of feeling neither fully formed nor a child, preceding the onset of young adulthood.

During young adulthood, individuals may engage in various sexual behaviors that reflect their need for intimacy and connection. These behaviors can range from casual dating to committed relationships, where individuals seek to establish trust, communication, and mutual respect with their partners. Exploring one's sexuality and preferences may also be a part of this stage, as individuals strive to understand themselves and their desires.

It is important to note that not everyone follows the same path when it comes to sexual behaviors during young adulthood. Some individuals may prioritize building strong emotional bonds before engaging in sexual activities, while others may be more open to casual encounters. Regardless of the specific behaviors, the underlying desire for connection and intimacy remains a central theme during this stage of development.

Intimacy within Erikson's framework extends beyond romantic love. It encompasses the exploration of one's sexuality and preferences, fostering emotional closeness with partners, and developing practical communication skills (Widman et al., 2018). Sexual behavior during young adulthood reflects this multifaceted pursuit of connection and can vary widely. Some individuals prioritize emotional intimacy before engaging in sexual activity, while others may be more open to casual encounters (Lyons et al., 2014). Vasilenko's (2022) longitudinal study underscores the impact of these choices on physical, mental, and social health outcomes.

Further research suggests intriguing demographic variations in sexual behavior. Cisgendered men, particularly between the ages of 25 to 29, tend to report more sexual partners than women (Vasilenko, 2014). Racial background also plays a role, with Black participants initiating sex earlier and having more partners overall, while White cisgendered men become more likely to have multiple partners by their mid-20s (Pflieger et al., 2013). Sexual minority youth also exhibit distinct behavioral patterns compared to their heterosexual counterparts (Goldberg, 2017). Despite these variations, the core theme of young adulthood remains the establishment of intimacy. This stage presents a crucial opportunity to solidify one's sense of self, achieved in the previous stage, and weave it into the rich tapestry of meaningful relationships. Understanding the complexities of intimacy during young adulthood allows researchers and mental health professionals to support individuals better in navigating this critical developmental phase.

DEVELOPING ATTRACTION TO SEXUAL PARTNERS

The development of attraction, specifically to sexual partners, is a complex process shaped by various influential factors, involving biological, psychological, and social elements. The biopsychosocial model explores the interconnection of biological, psychological, and socioenvironmental aspects of several different domains, but mainly of health, psychiatry, and human development (Borrell-Carrió et al., 2004). In the context of sexual attraction, biological aspects play a fundamental role, including hormonal influences such as testosterone, progesterone, estrogen, oxytocin, and vasopressin (Wang et al., 2019). These hormones are linked to sexual desire and arousal in individuals assigned male or female at birth (Exton et al., 2000; Wang et al., 2019).

For example, shifts in hormones across the menstrual cycle are associated with fluctuating sexual interest. One study which examined cisgendered women's attractiveness to their partner during ovulation and menstruation found a slight change (increase) in ratings of attractiveness of one's partners (Garza & Byrd-Craven, 2023).

Furthermore, one's hormonal medical history may significantly influence sexual attraction, arousal, and desire. Adrenaline also plays a significant role in sexual attraction. This is partly because the body undergoes similar physiological changes, such as increased heart rate and blood pressure, akin to the fight-or-flight response (Seshadri, 2016). Research has indicated that heightened levels of adrenaline can enhance perceptions of attractiveness in others (Seshadri, 2016).

Individuals experience sexual attraction for a variety of reasons. While biological and psychological factors are common factors for many individuals, they may play a lesser role or even be negligible for others.

Socioenvironmental elements, societal norms, influences from peers, and cultural expectations mold individuals' perceptions of attractiveness and impact their preferences regarding sexual partners (Hall, 2016). Cultural standards of beauty, desirability, and sexual imagery, as depicted in media (including social media) and prevalent culture, can shape individuals' benchmarks for attractiveness and sway their decisions regarding sexual partners (Gewirtz-Meydan & Spivak-Lavi, 2023).

Physical attraction to another person is often based on appearance (i.e., their body, eyes, hair, attire, and/or overall physical appearance). While some individuals may be attracted to specific physical features, personality traits, or sexual behaviors, based on their unique desires and fantasies, outward appearance or physical attractiveness is often the predominant factor influencing attraction (Karandashev & Fata, 2014).

Perceptions of attractiveness, however, can vary widely based on individual preferences and cultural norms. Although the concepts of sexual and physical attraction are closely linked, they are distinct concepts. *Sexual attraction* involves the desire to engage in sexual activities with a partner and is often accompanied by feelings of sexual arousal in their presence, or simply by thinking of one's sexual partner (Karandashev & Fata, 2014). *Physical attraction*, on the other hand, is a broader concept that encompasses various attractions based on physical appearance, often aesthetic in nature, without necessarily being sexual. While sexual attraction may encompass physical attraction, it specifically includes the sexual intimacy between romantic partners (Karandashev & Fata, 2014).

Although physical appearance may initially draw individuals to each other, factors such as personality, compatibility, social influences, and sexual chemistry play crucial roles in deepening attraction and forming intimate relationships. This includes shared values, interests, and beliefs that can deepen attraction as well.

Psychological processes, such as attachment styles, past experiences, and unconscious biases, can also impact attraction to sexual partners (Dosch et al., 2016; Nadelkov, 2015). For example, individuals with secure attachment styles may be drawn to partners who offer emotional security and intimacy, while those with anxious or avoidant attachment styles may have different patterns of attraction based on their relationship needs and fears (Dosch et al., 2016).

The *psychological* aspect of developing attraction encompasses how an individual perceives, remembers, thinks about, and imagines another person. It is suggested that psychological elements involve subjective perceptions, memories, thoughts, imaginings, and language, often biased toward favorability (Karandashev & Fata, 2014).

The *emotional* aspect of sexual attraction involves experiencing pleasurable feelings, physiological reactions, and a positive disposition when in the presence of one's partner. Emotions subjectively shape the perception of a sexual partner by accentuating certain physical traits while disregarding others (Karandashev & Fata, 2014). Attributes of a partner that align with our emotional and physical needs are cognitively assessed as desirable and may foster attraction.

In conclusion, the process of developing attraction toward sexual partners is intricate and fluid, shaped by a combination of biological, psychological, social, and cultural elements. While initial attraction may be sparked by physical appearance, factors like personality, compatibility, social context, and sexual chemistry are essential in strengthening attraction and fostering intimate connections.

ADULTHOOD AND OLDER ADULTHOOD SEXUALITY

Research on sexuality in older adults (over age 50) has moved away from a narrow medical perspective focused solely on limitations. Instead, a more comprehensive biopsychosocial approach acknowledges the influence of biological factors (health and illness) but also considers psychological aspects (attitudes and knowledge) and relationship dynamics (quality and satisfaction) on sexual function and experience (Carpenter & DeLamater, 2012).

This shift is crucial because past research often concentrated on a limited range of sexual activities, primarily focusing on sexual desire, erectile dysfunction, and the frequency of intercourse (Tiefer, 1996). This narrow definition medicalized sexuality and failed to capture the richness of sexual experience in later life. A broader definition that encompasses a wider range of activities (including solo and partnered masturbation and oral sex) and considers both objective and subjective aspects (frequency and satisfaction) is needed for a complete understanding of sexual well-being (Araujo et al., 2004; Laumann et al., 2006).

Fortunately, recent data from the United States suggests that sexual activity remains common among older adults, even with a biopsychosocial approach. Though sexual activity tends to decline with age, a significant portion of older adults remain sexually active. Laumann et al. (2007) found that 73% of respondents aged 57 to 64 reported sexual activity, dropping to 53% for those 65 to 74 and 26% for those 75 to 85. Studies like the National Survey of Sexual Health and Behavior (NSSHB) conducted in 2009 found that solo masturbation is frequent, with significant portions of men and women over 70 years old engaging in this practice (Herbenick et al., 2010). Oral sex with a partner is also relatively common, and the frequency of intercourse remains significant well into people's seventies (Herbenick et al., 2010; Schick et al., 2010). Having a partner and good health are the key factors influencing continued sexual activity (Karraker et al., 2011).

This emphasis on relationships connects to Erik Erikson's (1982) concept of generativity versus stagnation, a psychosocial stage during midlife (ages 40–65) that focuses on an adult's desire to leave a lasting impact on the world and the next generation. Sexuality can play a significant role in this stage (E. Erikson, 1982). Generativity manifests in various ways, including leaving a legacy, nurturing the next generation, and finding meaning in relationships (Bradley, 1997; McAdams & de St. Aubin, 1992). Sexuality within a committed relationship can be a powerful tool for nurturing those relationships and contributing to feelings of generativity (E. Erikson, 1982).

As life spans increase and older adults live healthier lives, maintaining sexual activity is likely to become even more important in the future. Understanding the complexities of sexuality in later life through a biopsychosocial lens can help us support healthy sexual expression and foster a sense of generativity for older adults.

Štulhofer et al. (2018) noted that navigating sexual aging presents challenges and variations. While health conditions and medications can impact sexual function, emotional and relational aspects of intimacy also remain crucial for older adults.

This becomes particularly relevant when considering Erikson's psychosocial theory (E. Erikson, 1982). In later life, we face the critical stage of *ego integrity* versus *despair*. Here, individuals embark on a life review, revisiting successes and missed opportunities. Those who achieve ego integrity accept their life path and find wisdom in their experiences (E. Erikson, 1982). Conversely, those struggling with ego integrity may experience despair, characterized by regrets, anxieties about death, and a sense of wasted time (E. Erikson, 1982). The quality of past relationships and a sense of purpose in life seem to be key factors influencing how one resolves this stage (E. Erikson, 1982). Sexual health and intimacy can be woven into the tapestry of life experiences. A fulfilling sexual life, particularly for those who remain active later in life, may contribute to a sense of purpose and acceptance within the context of ego integrity. Conversely, challenges faced with sexual aging may potentially contribute to feelings of despair, particularly if they are intertwined with broader anxieties about aging and mortality.

FACTORS IMPACTING SEXUAL DEVELOPMENT

TECHNOLOGY, SOCIAL MEDIA, AND PORNOGRAPHY

The influence of technology, social media, and pornography on sexual development is complex and can alter greatly based on individual encounters and societal contexts. As society continues to become technology dependent, technology and the internet provide unprecedented access to information about sexuality, including sexual health, sexual expectations, self-image, relationships, and pleasure. This can empower individuals to learn about their bodies and sexual practices, potentially contributing to a more informed approach or a skewed approach to sexual development.

Media portrayals of sex and relationships shape cultural attitudes and norms surrounding sexuality. Exposure to sexual content in movies, television, music, and the internet can influence perceptions of beauty, desire, and intimacy. Moreover, online platforms and social media play a growing role in shaping sexual identities and behaviors among adolescents and young adults (Coyne et al., 2019). Sexual content is a common feature in mainstream media within the United States. Not all sexual content on social media, however, is explicit; however, most sexual content can be presented in a soft and implicit manner (Landry et al., 2017). Exposure to such content may increase curiosity and arousal, leading to heightened sexual desire in some individuals (Smith et al., 2016).

As previously discussed, you might consider Erikson's stages of development in regard to social media and sexual identity. During the adolescence stage of *identity* versus *role confusion*, individuals begin to develop a sense of self. Developing a clear, coherent identity (including sexual identity) is necessary for forming close intimate relationships with others, without losing one's sense of self in the relationship (Mitchell et al., 2021). Furthermore, social media currently plays a significant role in sexual development during this critical stage as individuals may experience the role of confusion due to the impact of social media and development.

Social media platforms facilitate communication and interaction among peers, as well as sexual content, including images, videos, and discussions about sexuality. Exposure to peers' experiences, opinions, and norms through social media can influence how individuals perceive and navigate their own sexual development and identity. For example, the use of filters on social media, comparing oneself to peers, and cyberbullying in which body shaming takes place all promote unrealistic images of the body and self (Jiotsa et al., 2021). This can lead to individuals internalizing these viewpoints and standards as their own. Furthermore, these unrealistic images can contribute to the promotion of idealized body images and beauty standards, potentially affecting individuals' self-esteem and confidence in their bodies. Thus, this can influence how individuals perceive themselves sexually and their willingness to engage in sexual activities.

Research shows this can increase earlier initiation of sexual experimentation, specifically in adolescents, including risky sexual behavior (Coyne et al., 2019). These risky behaviors can consist of anonymous "hookups" arranged through dating apps, increased sexual activity, or the sharing of explicit content online.

The modern idea of hook-up culture in American society is known as sexual activity between two individuals who are not in a committed romantic relationship (Currier, 2013). Social media shapes hook-up culture by easily facilitating connection, normalizing casual sex, and influencing individuals' attitudes and behaviors related to sexual activity (Landry et al., 2017). Sexually risky behaviors increase the likelihood of sexually transmitted infections (STIs) and unintended pregnancies (Landry et al., 2017).

Images and narratives on social media and pornography may reinforce ideas about "toxic" masculinity and femininity, contributing to the normalization of unhelpful gender norms and gender scripts (Currier, 2013). Social media and pornography often perpetuate traditional gender roles and stereotypes through the portrayal of gendered behaviors, appearances, and roles. These platforms can also contribute to the sexualization and objectification of individuals, particularly women, through the dissemination of sexually suggestive content, imagery, comments, and messages. This can perpetuate harmful stereotypes about gender and sexuality, leading to the commodification of bodies and the reinforcement of power dynamics based on gender (Currier, 2013).

Research commonly finds there is a heavy emphasis on sex as casual, relatively risk-free, and as following strict gender scripts (Kirsch & Murnen, 2015). Gender roles contribute to the development of sexual scripts, which are specific narratives that prescribe how sexual interactions should unfold. These scripts often reflect traditional gender roles, portraying men as initiators and women as gatekeepers of sexual activity. Sexual behaviors are often reinforced by gendered scripts that promote these divisive and unequal ideals of femininity and masculinity (Bacchus, 2017). Individuals may internalize these scripts and enact them in their own sexual encounters, to their detriment.

According to the sexual double standard, early romantic and sexual experiences have different social repercussions based on gender. Gender-specific norms dictate acceptable numbers of sexual partners, circumstances for engaging in sexual activity (such as on a "first date," before marriage, or in a noncommittal relationship), and the perceived motives behind sexual behavior (such as men engaging in sex without emotional attachment, while women are expected to only have sex when in love). When women and men are judged differently for the same sexual behaviors, male sexual openness is often accepted or praised, while female openness can lead to reputational damage and a perceived loss of virtue (Kreager & Staff, 2009).

While gendered norms surrounding sexual conduct have existed for centuries, it is arguable that strong sexual double standards persist in contemporary, postsexual revolution U.S. society, particularly considering shifts in sexual norms spurred by the sexual revolution, social media, and feminist movements (Kreager & Staff, 2009). Consequently, negative perceptions of sexual permissiveness may lower the social desirability of engaging in sexual behavior, regardless of gender (Sævik & Konijnenberg, 2023).

Platforms such as social media and pornography allow for escapism and fantasy exploration, in which both may promote indiscriminate sexual activity and increased sexual desire as individuals seek fulfillment of these fantasies online. On the positive side, these platforms allow individuals a space to express, explore, and assert their sexuality in ways they may not be able to offline. It also provides resources in regards to seeking support and connections, which may elicit a more positive perception that can increase the desirability of sexual activity.

Unfortunately, pornography mostly showcases actors and actresses with exaggerated and often unattainable body shapes, such as highly muscular men and extremely slender and curvaceous women. Exposure to these depictions can prompt individuals to unfavorably compare themselves to these ideals, potentially developing disapproval of one's own body image, ultimately impacting self-esteem and self-sexual exploration (Gewirtz-Meydan & Spivak-Lavi, 2023). Moreover, pornography may perpetuate unrealistic expectations of sexual performance through the selection of extreme genitalia, and the frequency and intensity of sexual acts (Goldsmith et al., 2017). Individuals exposed to these portrayals may develop distorted views of one's self and their expectations of sex, including attitudes regarding sex within intimate relationships (Goldsmith et al., 2017; Poulsen et al., 2013), potentially leading to feelings of inadequacy regarding one's own sexual experiences.

In conclusion, social media and pornography play significant roles in shaping sexual development, contributing both opportunities and challenges. Understanding the prevalent impact on individuals' attitudes, behaviors, and relationships is essential for promoting healthy sexual development in this digital age.

CULTURAL AND FAMILIAL FACTORS

As previously discussed, there are many customs that govern sexual behavior development and transitions in relation to puberty and adulthood. There are also a variety of behaviors—outside of transitions into puberty—that affect one's sexual psychological development. Cultural and familial influences are two major factors that significantly impact sexual development and behavior. *Cultural* norms dictate acceptable sexual behaviors, expressions, and identities within a society. These norms are often transmitted through family, religion, media, and educational institutions. Furthermore, attitudes toward sex education, gender roles, and consent vary widely across religions, cultures, and family systems.

Familial relationships and dynamics significantly impact sexual development. Parental attitudes toward sex, communication patterns, and family structure shape children's understanding and exploration of sexuality (Sævik & Konijnenberg, 2023). Open communication and parental support can foster healthy sexual development, while restrictive or judgmental attitudes may lead to shame or confusion. This may include shame regarding sexual thoughts, exploration with others and self, and sexual identity.

Research indicates that *sexual shame* correlates with self-directed hostility, sexual and relational difficulties, body image dissatisfaction, aggression, hypersexuality, and sexual addiction (Volk et al., 2016). Through sexual shame, a higher level of self-consciousness is generated that can lead to a maladaptive trail of thoughts, attitudes, beliefs, and behaviors, such as reduced self-esteem (Sævik & Konijnenberg, 2023).

RELIGIOUS AND SPIRITUAL BELIEFS

Religious and spiritual beliefs often play a significant role in shaping attitudes toward sexuality and governing individual and relationship sexual development. Different religious traditions offer diverse perspectives on topics such as premarital sex, contraception, abortion, and LGBTQIA+ rights. Most religions enforce moral behavior in the context of heaven/hell, karma, or scriptures, and critically, contraception is often viewed, either overtly or indirectly, as a sin or moral misstep, where abstinence, particularly until marriage, may be the only morally acceptable choice with specific regards to sexual behaviors and sexual health (Glazer et al., 2023). Religious teachings may promote the idea of abstinence and chastity, providing frameworks for expected sexual conduct (Glazer et al., 2023). For instance, in some religious cultures, premarital sex may be stigmatized, while in more liberal societies, it may be accepted (Bacchus, 2017). Individuals and couples who separate from their childhood or family's religious backgrounds may experience shame and guilt in regard to their sexual behaviors into adulthood (Perry & Snawder, 2017).

FORMAL EDUCATION AND HEALTHCARE SYSTEMS

Formal education and healthcare systems play crucial roles in providing information, resources, and support related to sexual health and behavior (Hendry et al., 2018). Comprehensive sexual education can empower individuals with knowledge about consent, contraception, STIs, and healthy relationships. Access to healthcare services, including reproductive healthcare and counseling, is essential in the development of sexual behaviors by addressing sexual health needs (Sabia, 2006).

Sexual Citizenship

Hirsch and Khan (2020), noting that most sexual assaults on campus occur within the first 6 to 8 weeks of a student's arrival, have been researching the presence and prevention of sexual assault on college campuses. From their research they have developed the SPACE toolkit (Sexual Assault Prevention and Community Equity), which includes strategies on how to develop individuals into *sexual citizens*. Sexual citizens, who are made over time, utilize consent practices and work to understand, embrace, and improve equity and safety. Sexual citizens also work on their *sexual projects*, that is, answer for themselves what "sex is for" and explore various aspects of sexual activity consensually.

Hirsch and Khan (2020) particularly discuss and name geographical and space issues (*sexual geographies*) and institutional inequities that unwittingly promote increased power for some groups and individuals over other individuals, contributing to sexual assault. One example is how dorm rooms may have a desk, a single chair, and a single bed, making it difficult for potential romantic partners to determine where to sit. Or, typically only fraternities are allowed alcohol, controlling how sorority members access it. Their work offers many ideas to redistribute power more equitably, particularly in physical spaces, thereby reducing opportunities for sexual assault.

Go to www.sexualcitizens.com/space-toolkit to download the free SPACE toolkit to learn more about these prevention efforts.

INFORMAL SEXUAL EDUCATION STRATEGIES

Informal sexual education strategies that affect one's sexual development include covert and overt messages represented and enacted by peers, families, friends, and media. One's exposure to certain messages dictates our perception of what constitutes healthy sexual behaviors and development. Informal methods may often be subject to our own direction and impulses. For example, one of the ways in which ciswomen often obtain informal sexual education is through the search for sex-positive and feminist-informed information. Thus, they can experience a greater sense of power over their bodies and selves (Edwards, 2016).

PARENTAL SEXUAL CONSENT-FOCUSED EDUCATION

Research has found significant correlations in parental sexual consent education, healthier sexual attitudes, and perceptions of social norms with respect to sexual consent attitudes and behavior (MacDougall et al., 2022). Positive perceptions of social norms, liberal sexual attitudes, and parentally provided sexual consent education were associated with lower negative attitudes toward sexual consent and more consistent use of explicit sexual consent. Positive perceptions of social norms and less sexual experience were associated with more positive sexual consent attitudes (MacDougall et al., 2022).

Quality sexual health education at school and at home has been linked to several positive sexual health outcomes including increased knowledge, safer sex behaviors, increased testing for sexually transmitted infections, and decreased likelihood of unplanned pregnancy (Bourke et al., 2014; Somers & Paulson, 2000; Widman et al., 2016). Additionally, more extensive sexual health education from parents and school is associated with more positive attitudes toward use of sexual consent and more consistent use of sexual consent with sexual partners (MacDougall et al., 2022). However, most parents do not engage in in-depth discussions of sexual health topics with their children (MacDougall et al., 2022).

Research has also found that parent-adolescent communication impacts sexual behavior and development among adolescents, correlating with an increase in safer sex behaviors, particularly with ciswomen (Widman et al., 2016) compared to cismen (Bourke et al., 2014).

GENDER ROLES AND SEXUAL DOUBLE STANDARDS

In contemporary American society, there is a widespread belief in the existence of differential standards of sexual behavior for women and men. This phenomenon, known as the sexual double standard, entails the endorsement of heterosexual sexual encounters among boys and cismen, often leading to commendation and rewards, while similar behaviors among girls and ciswomen are met with derogation and social stigma (Kreager & Staff, 2009). Women are simultaneously sexualized and exploited through mainstream media and also shamed when expressing their sexuality more liberally, whereas cismen are generally rewarded and praised for their liberal practices and openness regarding their sexual behaviors.

Gender roles often dictate societal expectations for how individuals should behave sexually based on their gender. For example, traditional gender roles dictate that men are expected to act assertive and sexually dominant, while women are expected to act passive and sexually submissive (Lefkowitz et al., 2014). These expectations can influence individuals' sexual behaviors and preferences. Many cultures place a strong emphasis on male sexual performance and virility. Men may feel pressure to conform to societal standards of masculinity, which often include being sexually assertive, experienced, and successful in their sexual encounters (Bacchus, 2017). As previously mentioned, some cultures may uphold traditional ideals of female sexual purity and modesty. Women may face expectations to remain chaste before marriage and to exhibit restraint in expressing sexual desires or initiating sexual activity.

MIGRATION AND IMMIGRATION FAMILIAL FACTORS

Research indicates that within migrant communities, patriarchal values tend to prioritize cismen's authority in household decision-making and cultural institutions, posing various obstacles to ciswomen's expression of ethnic identity regarding sexual behavior (Bacchus, 2017). Within immigrant households, ciswomen are at the epicenter of reproducing traditions, and their sexual experiences are often sites where they both contest and conform to cultural expectations of femininity (Bacchus, 2017). A significant portion of sexual behavior research highlights the challenges faced by immigrant ciswomen and their American-born daughters as they navigate the tension between adhering to the cultural ideals of female purity and sexual restraint from their homeland, and their aspirations for sexual fulfillment, often associated with what is perceived as "American behavior" (Bacchus, 2017). Children of immigrant families often wait until they become adults, living outside of their home, to freely explore sexual behaviors that were previously impossible or challenging to pursue during adolescence (Bacchus, 2017).

This conflict can often lead to rebellion as individuals struggle to assimilate into American culture while trying to uphold their culture traditions, as many immigrant parents want to maintain their home culture with their household and children. "Losing virginity" in early adulthood is significant for some children of immigrants due to the strong emphasis placed on virginity within their families.

In conclusion, cultural, familial, spiritual/religious, and educational factors exert profound influences on sexual behavior and development. Understanding the interplay between these factors is essential for promoting healthy attitudes toward sexuality, sexual behaviors, fostering positive relationships, and addressing challenges related to sexual development.

THEORIES OF CHILDHOOD SEXUAL DEVELOPMENT

FREUD'S THEORY OF PSYCHOSEXUAL STAGES

Freud initiated and popularized the theory of psychosocial development. This theory organizes stages of children's development, aligning with their sensual and psychological experiences. Freud, in his 1905 groundbreaking paper called *Three Essays on the Theory of Sexuality*, discussed the beginning of sexual pleasure in childhood and the impact it has on our later sexual lives. While these stages are generally no longer considered relevant in addressing human sexual development, due to a wide range of criticism and outdated views on gender, it is interesting to learn about the earliest thinking of sexual development.

The psychosexual stages include the *oral stage* where the infant's focus is on sucking, a stage which Freud calls autoerotic and transitions into kissing being pleasurable when the child is an adult. The second stage is called the *anal stage* and takes place at the same time as toilet training. As the child begins to gain mastery over toilet training, the process can result in a conflict of wanting to have mastery over something. The third stage is the *phallic stage* where children begin to recognize their genitals, leading to curiosity and exploration. This is also the stage where children begin to recognize differences between their gender and/or genitals and other children's gender and/or genitals. The last stage is the *genital* stage, characterized by the *Oedipal* complex where children begin to connect with their love objects and desire intimacy toward that love object. Freud theorized that girls developed a love object in their father and boys identified a love object in their mother. Freud viewed these stages as complete, ending around 6 years old (Axelrod & Vriesema, 2023; Silverman, 2020).

ERIKSON'S PSYCHOSOCIAL STAGES

Other theorists have evaluated psychosexual stages from Erikson's psychosocial stages viewpoint. As discussed earlier in this chapter, Erikson's theory provides goals through which a therapist can help move someone from one stage to another. Akin to Freud's description of the psychosocial stages resulting in conflict, Erikson posited that developmental stages are initiated when we respond to a crisis, challenge, or turning point in our life cycles. The goal is to resolve this conflict and move forward (Knight, 2017).

For example, some challenges include developing intimacy and relationships with other people, as well as cultivating one's sense of self. Another example involves the "stage of intimacy versus isolation." If a person emerges, for example, from the "stage of intimacy versus isolation" learning the "lesson of isolation," this may impair their sexual efficacy and sexual confidence, potentially undermining their ability to be aroused or feel satisfied sexually. Individuals in sexual relationships with men with whom they shared a deep emotional bond often emphasize the importance of honesty and trust in their relationships, which influenced their sexual behavior as well as being involved in long-term relationships with their partners (Bacchus, 2017).

PERSONAL CONSTRUCT THEORY

Personal construct theory (Kelly, 1955), which is also concerned with psychosocial stages, is rooted in constructive alternativism. It posits that there is a defined reality, but that reality is subject to interpretation, and from this interpretation, we create our identities (Horley & Clarke, 2016). Because life events do not have clear cut meanings, we have to make meaning for ourselves. To make this meaning, we often assign polarizing views: good–bad; rich–poor; new–old. Viewing the world with these types of dichotomies, however, is not the most adaptive method of living. Personal construct theory encourages us to view the world with all the complexity, understanding that no experience is complete without some level of social construction and filtering through various contexts, personal lenses, and expectations.

From this theoretical perspective, sexuality can also be viewed with all its inherent complexities. For example, gender identification need not be limited to a female or male binary, but instead can be considered as nuanced and dynamic. This theory more fully considers the role of power in sexuality and sexual development. It honors examining the perspectives of both partners when identifying what is limiting their intimate connection. It allows for us to understand how and when people internalize social messages and how this internalization—along with biology and other factors—manifests in sexual identity and behavior.

Personal construct theory not only explores the integration between biology, psychology, and sexuality, but it moves away from dichotomy toward a complex and nuanced understanding of how sex and sexuality develop over the course of one's life. Its framework includes the expectations we have related to how people manifest their sexual desire and behaviors.

RELATIONAL MODEL

Moore (2018) presents a relational model for sexual development in children. In this framework, Moore (2018) focuses on the constructed binary and polar nature of power in parents and children. Children have historically been seen as inferior and undeveloped, whereas adults have been seen as superior and fully developed. The longstanding assumption that children in our contemporary society have no exposure to elements of sexuality in the world is inaccurate. The relational model encourages us to be realistic about the exposure children have to sexual content, ideas, and experiences.

There are two challenges to exclusively using the parent–child binary. First, the child must be seen as an opposite of the parent, and any similarities must be considered rare. As it pertains to sexuality, children who have some knowledge about sexuality would no longer be seen as innocent, and might even be considered as having developed abnormally. The second element suggests that children repress the memories of early sexual development and these memories resurface as adults. When memories resurface, they can cause anxiety for the adult due to the way in which the memories were initially repressed.

Another consideration from the relational sexual development perspective concerns the intentional actions people may take to hide children from learning about sex. This can result in unintended consequences such as these children growing up into adulthood with little understanding of sex. The authors note that adults and society generally try to protect children from accessing or gaining information about sexuality in any capacity. At the same time, children learn about sexuality by observation. It may be impossible to prevent children from realistically having little to no access to sexual information. And in fact, with the plethora of age-appropriate sex educational books and videos, it may behoove parents and adults to take the lead in providing healthy and boundaried information about sex. This can ultimately help promote a life-long development of healthy and empowered sexuality.

Case Study 4.1: Development Across the Life Span

James (50 years old) and Clara (46 years old) presented in treatment with orgasm and desire disorders. From gathering information and making connections, the therapist conjectured that James's orgasm issues emerged as a consequence of poor learning history in his family of origin as a child, a childhood abuse event, heavy teen pornography use, a bad relationship breakup during a critical developmental stage (mid-20s), and negative messages from society over the course of his life about gender roles and masculinity. Clara was raised in a strict religious environment which contributed to her view of gender roles. She experienced penetrative sexual assaults by two individuals as a teenager and was told at that time that it was her fault. Clara was married to an abusive man prior to marrying James. James noticed he was having orgasm problems as their relationship became more committed. The more intimacy there was developing between the couple, the more James was unable to be aroused by her, yet he maintained arousal toward other women. As this cycle continued, Clara found herself feeling unattractive, dejected, and uninterested in having sex.

The treatment included working with the couple to remove sexual activity from the table to relieve the pressure of sex and its role in the relationship. Individual therapy with both was conducted to improve Clara's self-concept, and to help both Clara and James recover from their abuse histories. Conjoint therapy was used to improve their attachment to one another, review their inherited values and beliefs from family-of-origin, negotiate workable values for the relationship, and to destigmatize intimacy for James. Because many of the issues and beliefs were indeed at different points in the developmental life span, the therapy addressed the use of psychosocial stages to help the couple acknowledge and resolve the conflicts at each stage in more appropriate ways.

SUMMARY

Cultivating healthy sexual development is a lifelong process. From the very beginnings of conception to old age, the integration of genetics and physical disposition, personality, family, cultural factors, religion/spirituality, environment, relationship experiences, societal messages, and many other factors shape who we are and the meanings we make about our sexual identity and well-being.

There are many ways in which we understand and express our sexuality. Integrating appropriate skill-building opportunities across the life span focusing on learning about one's body, communication, boundary setting, choices, sexual scripts, gender roles, and expression relates to more positive levels, experience, and expression of sexual health.

DISCUSSION QUESTIONS

- Discuss the interplay of hormones, genes, history, experiences, biology, and the environment in the context of sexual development.
- Critically evaluate the impact of abstinence-only education on sexual development, with a focus on its limitations and potential negative consequences.
- Examine the role of CSE in promoting healthy sexual development, and discuss its key components and potential impact on reducing risky behavior and improving sexual health among young people.
- Analyze the importance of effective communication in supporting healthy sexual development, considering its role in understanding consent, expressing sexual needs, and establishing boundaries, with reference to relevant research and literature.

LEARNING ACTIVITIES

CourseConnect

To access self-assessment questions and interactive, competency-based learning activities for this chapter, visit www.springerpub.com/courseconnect. See inside front cover and tear-out card for CourseConnect details.

ADDITIONAL RESOURCES

Additional resources are online and available at www.springerpub.com/courseconnect.

REFERENCES

Aatscha, P. A., Arbor, T. C., & Krishan, K. (2023, August 28). Embryology, sexual development. In *StatPearls* [Internet]. StatPearls Publishing. Retrieved July 18, 2024, from https://www.ncbi.nlm.nih.gov/books/NBK557601

Araujo, A. B., Mohr, B. A., & McKinlay, J. B. (2004). Changes in sexual function in middle-aged and older men: Longitudinal data from the Massachusetts Male Aging Study. *Journal of the American Geriatrics Society, 52*(9), 1502–1509. https://doi.org/10.1111/j.0002-8614.2004.52413.x

Arnett, J. J. (2000). Emerging adulthood: A theory of development from the late teens through the twenties. *American Psychologist*, 55(5), 469–480. https://doi.org/10.1037/0003-066x.55.5.469

Arnold, A. P. (2017). A general theory of sexual differentiation. *Journal of Neuroscience Research, 95*(1–2), 291–300. https://doi.org/10.1002/jnr.23884

Assarzadeh, R., Bostani Khalesi, Z., & Jafarzadeh-Kenarsari, F. (2019). Sexual self-efficacy and associated factors: A review. *Shiraz e-Medical Journal, 20*(11), e87537. https://doi.org/10.5812/semj.87537

Atrian, M. K., Dehnavi, Z. M., & Kamali, Z. (2019). The relationship between sexual self-efficacy and sexual function in married women. *Journal of Midwifery and Reproductive Health, 7*(2), 1683–1690. https://doi.org/10.22038/jmrh.2018.30672.1333

Axelrod, M. I., & Vriesema, C. C. (2023). Psychosexual stages and development. In S. Hupp and R. Wiseman, *Investigating pop psychology* (pp. 75–85). Taylor & Francis Group. https://doi.org/10.4324/9781003107798-9

Aydoğdu, F., Gürsoy, F., & Aral, N. (2021). An investigation into the relationship between self-perception and sexual development in children attending preschool education. *European Early Childhood Education Research Journal, 29*(6), 828–841. https://doi.org/10.1080/1350293X.2021.1968466

Bacchus, N. S. (2017). Shifting sexual boundaries: Ethnicity and premarital sex in the lives of South Asian American women. *Sexuality & Culture, 21*(3), 776–794. https://doi.org/10.1007/s12119-017-9421-2

Barseghyan, H., Délot, E., & Vilain, E. (2015). New genomic technologies: An aid for diagnosis of disorders of sex development. *Hormone and Metabolic Research, 47*, 312–320. https://doi.org/10.1055/s-0035-1548831

Barseghyan, H., Délot, E. C., & Vilain, E. (2018). New technologies to uncover the molecular basis of disorders of sex development. *Molecular and Cellular Endocrinology, 468*, 60–69. https://doi.org/10.1016/j.mce.2018.04.003

Batmaz, H., & Çelik, E. (2021). Sexual dissatisfaction and sexual self-efficacy: An examination of the role of sexual self-confidence as a mediator. *Journal of Men's Health, 18*(1), 008. https://doi.org/10.31083/jomh.2021.067

Bhandarkar, T. R. (1928). *Some aspects of ancient Indian culture.* Asian Educational Services.

Borrell-Carrió, F., Suchman, A. L., & Epstein, R. M. (2004). The biopsychosocial model 25 years later: principles, practice, and scientific inquiry. *Annals of Family Medicine, 2*(6), 576–582. https://doi.org/10.1370/afm.245

Bourke, A., Boduszek, D., Kelleher, C., McBride, O., & Morgan, K. (2014). Sex education, first sex and sexual health outcomes in adulthood: Findings from a nationally representative sexual health survey. *Sex Education, 14*(3), 299–309. https://doi.org/10.1080/14681811.2014.887008

Boustani, M. M., Frazier, S. L., & Lesperance, N. (2017). Sexual health programming for vulnerable youth: Improving knowledge, attitudes, and behaviors. *Children and Youth Services Review, 73*, 375–383. https://doi.org/10.1016/j.childyouth.2017.01.013

Bradley, C. L. (1997). Generativity–stagnation: Development of a status model. *Developmental Review, 17*(3), 262–290. https://doi.org/10.1006/drev.1997.0432

Bramble, M. S., Lipson, A., Vashist, N., & Vilain, E. (2017). Effects of chromosomal sex and hormonal influences on shaping sex differences in brain and behavior: Lessons from cases of disorders of sex development. *Journal of Neuroscience Research, 95*(1–2), 65–74. https://doi.org/10.1002/jnr.23832

Byers, E. S., Sears, H. A., & Hughes, K. (2018). Predicting mother–adolescent sexual communication using the integrative model of behavioral prediction. *Journal of Family Issues, 39*(5), 1213–1235. https://doi.org/10.1177/0192513X17698183

Carpenter, L. M., & DeLamater, J. (2012). *Sex for life: From virginity to viagra, how sexuality changes throughout our lives*. NYU Press.

Clark, L., & Stitzlein, S. M. (2016). Neoliberal narratives and the logic of abstinence only education: Why are we still having this conversation? *Gender and Education, 30*(3), 322–340. https://doi.org/10.1080/09540253.2016.1203883

Coyne, S. M., Ward, L. M., Kroff, S. L., Davis, E. J., Holmgren, H. G., Jensen, A. C., Erickson, S. E., & Essig, L. W. (2019). Contributions of mainstream sexual media exposure to sexual attitudes, perceived peer norms, and sexual behavior: A meta-analysis. *Journal of Adolescent Health, 64*(4), 430–436. https://doi.org/10.1016/j.jadohealth.2018.11.016

Currier, D. M. (2013). Strategic ambiguity: Protecting emphasized femininity and hegemonic masculinity in the hookup culture. *Gender & Society, 27*(5), 704–727. https://doi.org/10.1177/0891243213493960

Dosch, A., Rochat, L., Ghisletta, P., Favez, N., & Van der Linden, M. (2016). Psychological factors involved in sexual desire, sexual activity, and sexual satisfaction: A multi-factorial perspective. *Archives of Sexual Behavior, 45*(8), 2029–2045. https://doi.org/10.1007/s10508-014-0467-z

Edwards, N. (2016). Women's reflections on formal sex education and the advantage of gaining informal sexual knowledge through a feminist lens. *Sex Education, 16*(3), 266–278. https://doi.org/10.1080/14681811.2015.1088433

Erikson, E. H. (1950). *Childhood and society*. Norton.

Erikson, E. H. (1968). *Identity, youth and crisis*. W. W. Norton & Company.

Erikson, E. H. (1982). *The life cycle completed*. W. W. Norton & Company.

Erikson, J. (1997). *The life cycle completed* (Extended version). W. W. Norton & Company.

Exton, N. G., Chau Truong, T., Exton, M. S., Wingenfeld, S. A., Leygraf, N., Saller, B., Hartmann, U., & Schedlowski, M. (2000). Neuroendocrine response to film-induced sexual arousal in men and women. *Psychoneuroendocrinology, 25*(2), 187–199. https://doi.org/10.1016/S0306-4530(99)00049-9

Finkelhor, D., Shattuck, A., Turner, H. A., & Hamby, S. L. (2014). The lifetime prevalence of child sexual abuse and sexual assault assessed in late adolescence. *Journal of Adolescent Health, 55*(3), 329–333. https://doi.org/10.1016/j.jadohealth.2013.12.026

Freud, S. (1905). *Three essays on the theory of sexuality* (standard ed., VII). The Hogarth Press.

Garza, R., & Byrd-Craven, J. (2023). The role of hormones in attraction and visual attention to facial masculinity. *Frontiers in Psychology, 14*, 1067487. https://doi.org/10.3389/fpsyg.2023.1067487

Gewirtz-Meydan, A., & Spivak-Lavi, Z. (2023). The association between problematic pornography use and eating disorder symptoms among heterosexual and sexual minority men. *Body Image, 45*, 284–295. https://doi.org/10.1016/j.bodyim.2023.03.008

Ghaffari, A., & Feizollahe Vahid, A. (2020). Comparing the effectiveness of sexual skills training and communication skills training on the sexual attitudes of married women. *Research and Development in Medical Education, 9*(1), 3. https://doi.org/10.34172/rdme.2020.003

Gillespie, B. J. (2017). Sexual synchronicity and communication among partnered older adults. *Journal of Sex & Marital Therapy, 43*(5), 441–455. https://doi.org/10.1080/0092623X.2016.1182826

Glazer, E., Valdez, E., DeBlauw, J. A., & Ives, S. J. (2023). An analysis of the impact of religious affiliation and strength of religiosity on sexual health practices of sexually active female college students. *International Journal of Environmental Research and Public Health, 20*(22), 7075. https://doi.org/10.3390/ijerph20227075

Goldfarb, E. S., & Lieberman, L. D. (2021). Three decades of research: The case for comprehensive sex education. *Journal of Adolescent Health, 68*(1), 13–27. https://doi.org/10.1016/j.jadohealth.2020.07.036

Goldberg, S. K. (2017). Patterns, predictors, and consequences of sexual initiation among sexual minority youth [ProQuest Information & Learning]. In Dissertation Abstracts International: Section B: The Sciences and Engineering (Vol. 78, Issue 2–B(E)).

Goldberg, S. K. (2017). Patterns, predictors, and consequences of sexual initiation among sexual minority youth [Doctoral dissertation, University of North Carolina at Chapel Hill]. Carolina Digital Repository. https://cdr.lib.unc.edu/concern/dissertations/g732db159

Goldsmith, K., Dunkley, C. R., Dang, S. S., & Gorzalka, B. B. (2017). Pornography consumption and its association with sexual concerns and expectations among young men and women. *Canadian Journal of Human Sexuality, 26*(2), 151–162. https://doi.org/10.3138/cjhs.262-a2

Hall, J. A. (2016). Interpreting social-sexual communication: Relational framing theory and social-sexual communication, attraction, and intent. *Social-Sexual Communication, 42*(1), 138–164. https://doi.org/10.1111/hcre.12071

Heard, E., Auvaa, L., & Pickering, C. (2015). Love bugs: Promoting sexual health among young people in Samoa. *Health Promotion Journal of Australia, 26*(1), 30–32. https://doi.org/10.1071/HE14055

Hendry, N. A., Brown, G., Carman, M., Ellard, J., Wallace, J., & Dowsett, G. W. (2018). Untangling the conflation of "young adults" and "young people" in STI and sexual health policy and sex education. *Sex Education, 18*(5), 527–540. https://doi.org/10.1080/14681811.2018.1434069

Herbenick, D., Reece, M., Schick, V., Sanders, S. A., Dodge, B., & Fortenberry, J. D. (2010). Sexual behavior in the United States: Results from a national probability sample of men and women ages 14-94. *The Journal of Sexual Medicine, 7*(Suppl. 5), 255–265. https://doi.org/10.1111/j.1743-6109.2010.02012.x

Hesapcioglu, S. T., Aktepe, E., Ozyay, F., Kaytanli, U., Ozmen, S., Tural, D. A., & Kose, S. (2017). The relationship between children's masturbation behavior and their mothers' temperament and character dimensions: A case-control study. *Psychiatry and Behavioral Sciences, 7*(1), 20. https://doi.org/10.5455/jmood.20170214110054

Hirsch, J. S., & Khan, S. (2020). *Sexual citizens: Sex, power, and assault on campus.* W. W. Norton.

Horley, J., & Clarke, J. (2016). *Experience, meaning, and identity in sexuality* (pp. 35–70). Palgrave Macmillan. https://doi.org/10.1057/978-1-137-40096-3_2

Jiotsa, B., Naccache, B., Duval, M., Rocher, B., & Grall-Bronnec, M. (2021). Social media use and body image disorders: Association between frequency of comparing one's own physical appearance to that of people being followed on social media and body dissatisfaction and drive for thinness. *International Journal of Environmental Research and Public Health, 18*(6), 1–14. https://doi.org/10.3390/ijerph18062880

Kann, L., McManus, T., Harris, W. A., Shanklin, S. L., Flint, K. H., Queen, B., Lowry, R., Chyen, D., Whittle, L., Thornton, J., Lim, C., Bradford, D., Yamakawa, Y., Leon, M., Brener, N., & Ethier, K. A. (2018). Youth risk behavior surveillance—United States, 2017. *Morbidity and Mortality Weekly Report. Surveillance Summaries, 67*(8), 1–114. https://doi.org/10.15585/mmwr.ss6708a1

Karandashev, V., & Fata, B. (2014). Change in physical attraction in early romantic relationships. *Interpersona: An International Journal of Personal Relationships, 8*(2), 257–267. https://doi.org/10.5964/ijpr.v8i2.167

Karraker, A., Delamater, J., & Schwartz, C. R. (2011). Sexual frequency decline from midlife to later life. *The Journals of Gerontology. Series B, Psychological Sciences and Social Sciences, 66*(4), 502–512. https://doi.org/10.1093/geronb/gbr058

Keniston, K. (1971). *Youth and dissent: The rise of a new opposition.* Harcourt Brace Jovanovich.

Kirsch, A. C., & Murnen, S. K. (2015). "Hot" girls and "cool dudes": Examining the prevalence of the heterosexual script in American children's television media. *Psychology of Popular Media Culture, 4*(1), 18–30. https://doi.org/10.1037/ppm0000017

Knight, Z. G. (2017). A proposed model of psychodynamic psychotherapy linked to Erik Erikson's eight stages of psychosocial development. *Clinical Psychology and Psychotherapy, 24*(5), 1047–1058. https://doi.org/10.1002/cpp.2066

Kreager, D. A., & Staff, J. (2009). The sexual double standard and adolescent peer acceptance. *Social Psychology Quarterly, 72*(2), 143–164. https://doi.org/10.1177/019027250907200205

Lamb, S., & Gilbert, J. (Eds.). (2018). *The Cambridge handbook of sexual development: Childhood and adolescence.* Cambridge University Press.

Landry, M., Turner, M., Vyas, A., & Wood, S. (2017). Social media and sexual behavior among adolescents: Is there a link? *JMIR Public Health and Surveillance, 3*(2), e28. https://doi.org/10.2196/publichealth.7149

Laumann, E. O., Paik, A., Glasser, D. B., Kang, J. H., Wang, T., Levinson, B., Moreira, E. D., Jr, Nicolosi, A., & Gingell, C. (2006). A cross-national study of subjective sexual well-being among older women and men: Findings from the Global Study of Sexual Attitudes and Behaviors. *Archives of Sexual Behavior, 35*(2), 145–161. https://doi.org/10.1007/s10508-005-9005-3

Lefkowitz, E. S., Shearer, C. L., Gillen, M. M., & Espinosa-Hernandez, G. (2014). How gendered attitudes relate to women's and men's sexual behaviors and beliefs. *Sex and Culture, 18*(4), 833–846. https://doi.org/10.1007/s12119-014-9225-6

Levinson, D. J. (1978). *The seasons of a man's life.* Ballantine Books.

Lindau, S. T., Schumm, L. P., Laumann, E. O., Levinson, W., O'Muircheartaigh, C. A., & Waite, L. J. (2007). A study of sexuality and health among older adults in the United States. *The New England Journal of Medicine, 357*(8), 762–774. https://doi.org/10.1056/NEJMoa067423

Lyons, H. A., Manning, W. D., Longmore, M. A., & Giordano, P. C. (2014). Young adult casual sexual behavior: Life course specific motivations and consequences. *Sociological Perspectives, 57*(1), 79–101. https://doi.org/10.1177/0731121413517557

MacDougall, A., Craig, S., Goldsmith, K., & Byersb, E. S. (2022). Sexual consent attitudes and behaviour: Associations with sexual health education, sexual consent education, and sexual attitudes. *The Canadian Journal of Human Sexuality, 31*(2), 185–197. https://doi.org/10.3138/cjhs.2021-0057

Martino, S. C., Elliott, M. N., Corona, R., Kanouse, D. E., & Schuster, M. A. (2008). Beyond the "big talk": The roles of breadth and repetition in parent-adolescent communication about sexual topics. *Pediatrics, 121*(3), e612–e618. https://doi.org/10.1542/peds.2007-2156

McAdams, D. P., & de St. Aubin, E. (1992). A theory of generativity and its assessment through self-report, behavioral acts, and narrative themes in autobiography. *Journal of Personality and Social Psychology, 62*(6), 1003–1015. https://doi.org/10.1037/0022-3514.62.6.1003

McKay, E. A., Placencio-Castro, M., Fu, M. R., & Fontenot, H. B. (2022). Associations between sex education types and sexual behaviors among female adolescents: A secondary data analysis of the national survey of family growth 2011–2019. *Sexuality Research & Social Policy, 19*(3), 922–935. https://doi.org/10.1007/s13178-021-00664-w

Mead, M. (1928). *Coming of age in Samoa: A psychological study of primitive youth for Western civilization*. William Morrow & Company.

Mitchell, L. L., Lodi-Smith, J., Baranski, E. N., & Whitbourne, S. K. (2021). Implications of identity resolution in emerging adulthood for intimacy, generativity, and integrity across the adult lifespan. *Psychology and Aging, 36*(5), 545–556. https://doi.org/10.1037/pag0000537

Moore, A. (2018). Toward a central theory of childhood sexuality: A relational approach. In S. Lamb & J. Gilbert (Eds.), *The Cambridge handbook of sexual development* (pp. 35–53). Cambridge University Press. https://doi.org/10.1017/9781108116121.003

Musavi, M., Rahimzadeh, M., Tabaghdeh, M. H., & Saeieh, S. E. (2024). The effect of sexual education on the postpartum women's sexual self-confidence and self-efficacy: A theory-based intervention. *BMC Pregnancy Childbirth, 24*(1), 64. https://doi.org/10.1186/s12884-024-06255-y

Nadelkov, C. (2015). Physical, unconscious, and non-physical factors of attraction. *Journal of Student Research, 4*(2), 1–6. https://doi.org/10.47611/jsr.v4i2.233

Orlofsky, J. L., Marcia, J. E., & Lesser, I. M. (1973). Ego identity status and the intimacy versus isolation crisis of young adulthood. *Journal of Personality and Social Psychology, 27*(2), 211–219. https://doi.org/10.1037/h0034787

Perry, S. L., & Snawder, K. J. (2017). Pornography, religion, and parent–child relationship quality. *Archives of Sexual Behavior, 46*(6), 1747–1761. https://doi.org/10.1007/s10508-016-0927-8

Pflieger, J. C., Cook, E. C., Niccolai, L. M., & Connell, C. M. (2013). Racial/ethnic differences in patterns of sexual risk behavior and rates of sexually transmitted infections among female young adults. *American Journal of Public Health, 103*(5), 903–909. https://doi.org/10.2105/AJPH.2012.301005

Poulsen, F. O., Busby, D. M., & Galovan, A. M. (2013). Pornography use: Who uses it and how it is associated with couple outcomes. *Journal of Sex Research, 50*(1), 72–83. https://doi.org/10.1080/00224499.2011.648027

Richardson, G. B., Barbaro, N., Nedelec, J. L., & Liu, H. (2023). Testing environmental effects on age at menarche and sexual debut within a genetically informative twin design. *Human Nature (Hawthorne, N.Y.), 34*(2), 324–356. https://doi.org/10.1007/s12110-023-09451-5

Rogol, A. D., Roemmich, J. N., & Clark, P. A. (2002). Growth at puberty. *Journal of Adolescent Health, 31*(6), 192–200. https://doi.org/10.1016/s1054-139x(02)00485-8

Sabia J. J. (2006). Does sex education affect adolescent sexual behaviors and health? *Journal of Policy Analysis and Mmanagement, 25*(4), 783–802. https://doi.org/10.1002/pam.20208

Sævik, K. W., & Konijnenberg, C. (2023). The effects of sexual shame, emotion regulation and gender on sexual desire. *Scientific Reports, 13*(1), 4042. https://doi.org/10.1038/s41598-023-31181-y

Santelli, J. S., Grilo, S. A., Lindberg, L. D., Speizer, I. S., Schalet, A., Heitel, J., Kantor, L. M., McGovern, T., Ott, M. A., Lyon, L. E., Rogers, J., Heck, C. J., & Mason-Jones, A. J. (2017). Abstinence-only-until-marriage policies and programs: An updated position paper of the Society for Adolescent Health and Medicine. *The Journal of Adolescent Health, 61*(3), 400–403. https://doi.org/10.1016/j.jadohealth.2017.06.001

Schick, V., Herbenick, D., Reece, M., Sanders, S. A., Dodge, B., Middlestadt, S. E., & Fortenberry, J. D. (2010). Sexual behaviors, condom use, and sexual health of Americans over 50: Implications for sexual health promotion for older adults. *Journal of Sexual Medicine, 7*(Suppl. 5), 315–329. https://doi.org/10.1111/j.1743-6109.2010.02013.x

Schwanz, L. E., & Georges, A. (2021). Sexual development and the environment: Conclusions from 40 years of theory. *Sexual Development, 15*(1–3), 7–22. https://doi.org/10.1159/000515221

Scull, T. M., Dodson, C. V., Geller, J. G., Reeder, L. C., & Stump, K. N. (2022). A media literacy education approach to high school sexual health education: Immediate effects of media aware on adolescents' media, sexual health, and communication outcomes. *Journal of Youth and Adolescence, 51*(4), 708–723. https://doi.org/10.1007/s10964-021-01567-0

Sell, K., Oliver, K., & Meiksin, R. (2023). Comprehensive sex education addressing gender and power: A systematic review to investigate implementation and mechanisms of impact. *Sexuality Research & Social Policy, 20*(1), 58–74. https://doi.org/10.1007/s13178-021-00674-8

Senior, K., & Chenhall, R. (2016). More than "just learning about the organs": Embodied story telling as a basis for learning about sex and relationships. In L. Allen & M. L. Rasmussen (Eds.), *The Palgrave handbook of sexuality education* (pp. 95–114). Palgrave Macmillan UK. https://doi.org/10.1057/978-1-137-40033-8_5

Seshadri, K. (2016). The neuroendocrinology of love. *Indian Journal of Endocrinological Metabolism, 20*(4), 558–563. https://doi.org/10.4103/2230-8210.183479

Silverman, D. K. (2020). Psychosexual stages of development (Freud). In V. Zeigler-Hill & T. K. Shackelford (Eds.), *Encyclopedia of personality and individual differences* (pp. 1–5). Springer International Publishing. https://doi.org/10.1007/978-3-319-28099-8_1417-1

Simsek, N., Evli, M., Uzdil, N., Albayrak, E., & Kartal, D. (2020). Body image and sexual self-confidence in patients with chronic urticaria. *Sexuality and Disability, 38*(1), 147–159. https://doi.org/10.1007/s11195-019-09610-6

Smith, L. W., Liu, B., Degenhardt, L., Richters, J., Patton, G., Wand, H., Cross, D., Hocking, J. S., Skinner, S. R., Cooper, S., Lumby, C., Kaldor, J. M., & Guy, R. (2016). Is sexual content in new media linked to sexual risk behaviour in young people? A systematic review and meta-analysis. *Sexual Health, 13*(6), 501–515. https://doi.org/10.1071/SH16037

Somers, C. L., & Paulson, S. E. (2000). Students' perceptions of parent–adolescent closeness and communication about sexuality: Relations with sexual knowledge, attitudes, and behaviors. *Journal of Adolescence, 23*(5), 629–644. https://doi.org/10.1006/jado.2000.0349

Štulhofer, A., Hinchliff, S., Jurin, T., Carvalheira, A., & Træen, B. (2018). Successful aging, change in sexual interest and sexual satisfaction in couples from four European Countries. *European Journal of Ageing, 16*(2), 155–165. https://doi.org/10.1007/s10433-018-0492-1

Tiefer, L. (1996). Towards a feminist sex therapy. *Women & Therapy, 19*(4), 53–64. https://doi.org/10.1300/J015v19n04_07

Turner, V. W. (1967). *The forest of symbols: Aspects of Ndembu ritual.* Cornell University Press.

Turner, V. W. (1969). *The ritual process: Structure and anti-structure.* Aldine Pub. Co.

van Gennep, A. (1909). *Les rites de passage.*

Vasilenko S. A. (2022). Sexual behavior and health from adolescence to adulthood: Illustrative examples of 25 years of research from add health. *The Journal of Adolescent Health, 71*(6 Suppl.), S24–S31. https://doi.org/10.1016/j.jadohealth.2022.08.014

Vasilenko, S. A., & Lanza, S. T. (2014). Predictors of multiple sexual partners from adolescence through young adulthood. *The Journal of Adolescent Health, 55*(4), 491–497. https://doi.org/10.1016/j.jadohealth.2013.12.025

Verbeek, M. C., Luijk, M., Weeland, J., & van de Bongardt, D. (2023). Male adolescents with mild intellectual disabilities: Normative sexual development and factors associated with sexual risks. *Sexuality and Disability, 41*(4), 769–784. https://doi.org/10.1007/s11195-023-09814-x

Volk, F., Thomas, J., Sosin, L., Jacob, V., & Moen, C. (2016). Religiosity, developmental context, and sexual shame in pornography users: A serial mediation model. *The Journal of Treatment & Prevention, 23*(2–3), 244–259. https://doi.org/10.1080/10720162.2016.1151391

Wang, Y., Wu, H., & Sun, Z. S. (2019). The biological basis of sexual orientation: How hormonal, genetic, and environmental factors influence to whom we are sexually attracted. *Frontiers in Neuroendocrinology, 55*, 100798. https://doi.org/10.1016/j.yfrne.2019.100798

Widman, L., Choukas-Bradley, S., Noar, S. M., Nesi, J., & Garrett, K. (2016). Parent-adolescent sexual communication and adolescent safer sex behavior: A meta-analysis. *JAMA Pediatrics, 170*(1), 52–61. https://doi.org/10.1001/jamapediatrics.2015.2731

Widman, L., Golin, C. E., Kamke, K., Burnette, J. L., & Prinstein, M. J. (2018). Sexual assertiveness skills and sexual decision-making in adolescent girls: Randomized controlled trial of an online program. *American Journal of Public Health, 108*(1), 96–102. https://doi.org/10.2105/AJPH.2017.304106

Yazdkhasti, M., Molaeinezhad, M., Tarrahi, M. J., Karahmadi, M., & Salimi, H. (2023). Investigating the relationship between early maladaptive schemas and sexual self-confidence and sexual self-efficacy in individuals with gender dysphoria. *Advanced Biomedical Research, 12*(1), 232–232. https://doi.org/10.4103/abr.abr_443_22

CHAPTER 5

Considering Gender With All Clients

Michelle M. Marchese

LEARNING OBJECTIVES

- Understand how gender socialization can impact clients of all genders in regard to access to services, affect, behavior, and ability to relate to parts of self.
- Use the lens of gender to support clients in a range of mental health goals and in softening learned defenses.
- Review current language in regard to working therapeutically with transgender, nonbinary, and gender-diverse communities.

INTRODUCTION

All gender identities come with stories, roles, and expectations that may or may not align with someone's personal experience and varying degrees of comfort and discomfort. Gender is such a ubiquitous force that some people are not even aware that they have internalized these stories, roles, and expectations, and/or have not had a place where they can unpack their own gender and the narratives of gender that have been thrust upon them.

I once had a clinical supervisor tell me, "Your clients can only go where you are willing to go." This does not mean that you have to question your gender or have everything figured out about your own gender. However it is important to recognize how gender operates—and how your gender operates—so you can understand how it might be working—or not working—for your clients. As you go through this chapter, please keep in mind that gender is different for each person and that everything discussed here will not necessarily apply to each client of a particular gender that you encounter.

I have worked in highly gendered clinical settings: a Veterans Administration milieu program that primarily served cisgender men; an eating disorder clinic at a historically women's liberal arts college as the director of counseling; and in an independent practice in the vibrant and active feminist, queer, and transgender communities of Northampton, Massachusetts. This clinical background has informed much of the information in this chapter. Within these different settings, I have heard clients use gender to minimize their mental health symptoms and their experiences. For example, I have heard women survivors of incest say, "I can't have PTSD, I'm not a guy who went off to war." Veteran men have said to me, "I went to war, but that's not as horrible as being a woman who is raped." A transgender woman admitted, "My experience is not so bad because I mostly pass [read as cisgender]; it would be much worse if I were nonbinary." A young transman initially focused on depression as his presenting problem when he instead experienced dissociation caused by high anxiety—his response was, "I always think of anxiety as feminine—my mom had it—it feels hard to accept [and address] this."

Now that I have explained why you should consider gender in your practice, here are some of the ways to operationalize gender in your work with your clients:

1. Point out how gender expectations and norms affect your client's behavior, emotions, and thoughts. This can be a means of externalizing common obstacles to health such as blame, shame, and guilt.
2. Explore how gender expectations train people to behave with certain tendencies, as this may help clients understand how behaviors may or may not make the most sense for their life and situation.
3. Watch for the impact of gender norms on the inhibition of certain emotional expressions like anger, powerlessness, and fear, and explore this with your client so that they may better access those feelings.
4. Examine how your client's socialization constructs include a hierarchical, gender-based understanding of relative human "value" and "trustworthiness." This, in turn, can help a client make sense of unhelpful/harmful ways that others have reacted to them, especially when they were particularly vulnerable or needing support.
5. It is important to note that there may also be a source of conflict for individuals between their gender and other social identities like race, ethnicity, physical or mental ability, age, socioeconomic class status, sexual orientation, and marital status, among others. Challenges arising from these intersections may contribute to (a) options that a client imagines for themselves, (b) effects regarding the pressure they put on themselves, and/or (c) interference with their ability to engage in self-compassion. I invite you to imagine how the intersection of gender and other social identities may come up in work with clients such as a retired Black veteran man who now must use a wheelchair as a result of an injury during active service; a single, White woman who was homeless during a devastating hurricane; a young Indian woman, recently matched with a husband, now diagnosed with invasive breast cancer; or a Chinese nonbinary person who has been emotionally terrorized by their affluent family of origin.

This chapter is organized into three sections: working with (a) women, (b) men, and (c) **T**ransgender/nonbinary/**G**ender expansive or fluid/genderqueer/**D**iverse (referred to in the rest of the text as TGD) people. This chapter is by no means exhaustive of the ways that gender impacts individuals, systems, the context of mental health, or the ways to address gender in the context of treatment. However, my hope is that it adds some dimension to the important work you do with each and every one of your clients.

Perhaps many of the suggestions I make here are already being integrated into your framework—and I would be thrilled to know that this is the case! Still, continuing to think about clinical interventions within the context of gender, and utilizing humility about the culture and experiences of any of your clients, will always further enhance your practice.

WHAT IS GENDER?

Theorists in many fields still debate the concept of gender identity. Aristotle planted the seeds of a biological deterministic view of gender, and more recently Judith Butler proposed that gender is merely a performance (Bodnar, 2018; Butler, 1993). We now tend to understand gender as a social construct, meaning that a gender identity is not dictated by biology, but is instead prescribed by the culture someone lives in as a series of behaviors, preferences, presentations, abilities, roles, tasks, and emotional expressions.

People tend to confuse or try to connect the concepts of *sex* with *gender*. Let us look closely at this: In the United States, a parent gets an ultrasound at about 18 weeks of cells growing in a uterus. A technician squints at some pixels thought to represent external genitalia and declares that the cells are "a boy" or "a girl," and this leads people to lay out a myriad of gender-based expectations and limits that will last a lifetime. This scenario can also happen at birth. Babies can also be born *intersex* and possess "atypical" genital characteristics or reproductive organs. Since the 1950s, "gender normalizing" surgeries have been frequently performed at birth with and without parental consent—and, of course, without the consent of the child (Creighton, 2001).

However, what do a baby's perceived genitals have to do with the kinds of clothes they may like to wear, their favorite colors, the kinds of jobs they might be drawn toward, the division of domestic and emotional labor in their homes, or their relationship with anger? When people start to tie gender to bodies, the argument falls apart. If gender is related to body parts, what does this mean for women who have had mastectomies, hysterectomies, or oophorectomies? Similarly, if we determine gender based on genetic markers, what about the thousands of people born with more or less than the prevalent 46 chromosomes? Sometimes people will argue that hormone levels explain gender norms; what implication does this have for younger and older people (people who have different hormone levels due to their developmental age), or people on hormone blockers due to cancer (Burstein et al., 2019; Senefeld et al., 2020)? We all know plenty of people who, even though they feel that their gender aligns with the sex they were assigned or assumed at birth, do not conform to gender norms. Many are students, clinicians, and therapists reading this book.

It may be easier to see how gender is constructed socially when we look outside of our immediate culture and notice differences in the expectations for, and attitudes about, genders. For example, women were prohibited from wearing pants throughout much of European history. Many transgender people are recognized and named within their cultures such as the *hijura* of India and Pakistan, the *kathoey* of Thailand, and *muxe* of Mexico; it was the influence of British colonization that introduced judgment and discrimination of people with these genders (Chang et al., 2018). Similarly, most indigenous North American (or Turtle Island) communities recognize and accept the *Two-Spirit* gender role, in addition to the roles of women and men (Ristock et al., 2010). In Israel, all citizens regardless of gender must register for the Israeli Army. You may observe that some of these examples reference the past, but the introduction of time only further confirms the point of gender being socially constructed, because this means that gender roles were created by the culture *of that time* and that our current culture *no longer* recognizes those distinctions.

Because gender roles, expectations, and stories are socially constructed, it becomes important to understand how each individual feels in relation to these social narratives. Even the person who seems to most strictly conform to a culture's gender norm probably has moments where something about their gender role does not feel 100% right for them.

BASIC LANGUAGE CONCEPTS

Our language is constantly evolving. For example, your great-grandparents may think of "slides" as a photographic image on a piece of glass. Your parent may think of "slides" as an individual piece of photographic film, inserted into a projector, and viewed at a much larger capacity on a blank wall. Currently, a college undergraduate student may use "slides" to denote a series of text-based images posted online via social media or used on a computer in a PowerPoint presentation. In the same way, our language regarding gender is constantly changing—and fast. In fact, some of the language I employ in this chapter may soon be out-of-date. It is important to keep this in mind and stay curious, especially when working with people whose gender is different from yours or who are at different life stages. **Box 5.1** illustrates some of the gender-related terms I use in this chapter and with which you may or may not be familiar. These definitions stem from literature created by TGD individuals and communities; affirming organizations that serve them, such as the World Professional Association for Transgender Health (WPATH); my professional experience working with TGD clients for over 15 years; and my personal experience of being non-binary within queer communities (Chang, 2017; GLAAD, 2022; Shlasko & Hofius, 2017; WPATH, 2022). Keep in mind that terms referring to individuals should be first used by the persons themselves.

BOX 5.1. GENDER-RELATED TERMINOLOGY

Assigned-Sex-at-Birth, Assigned-Male-at-Birth, Assigned-Female-at-Birth (or AMAB or AFAB): The sex marker, usually male or female, declared at someone's birth according to their perceived external genitalia. Many legal documents will refer to this marker. Some sex educators and activists also use the term "sex assumed at birth" to denote the actual complexity and variety of marker and feature combinations.

Gender Identity: The internal, felt sense of an individual's gender. You cannot tell someone's gender identity just from looking at them, even if you think you can!

Gender Presentation or Expression: The outward mannerisms, accessories, or ways of relating and communicating that people tend to describe as "masculine" or "feminine." This does not have to align with someone's internal sense of their gender.

Gender Binary: The idea that there is only the two distinct, opposite gender categories of "male" and "female."

Transgender (or trans): Someone who moves from living their life as one gender to another. This transition may or may not incorporate physical, social, or legal changes. Many people no longer use "transsexual," so avoid this term unless the person claims this identity. For example, some older trans people who have been through physical transition use this term to denote the difference between themselves and trans people who have not engaged in any physical changes in regards to their gender.

Gender-Diverse: A term that can encompass a range of gender identities that do not fall under binary gender definitions.

Gender Nonconforming: Used for people who identify as either "male" or "female" but who present in ways that do not conform to traditional gender roles.

Nonbinary: Someone who does not identify as either or entirely "man" or "woman." A nonbinary identity can fall under either the categories of "gender-diverse" or "transgender," or both. Can be shortened to "ENBY" but not "NB," as the latter means non-Black.

Cisgender: A person whose gender identity aligns with their sex assigned at birth. Someone who is not trans.

Gender Pronouns: All personal pronouns are gender pronouns. "They/them" is a common gender/neutral pronoun for a singular person. Some people use no pronouns. Other pronouns people may use include: ze/zir/zirs or ze/hir/hirs.

Gender Dysphoria: This is a diagnosis in the *Diagnostic and Statistical Manual of Mental Disorders* (5th ed.; *DSM-5*; American Psychiatric Association, 2013) that is often used to have someone's gender-affirming care covered by insurance. Being transgender is not a psychiatric disorder.

Gender Critical and TERF (Trans-Exclusionary Radical Feminists): Anti-trans activists who exclude trans women from women's spaces and who attempt to limit trans people to designations related to their gender assigned at birth only.

GENDER SELF-REFLECTION EXERCISE FOR CLINICIANS

There are many ways that we have been socialized to understand gender and the gender identities of those around us. To be gender-affirming to all of our clients, and to avoid replicating forced gender expectations of any individual, it is important to unpack our own relationship to gender. By understanding how the mechanisms of gender work within ourselves, we are more likely to see how they work for and against our clients. This type of personal reflection and deconstruction demands more than just considering these few questions, but they may provide an entry point for further exploration (see **Box 5.2**).

BOX 5.2. GENDER SELF-REFLECTION QUESTIONS

- When you were a child, what kinds of messages did you receive about how you should dress, how you should act, or how others should treat you that were related to your assigned gender at birth?
- Who were the people who communicated these messages to you? What kinds of power did they hold over you? Were they teachers, parents, peers, celebrities?
- Did you ever receive praise for conforming to gender roles or expectations?
- What happened when you did not conform to gender expectations?
- Have there been sexual or affective expectations of you because of your gender?
- Are there ways that you have communicated to others when they are or are not conforming to normative gender roles? Example: Have you joked about someone's gender or gender presentation?
- How did your gender play or not play a role in your choice to become a therapist / clinician?
- How do different clients of all genders react to your gender?
- How are clinicians of different genders treated in your clinical setting? Are they paid differently? Do you notice any connections between their gender and the power they hold in your setting?
- Are there assumptions you have about your clients of any genders, especially in regards to them needing mental health treatment? Have you noticed that some genders seem to be given certain diagnoses more than others? What have or have you not noticed about the gender of clients who have been previously diagnosed with bipolar disorder, borderline personality disorder, posttraumatic stress disorder (PTSD), acute stress disorder, narcissistic personality disorder, or dissociative identity disorder, among others?
- Do you notice the physical or fashion attributes of clients of particular genders more than you do those of other genders? Do you expect clients to present to you a certain way according to their gender? If a client does not conform to your idea of their gender, does this make you wonder about them diagnostically?
- What theoretical models have you been trained in or have you been drawn toward? What has been their view on clients of different genders? Did any of these models particularly pathologize women or transgender people? Were they initially conceptualized by men, women, or a TGD individual?

These questions were inspired by a similar exercise in the excellent book, *A Clinician's Guide to Gender-Affirming Care,* by Chang et al. (2018).

THERAPY WITH WOMEN*

The psychological field has been tainted by gender values and ideas since it was birthed by a man. Sigmund Freud famously treated cisgender women who were thought to suffer from something called *hysteria*. He subsequently published a paper in 1896 called *The Etiology of Hysteria*, in which he recognized that most of his patients reported what we now call sexual assault and incest. His findings threatened the power of the cisgender men who perpetrated these crimes. In deference to that power, and to shield himself from the consequences of highlighting traumas steeped

* I use the term *women* here to apply to both cisgender and transgender women. However, I currently often use the term *femme* because this term can include queer or nonbinary people who do not identify as a woman or a girl but who present in a "feminine" manner and, as a result, may all experience similar effects of gender bias.

in gender bias, Freud abandoned his "seduction theory" (Herman, 1992; Masson, 1984). Instead of describing the etiology of hysteria symptoms as stemming from sexual trauma, he proposed that they were caused by graphic, upsetting "fantasies" that were a result of deficits in psychosexual development (Jahoda, 1977).

Many master's and doctoral level programs in psychology and social work, as well as prestigious psychoanalytic training programs, still teach Freud's theories. Despite the fact that our field has critiqued the mechanics of Freud's original theories, the profession has not fully disentangled gender bias from the field of psychology. If the foundation of psychological history is rife with gender bias, how might that bias have remained in some form in more modern theories, or through the work of respected teachers and experienced trainers?

Fast-forward to the present.

Women are a third less likely to report trauma than men; however, they are two times as likely to develop PTSD and four times as likely to develop chronic PTSD than men (Kimerling et al., 2013; Tolin & Foa, 2006). (While transgender women and transgender men may have been included in those large categories of gender in the literature, TGD individuals are not referenced in this research.) This rate discrepancy is not because of something inherent in women that makes them more susceptible to trauma or PTSD, but instead has to do with various social and cultural factors, including the fact that women are more often victims of interpersonal violence (Centers for Disease Control and Prevention [CDC], 2024b). One type of interpersonal violence, sexual assault, is more likely to cause PTSD than other traumatic experiences (DiMauro & Renshaw, 2021). Our culture tends to blame victims, especially women (Kennedy & Prock, 2018). Blaming the victim works to minimize the effects and symptoms of trauma of the one who was harmed in order to preserve a sense of control in the face of upsetting events. *Rape culture* is a term used to describe the pervasive particular cultural messages, in the context of interpersonal sexual violence, that seek to normalize rape and blame women for the violence perpetrated against them (Connell & Wilson, 1974). Victim-blaming may keep them from getting help because they do not "deserve" it, which can further exacerbate symptoms.

With other mental health conditions, there continues to be a gender gap. Of note, most of the research cited here does not include TGD people in their statistics. Boys are twice as likely to receive an attention deficit hyperactivity disorder (ADHD) diagnosis than girls (CDC, 2024a). Twice as many women are diagnosed with depression than men (Villarroel & Terlizzi, 2020). The majority of women diagnosed with autism spectrum disorder (80%) did not have their condition recognized until they were over 18 years of age (UCLA Health, 2023). As you read through this chapter, consider how some of the issues around gender norms and expectations may play a part in many of these discrepancies.

Some mental health issues related to depression, anxiety, sleep difficulties, sexual function, and "productivity" can be affected by physical changes across the life span. Being familiar with women's health issues around pregnancy, endometriosis, premenstrual conditions, menopause, and elder aging may help you make appropriate referrals to physical health providers so that your client does not continue to suffer without a full spectrum of help.

ACCESS ISSUES

Decades of economic inequality also may impede a woman's ability to pay for or take time off to attend therapy sessions, inequalities that are even more exaggerated for women who are BIPOC (Black, Indigenous, and People of Color; Wingfield, 2020). Since insurance is frequently tied to employment in the United States, unregulated work, such as sex work, further decreases access to treatment for women who labor in those fields. While insurance is available through the Affordable Care Act, there is a vast difference in deductible amounts and access to providers based on state policy choices (Sharer & Lukens, 2024). Women still shoulder the brunt of childcare, highlighted by the COVID-19 pandemic (Kenny & Yang, 2021). This constrains the time and resources some women may have to seek out and engage in therapy.

INTERACTION WITH LEGAL SYSTEMS

While interpersonal violence is unfortunately perpetrated against people of all genders, as mentioned previously, women report the highest rates of sexual and interpersonal victimization (CDC, 2024b). If survivors engage in the legal system as a result of this violence, they may experience structural or individual gender bias from local police departments, school administrators, hospitals, and human resource departments. As a result, your client may not only suffer from the initial trauma, but also may suffer from trauma related to how they were treated at the police station, what was said during a medical exam at the hospital, how their college has treated similar cases in the past, or even how governmental officials, as highly placed as the U.S. Supreme Court bench, are not fully investigated after allegations of assault have been made public.

This has two implications for treatment.

One, you may need to ask your client about the initial experience of violence, as well as identify subsequent traumatic interactions with institutions that were supposed to have supported your client.

- *Example:* If you are treating a traditional-aged college student who has survived a rape, together you will process the rape, but you also might need to process the school administration's suggestion to not pursue legal consequences, or her lawyer's insinuation that her drinking or clothing choices were the reasons your client was assaulted.

Two, your client may not even recognize these instances of bias and instead internalize the negative messages experienced. Helping your client externalize and restructure her beliefs and judgments about the traumatic event needs to be part of the treatment.

- *Example:* If this client internalized the idea that it was her fault that she was assaulted because she had been drinking, helping her understand how gender bias contributed to that belief may aid your client in no longer continuing to blame herself. This, in turn, may allow your client to access more adaptive beliefs related to her value and/or the values of gender equality. This new understanding may permit identification of resources that she either felt she did not deserve (when she believed the assault was "her fault") or resources that can represent gender liberation.

EMOTIONAL AND BEHAVIORAL CONSIDERATIONS

People are taught what emotions are socially acceptable for them according to their gender via social and institutional interactions and media (Kennedy-Root & Denham, 2010). This can show up in treatment sessions with women in particular ways. I will highlight two examples of such emotions: anger and disgust.

Anger

In the United States, *anger* is an emotion that many people who are socialized as female are often not comfortable expressing. They are told, "Anger is not productive," "Your anger hurts other people," "All anger is bad." Showing anger contradicts the cultural expectations that women and girls should be caretakers and peacemakers. In fact, our culture has a negative and offensive term for women and girls who express anger—*bitch*—yet there is no equivalent of this term for male subjects.

Since your client may not know how to engage with her anger, she may instead overidentify with other emotions such as fear, sadness, the experience of having autonomy blocked (powerlessness), guilt, or shame. I encourage you and your client to get curious about her lack of anger and explore how it may be impacting her other feelings.

All of this may also mean that the only "acceptable" way for her to express anger is to turn it against herself. Anticipate ways this may creep into treatment:

- Anger turned against the self can show up as symptoms such as self-harm, disordered eating, suicidal thoughts, stomach pains and headaches, and perfectionist behavior.

- You may need to offer specific psychoeducation to normalize anger, explain its function, and model healthy expression.
- A client might not recognize sensations of anger because she has never been allowed to have them.
- You may need to reorient your client toward anger. She may benefit from validation of her anger and/or an invitation to unpack her cultural or familial messages about anger.
- A client may struggle to feel anger because she feels guilty about feeling it in the first place.
- Share information about how people tend to somatically feel anger in their head, chest, or hands. This may help her start to connect with her sensations of anger even if she is defended cognitively.

Be sure to always consider the intersection of other social identities in relation to emotions. For example, Black women are often stereotyped as "angry" (Ashley, 2014). This pejorative trope could impact your client's ability to express anger, and depending on *your* race, it may impact her ability to express it to *you*.

Disgust

I have also found the emotion *disgust* to be implicated in gender socialization. Disgust is an emotion that has a particularly strong, negative, somatic charge to it. As a result, both clients and clinicians may find themselves avoiding digging into this emotion. However, disgust can be an integral part of sexual and interpersonal violence, medical issues, experiences of depression or anxiety related to eating and body image, or sensation sensitivity related to neurodiversity.

In addition to protecting herself, a woman may be inclined to shield you, her clinician, from her disgust or aspects of her experiences that are disgusting. While some of this may be a manifestation of the classic avoidance response to traumatic material, it also may be tied to shame from victim-blaming, as well as socialized behaviors to caretake and prioritize the comfort of others, even at your client's own expense. Consider ways to bring up and normalize disgust for your client:

- Assess for caretaking behaviors in your client.
- Talk to your client about how she might avoid or hide content because she thinks it may upset you. Always reassure your client that this is not necessary.
- Suggest disgust as a possible emotion she may feel when exploring affective reactions.
- Ask about emotions associated with nauseous feelings. Disgust is often characterized by an obvious, particular facial expression. If you notice even a flicker of that across your client's face, bring attention to it.

Another aspect of disgust is that, like anger, it can be easily turned toward the self. Pay attention to the language your client uses such as, "I was disgusted with myself." This could be a clue to explore internalized judgments about the self and process disgust about other experiences.

In addition to emotions, gender socialization affects behaviors. One of these behaviors is caretaking, which was mentioned previously. A related behavior is the act of saying "no." The first thing that might come to your mind after reading that statement is the historical phenomenon of "no" in the context of sexual consent. This context has served to render a woman's "no" as meaningless, not to be respected or believed. That context also highlights how women are conditioned in general to *not* say "no" to others in order to keep the peace or because her needs are valued less than the needs of others. The behavior of saying "no" has implications in the treatment of sexual trauma, and it affects our clients' abilities to set healthy boundaries, which has a wide array of mental health implications. It can also play into the tendency to be a people-pleaser. Examples of how this may appear in treatment follow:

- A client who often misses sessions due to obligations in her personal and professional life. It can also mean that it is not enough simply to ask for your client's consent to treatment. You must normalize her opinions and her choice to speak up if something in the treatment is not feeling helpful, and reassure her that this is in fact what you want.

- Your client may need some additional permission from you to communicate when she needs a shift in the present therapy session or trajectory.
- What is probably most obvious is that your client might struggle with the idea that she did or did not say "no" during interpersonal violence. She may also be judgmental of the fact that she *froze* during an upsetting event or that she *fawned* (utilized people-pleasing behaviors) over a perpetrator. Sharing explanations on how she may have been taught to not occupy physical or emotional space, and to diffuse the negative feelings of others, may facilitate healing.
- Other people in her life may react to her growth and changes—especially if she is setting up more boundaries or is less available to their needs. Treatment may need to focus on continuing to hold new boundaries or creating new relationships.
- She may be so used to attending to others that she has trouble with *interoception* (tuning into and recognizing her own bodily sensations). This may mean that somatic-based interventions need additional scaffolding.

THERAPY WITH MEN*

In general, men do not face the same issues of pay inequity, cultural pressures to be the primary caretaker of children and families, legal bias, and assumptions about their blame as women. (Although, again, race, age, socioeconomic class, ability, and other social identities can complicate this picture.) To return to the history of psychology, half of the cases Freud published centered on male patients, and male psychoanalysts were expected to be in treatment themselves throughout their careers. So, why are men accessing therapy at lower rates, and quitting therapy at higher rates? And how might gender impact how many men engage with therapy?

ACCESS ISSUES

While cisgender men do not face the same structural issues of access that women or TGD clients do, they do struggle to start and complete treatment (Shiner et al., 2017). Part of this is due to stigma around men needing or seeking help (Sagar-Ouriaghli et al., 2019). Furthermore, many men are not acculturated to the language around therapy and the emotional activities inherent in it. Rather, certain expectations regarding the domination of others and one's environment, toughness, physical force and violence, aggression, blaming others, being independent, and not showing emotions are all messages that boys and men receive from parents, media, peers, family, lovers, and people in authority such as doctors or the police (Seidler et al., 2016).

While there is a spectrum of these narratives and the ways that individual men identify with them, some people refer to the constellation or phenomenon of these negative expectations as *toxic masculinity,* a term originating from men involved in the self-help movement of the 1970s. Toxic masculinity includes qualities that some cultures attribute to masculinity that are harmful to the man who exhibits them and to the people around him. The function of toxic masculinity is to keep and to consolidate power for men by devaluing qualities deemed to be "feminine," such as emotional sensitivity, tenderness, emotional connection, and warmth. However, while toxic masculinity works to hold on to certain kinds of interpersonal power, it denies the subject loving, mutual, supportive, affective experiences and relationships.

Yet research shows that men are struggling. In 2021, men were more than 4 times as likely as women to commit suicide (Garnett et al., 2023). However, in 2022, men reported an average of any mental illness (AMI) 6.7% lower than women (National Institute of Mental Health [NIMH], 2024). To report illness, someone most likely must be connected to mental health

---

* I use the term *men* here to apply to both cisgender and transgender men. However, the term *masc* can also include queer or nonbinary people who do not identify as a man or a boy but who present in a "masculine" manner and, as a result, may all experience similar effects of gender bias.

psychoeducation and services, and yet men continue to lag in accessing mental health treatment (NIMH, 2024).

Since men may not have been socialized to seek help, they may first encounter therapy tied to their employment in some way. Some examples of this are services provided by the Department of Defense or Veterans Affairs, or through employee assistance programs (EAP). These providers and programs tend to offer time-limited, brief services. Due to the nature of this, a focus on outcomes and prescribed processes is common, and, as a result, may not allow the opportunity for acculturation to therapy or titrated experimentation with, and exploration of, emotions and acts of vulnerability.

Another way that men may find themselves in therapy is through referrals from other health providers. The steps between a suggestion during a routine health exam and a connection to an individual therapist, combined with the variables of stigma and lack of acculturation, create layers of barriers.

Additionally, issues around a therapeutic gender "match" seem notably heightened for many men (Shiner et al., 2017). If a man is working with a female clinician, he may feel the need to adhere to prescribed gender roles and expectations or may assume that she will not grasp the intricacies of his gender experiences. If he works with a male clinician, he may worry about being emotionally vulnerable to another man who may judge him for his emotional reactions. In fact, some research shows that men are more likely to quit therapy if working with a male clinician (Shiner et al., 2017). If he works with an "out" transgender or nonbinary clinician, any of these previous issues, plus gender insecurity or fears about homosexuality (homophobia), could arise.

EMOTIONAL AND BEHAVIORAL CONSIDERATIONS

Considering that our culture can communicate messages that masculinity requires a stoic posture, it comes as no surprise that many men may deal with some level of *alexithymia*, or difficulty feeling and expressing emotions (Sullivan & Brown, 2015). This may require you to be more directive and specific when assessing emotional experiences and symptoms, as well as in your explanations of the therapeutic process. You may also need to prioritize explicit psychoeducation on emotions, thoughts, and behaviors; work to restructure stigma about engaging in therapy; and identify positive resources that showcase masculinity and emotionality.

Whereas women tend not to be encouraged to feel or express anger, for many men the only feeling they have been socialized to own is anger (Chaplin, 2015). This is because anger can take forms that preserve the dominance and insensitivity inherent in toxic masculinity. Many men feel a range of emotions but have learned to unconsciously translate all of them into anger (Chaplin, 2015). This has implications in avoiding other negative emotions like grief or loneliness. Interventions that reorient, validate, and normalize other emotions, as well as ones that direct to other somatic sensations, may be useful. Some men who do not engage with anger for a variety of reasons may experience shame or self-judgment due to not aligning with a cultural masculine ideal.

Since many men are socialized to express anger and to avoid accountability through aggression, it may be particularly challenging for them to process feelings of vulnerability, fear, weakness, fear of losing autonomy (powerlessness), and shame. Digesting these emotions may come with the secondary grief of losing the idea of the man he thought he was, that his parents wanted him to be, or who is attractive to his partner. Make sure to help your client see the benefits of a full emotional life and discuss how many people value a man who can be supportive, take responsibility, and connect on emotional levels. Resources or references to positive male role models may be helpful here. Some of the ones I use include Coach Eric Taylor from the TV show *Friday Night Lights*, T'Challa from the *Black Panther* film, Lieutenant Commander Paul Stamets from *Star Trek Discovery*, Atticus Finch from the book *To Kill a Mockingbird*, or Randall Pearson from the TV show *This Is Us*.

Therapeutic work might revolve around practicing emotional reactions besides anger or learning to express anger in ways that are not harmful to the client or those around him. It also may be about cultivating compassion for himself and others and practicing vulnerability around personal needs in future relationships and situations.

MALE SURVIVORS OF INTERPERSONAL VIOLENCE

When people imagine victims of physical, sexual, or emotional abuse, the first image that comes to mind is probably not one of a man. Yet in the United States, one in four men have survived some form of sexual violence (CDC, 2024c). Rates of sexual abuse of boys by members of the clergy are in the tens of thousands (Fitzgibbons & O'Leary, 2011). Mens' experiences of interpersonal violence tend to be erased due to some of those previously mentioned toxic masculinity issues. Fear of minimization, being mocked, or not being believed can silence boys and men who experience this kind of trauma (Briere & Elliot, 2003).

How can your work not collude with the erasure of these men's experiences? What language about survivors can you use on your website to be inclusive of male survivors? Do you ask about all kinds of interpersonal violence for each of your clients, no matter their gender? Do you know where to find resources for referrals, additional professional supports, and books and articles that you can give to these clients? Many of these male survivors struggle with loneliness and shame due not only to the initial trauma but also to the cultural response—or lack thereof—to their experiences. As a result, group modalities may be transformative, and examples of this can include group meetings that focus on resourcing sessions for men, groups focusing on the future, or group EMDR (G-TEP) that would allow clients to process in a community of other male survivors.

In addition to issues of erasure and alienation, male survivors may have fears about what their traumatic experiences mean about their gender identity or sexual orientation. This is because being a victim of interpersonal violence is the antithesis of embodying certain toxic masculine ideals. While you may truly work with clients who have survived interpersonal violence, and who are also questioning their gender or sexual identities (while being assigned/assumed male at birth), be careful not to validate incorrect causal relationships between those things for your clients.

THERAPY WITH TRANSGENDER AND GENDER-DIVERSE CLIENTS

I highly recommend Dr. Sand C. Chang's chapter entitled, "EMDR Therapy as Affirmative Care for Transgender and Gender Nonconforming Clients" in Mark Nickerson's book *Cultural Competence and Healing Culturally Based Trauma with EMDR Therapy* (2017). Some of the information discussed here may overlap with some of the material found in that chapter; however, Chang's work provides a wealth of information far beyond what I can present here.

Transgender, gender-diverse, and nonbinary clients may seek therapy for a variety of concerns. TGD people are at a higher risk for trauma, depression, and anxiety due to discrimination in many contexts of their lives (Atteberry-Ash et al., 2021; Clements-Nolle et al., 2006; Edelman, 2011; Nadal et al., 2010). As a result, individuals may be experiencing mental health symptoms for events related to their gender identity, such as being estranged from family members, bullying, workplace discrimination, medical trauma, religious trauma, and interpersonal violence. Eating disorder rates are higher for queer and trans individuals, as is substance use posttrauma for youths (Nagata et al., 2020; Simmons & Suaréz, 2016).

However, being TGD is itself not traumatic or a mental illness, and not all TGD people find aspects related to their gender, legal, social, or physical transition connected to mental health symptoms. Instead, TGD people might be seeking services for the same reasons as cisgender clients. However, as with all other genders, I encourage you to be curious about how the experience of gender may impact your TGD client's experiences or their relationship to those experiences. If you are cisgender, please approach this part of the chapter knowing that you may already have TGD people as your clients, even if they are not out to you, and that TGD people may also already be your clinical colleagues.

ACCESS ISSUES

TGD clients have faced high rates of discrimination and harm by the mental health field due to anti-trans bias and ignorance (Campbell & Arkles, 2016; Chang et al., 2018). As a result, they may avoid mental health treatment (Chang et al., 2018). Keeping this history in mind, work to create trust and believe your clients, even if they report negative experiences with one of your beloved peers. Know that you might need to help your client process interactions they have had with previous providers.

Challenges with insurance if or when someone has not legally changed their name, or insurance that is provided by a family member who does not know your client is TGD, creates barriers to treatment. To manage some of these barriers, be thoughtful and collaborate with your client about how to bill and document services. Discuss ahead of time about how to coordinate with other providers, agencies, or family members.

Structural oppression such as homelessness, poverty, unemployment, and police brutality hinder not only the availability of services for TGD clients, but also the opportunity to choose providers based on their gender-affirming capabilities. Some of the considerations listed under "Interaction With Legal Systems" in the section on "Therapy With Women" may be applicable to consider in the context of some TGD identities. Not all TGD people will transition physically, socially, or legally. Some of this is due to personal choice, the cost and challenges associated with some changes, and current legal challenges to accessing gender-affirming care.

Understand the limits of your knowledge and seek out resources that you can share with your TGD clients. Take care to continue to educate yourself and shift your practice to recognize TGD identities in the first interaction someone has with you or your practice.

To that end, I encourage you to change your intake paperwork to be inclusive of all genders (see **Box 5.3**). This means not assuming anything related to gender with any of your clients. You may find that some of your cisgender clients question you about this, but I find explaining at the start of any intake that, "I am going to ask you questions that I ask everyone who first comes into my office. Some of them may seem obvious to you, but I just don't want to assume anything about anyone," alleviates many tensions. Many of my suggestions seem simple once you read them, but I have found that clinicians often ask me how to specifically operationalize these ideas into questions.

PRACTICING LANGUAGE

I referred to gender pronouns earlier, but nouns can also be gendered. You do not have to erase all gendered nouns from your language, but it is helpful to know some gender-neutral substitutes and to practice using them when you do not specifically know someone's gender (see **Box 5.4**).

BOX 5.3. SOME SUGGESTIONS FOR GENDER-INCLUSIVE INTAKE QUESTIONS

For all clients:

- What is your name?
- What is your gender identity? *(With no predetermined categories listed)*
- What are your pronouns?
- What has your experience been like working with other mental health providers?

For TGD clients:

- Are you "out" about your gender identity to other providers I will be communicating with to coordinate care? *(Make sure to protect their privacy and honor their choices.)*
- Does your insurance have another name on it? *(Do NOT ask things like: What is your REAL name or the name you were given. This is considered offensive.)*
- How do other people in your life react to your gender identity? Who is supportive? Who isn't?

BOX 5.4. GENDER-NEUTRAL NOUNS

sister or brother … try SIBLING
niece or nephew … try NIBLING
girlfriend or boyfriend … try PARTNER, DATE, or SIGNIFICANT OTHER
husband or wife … try any of the above or SPOUSE
alumnae, alumnus … try ALUM
mother or father … try PARENT

I have found that some clinicians who are not part of the LGBTQI2 (Lesbian, Gay, Bisexual, Transgender, Queer/Questioning, Intersex, Two-Spirited) community, and even some who are, have trouble with changing names, nouns, and pronouns for their clients. That is likely because they do not often get a chance to practice. The following two short case vignettes provide you with such a practice opportunity (see **Box 5.5**).

EMOTIONAL AND BEHAVIORAL CONSIDERATIONS

TGD people are susceptible to the cultural messages that other genders face. So, while there are specific considerations for supporting TGD clients, also know that, for example, when working with a transgender woman, issues previously discussed about women need to be held

BOX 5.5. CASE VIGNETTES

Practice changing this client's name, pronouns, and gendered nouns to the two suggestions that follow.

1. **Imagine that your client Jason has transitioned to Halie, a transgender woman who uses she/her pronouns.**
   Jason is a 24-year-old, White, cisgender man from Amherst, Massachusetts. He is an alumnus of a local liberal arts college and works as a mechanical engineer. He presented to treatment due to long-standing issues with acute anxiety and panic. He states that he wants to work on these symptoms so that he can more fully commit to his wife and "be a good husband."

   …

   Halie is a 24-year-old, White, transgender woman from Amherst, Massachusetts. She is an alumna of a local liberal arts college and works as a mechanical engineer. She presented to treatment due to long-standing issues with acute anxiety and panic. She states that she wants to work on these symptoms so that she can more fully to commit to her wife and "be a good wife."
2. **Here is another example. Imagine that your client Aika has transitioned to Asao, a nonbinary person who uses they/them pronouns.**
   Aika is an 18-year-old, cisgender female, Japanese international first-year student who recently graduated from boarding school in upstate New York. She currently majors in contemporary ballet. She is estranged from her family due to parental emotional abuse and wonders what family obligations she has as an elder sister to her five brothers.

   …

   Asao is an 18-year-old, nonbinary, Japanese international first-year student who recently graduated from boarding school in upstate, New York. They currently major in contemporary ballet. They are estranged from their family due to parental emotional abuse and wonder what family obligations they have as an elder sibling to their five brothers.

in mind: This is because transgender men are men, and transgender women are women. However, navigating gender roles and norms can be complicated when someone has been raised as one gender and is now living as another gender. They may even feel at the mercy of *all* gender roles and norms at different times of their lives, especially during "coming out" or transitioning periods, or if they are gender-expansive or gender-fluid. Feelings related to "passing"—meaning, how much someone is perceived as cisgender—may impact someone's relationship to emotions and behaviors.

GENDER DYSPHORIA AND IMPLICATIONS FOR DISSOCIATION

Dissociation can be an adaptive strategy to cope with *gender dysphoria* (distress that someone feels when their gender identity does not align with the sex they were assigned at birth or with their body), navigating between places where they are "out" and "not out" about their gender identity, and environments steeped in trans bias. Trauma therapists and clinicians are trained to screen for trauma-related dissociation because this type of dissociation can interfere with treatment or can retraumatize clients during the general phase two of a three-phase trauma-healing model (Herman, 1992; Schauer & Elbert, 2010). However, the most widely used dissociation measure, *The Dissociative Experiences Scale II*, does not distinguish among these types of dissociation and, as a result, does not account for the divergent meanings of certain questions. For example, the statement "Some people have the experience of looking into a mirror and not recognizing themselves" can have different meanings for people with trauma-related dissociation and people who are in various stages of physical, social, or legal transitioning. In the latter case, a positive answer may not mean that they suffer from dissociation or that their dissociation could impact trauma processing, but instead refers to the way their gender identity does not correspond to how they look right now. Note that not all TGD individuals experience gender dysphoria, and that since 2019 the World Health Organization no longer considers gender dysphoria a mental health disorder.

Therefore, talk to your client about dissociation in relation to their gender dysphoria, identity, or fluidity. If you assess for dissociation, and they give higher scores to questions on the scale, ask them more about the context of their answers. Assess to see if gender dysphoria or gender fluidity plays a part in their answers or not.

If your client does dissociate to manage gender dysphoria, you will still want strategies and coping skills to help them manage the dissociation. Some of these can be helpful if your client has, for example, just returned from an unsafe situation, or has not been able to be "out" all day until they settle into your office or with you via telehealth. Orienting them to a safer, present moment can then be helpful. However, many times if someone is feeling a higher level of bodily discomfort due to gender dysphoria, orienting to the current distressing moment is not helpful.

I suggest talking to clients about how you both can work to decrease this kind of dissociation in sessions. It is important to note that this dissociation may be highly adaptive for your client's situations or environments, so your goal is not to necessarily eliminate the dissociation completely, but to support your clients in having more control over it. Some examples of what problem-solving this dissociation with clients can look like include:

- A transgender man wears a restrictive binder to smooth out the appearance of his chest. By the time we have our session at the end of the day, the binder is causing physical pain that reminds him about his discomfort with his body. This is hard to ignore and the client finds himself dissociating to cope with this. As a result, we change his appointment time to first thing in the morning when he is more physically comfortable.
- A transgender woman works alone at home as a software engineer. Her family of origin is not accepting of her gender identity. Her being "out" to me does not alleviate the stress caused by the lack of experiences of feeling seen as a woman in general. This stress causes her to dissociate. As we explore this together, she recognizes that she feels the best about herself at

the gym where she can see herself in the mirror running on the treadmill with her ponytail swinging behind her. As a result, she plans workouts before our therapy, and if she feels gender dysphoria coming on, she strokes her long ponytail to reorient to the positive feelings from her gym session.

- A nonbinary client tells me that their gender dysphoria is heightened each month during their menstruation cycle. As a result, we track their cycle and use this information to understand their emotional reactions in and outside the session those weeks.

RESOURCING, IMAGERY, AND PARTS CONSIDERATIONS

Although guiding clients to imagine themselves as a child can be therapeutically powerful and an integral part of many interventions and related therapies, you must talk to your TGD client before engaging in these activities (Chang et al., 2018). For some people, seeing themselves as a younger person presenting in a gender that they do not identify with is extremely painful. For other people, it may be clinically appropriate to invite them to imagine themselves as a child, presenting as their true gender identity even if they were not able to embody this at that time. Still other clients may not imagine their child-self looking different, but may want you to use either their current name and pronouns, or to use their name and pronouns assigned at birth. Discuss all of these possibilities with your client when beginning these types of parts work interventions. Of note, should TGD clients decide to use different names and pronouns for a younger self, this does not imply "alters" or "multiple personalities."

Relatedly, be thoughtful about the genders of your client's resources that you may use in imagery exercises. Suggest specific figures that might bring the comfort of recognizing and accepting their gender, or may even mirror their identity. When choosing resource figures culled from their life experiences, make sure those figures are not contaminated by any anti-trans bias from other interactions.

I wholeheartedly encourage you to check out one of the best resourcing interventions developed by a nonbinary therapist for TGD clients. It is called the "Future Empowered Self" and can be found in the Sand C. Chang chapter referenced at the start of this section.

SOMATIC INTERVENTION CONSIDERATIONS

Now that you have read about gender dysphoria and how it relates to discomfort with one's body, carry this information over to your consideration whenever you bring attention to bodily sensations or use the body for grounding or regulation skills. First, talk with your client ahead of time about the practice and the utility of bringing attention to their body (Chang, 2017). During this conversation, you might explore ways to make this attention more comfortable. However, accept that some TGD people may have days when this kind of attention is not an option; for others, it may never be an option (Chang, 2017).

Next, get consent for somatic work each and every session you might engage in body-based work (Chang, 2017). You may get consent from a client to focus on their body one day, but dysphoria may be higher the next day for a variety of reasons, so always check in with your clients.

Another issue with somatic work is that there may continue to be physical discomfort for your TGD client that is not related to their emotional experiences. This discomfort may remain because it is a result of a recent gender-affirming medical procedure or a garment used to contour certain physical characteristics. It is therefore important not to assume that certain bodily tension is related to the therapy work you are engaging in during sessions.

Finally, TGD folks tend to be physically scrutinized in many situations (Chang et al., 2018). Others may attempt to figure out an individual's gender according to how their body looks, or they may be overly curious when they notice physical changes. Either way, this translates into the importance of checking in with your TGD clients and being sensitive to what body-based attention is best for them in a psychotherapy context.

SEXUAL HEALTH CONSIDERATIONS WITH TRANSGENDER AND GENDER-DIVERSE CLIENTS

When discussing sexual health with your TGD clients, please ask about the kind of language they use. Like your cisgender clients, your TGD clients may use a range of words to describe their body parts and what pleasure or pain they experience in their bodies. However, words that you may be comfortable using with your cisgender clients could be invalidating, misgendering, and, at worst, triggering for your TGD clients. You will want to let your client be in control of the language used in session, as you would with all of your clients. Since you are in a position of power as a clinician, it is important to use this power to show sensitivity and anticipate challenging conversations. Do this by inquiring about language right away by using simple questions such as:

"Are there words that you would like me to use or not use when referring to your body or talking about sex?"

At the same time, as previously mentioned, many TGD individuals have the experience of having their body scrutinized by others due to curiosity, so only explore their sexual health after they have consented to talk about this with you.

There are some particular considerations to keep in mind about your TGD clients' sexual health if they are in the process of physically transitioning. While someone can anticipate some common changes when starting hormone replacement therapy (HRT) or after some gender-affirming surgeries, every person is unique, so it is necessary to check in with your individual client without relying also on them to educate you on the basics of these experiences. To this end, it will be essential to refer to the latest research on how primary and secondary sex characteristics can change when someone is new to HRT, especially since some of your clients may be surprised about these changes, too, as all medical providers do not always provide detailed information about what to expect.

Issues related to gender dysphoria, in addition to hormones or surgeries, can potentially affect your client's interest in sex, and even who they are attracted to sexually. You may find your clients talking about "a second puberty," a desire to experiment and explore different gender roles in the context of sex, or a curiosity about other sexual orientations and those orientations' cultures around sex. The latter two may also emerge if your client is newly single or exploring polyamory after transitioning. In any situation, do not jump to gendered or binary conclusions about any of these changes. As we all know, change is often anxiety producing, so encourage your client to allow themselves the freedom to play and experiment!

SUMMARY

Gender impacts all people, regardless of their gender identity. Gender can be a source of pleasure or terror, with a wide range of experiences in between. Considering the effects of gender on every client, and talking with any of them about gender when appropriate, can encourage and deepen any therapy intervention. I encourage you to seek out consultation and explore how gender may be operating in regard to transference and countertransference, whether or not you share gender identities with your client. If gender is affecting how you and your client connect, perhaps seek supervision with a consultant of a gender different from your own, or one that aligns with the client you want to discuss. Gender is different for each person, so all issues and concepts will not apply to each person who identifies with a particular gender. This chapter is far from exhaustive in its exploration of gender and therapy; my hope is that you continue to not only expand your knowledge and comfort on this therapeutic topic, but also to expand the rules of gender expression of liberation for all.

DISCUSSION QUESTIONS

- How have gender role expectations been communicated to you, and how have you felt about those messages?
- When you think of the words *man*, *male*, or *boy*, what stereotypes come to mind?

- When you think of the words *woman*, *female*, or *girl*, what stereotypes come to mind?
- When you think of a TGD person, what stereotypes come to mind?
- How have you personally experienced or witnessed how the stereotypical female/male gender binary has limited you in your full experience of being human, or limited someone close to you?
- What are some strategies you can adopt today to increase gender-affirming inclusiveness in your work with all genders?

LEARNING ACTIVITIES

CourseConnect

To access self-assessment questions and interactive, competency-based learning activities for this chapter, visit www.springerpub.com/courseconnect. See inside front cover and tear-out card for CourseConnect details.

ADDITIONAL RESOURCES

Additional resources are online and available at www.springerpub.com/courseconnect.

REFERENCES

American Psychiatric Association. (2013). *Diagnostic and statistical manual of mental disorders* (5th ed.). https://doi.org/10.1176/appi.books.9780890425596

Ashley, W. (2014). The angry Black woman: The impact of pejorative stereotypes on psychotherapy with Black women. *Social Work in Public Health, 29*(1), 27–34. https://doi.org/10.1080/19371918.2011.619449

Atteberry-Ash, B., Kattari, S. K., Harner, V., Prince, D. M., Verdino, A. P., Kattari, L., & Park, I. Y. (2021). Differential experiences of mental health among transgender and gender-diverse youth in Colorado. *Behavioral Sciences, 11*(4), 48. https://doi.org/10.3390/bs11040048

Bodnar, I. (2018). Aristotle's natural philosophy. In E. N. Zalta (Ed.), *The Stanford encyclopedia of philosophy* (Spring ed.). https://plato.stanford.edu/archives/spr2018/entries/aristotle-natphil

Briere, J., & Elliot, D. M. (2003). Prevalence and psychological sequels of self-reported childhood physical and sexual abuse in a general population sample of men and women. *Child Abuse & Neglect, 27*, 1205–1222. https://doi.org/10.1016/j.chiabu.2003.09.008

Burstein, H. J., Lacchetti, C., Anderson, H., Buchholz, T. A., Davidson, N. E., Gelmon, K. A., Giordano, S. H., Hudis, C. A., Solky, A. J., Stearns, V., Winer, E. P., & Griggs, J. J. (2019). Adjuvant endocrine therapy for women with hormone receptor-positive breast cancer: ASCO clinical practice guideline focused update. *Journal of Clinical Oncology, 37*(5), 423–438. https://doi.org/10.1200/JCO.18.01160

Butler, J. (1993). *Bodies that matter: On the discursive limits of "sex."* Routledge Classics.

Campbell, L. F., & Arkles, G. (2016). Ethical and legal concerns for mental health professionals. In A. A. Singh & L. M. Dickey (Eds.), *Affirmative counseling and psychological practice with transgender and gender nonconforming clients* (pp. 95–118). American Psychological Association.

Centers for Disease Control and Prevention. (2024a, November 19). *Attention-deficit / hyperactivity disorder (ADHD): Data and statistics on ADHD.* https://www.cdc.gov/adhd/data/index.html

Centers for Disease Control and Prevention. (2024b, May 16). *Intimate partner violence prevention: About intimate partner violence.* https://www.cdc.gov/intimate-partner-violence/about/index.html

Centers for Disease Control and Prevention. (2024c, May 16). *Intimate partner violence, sexual violence, and stalking among men.* https://www.cdc.gov/intimate-partner-violence/about/intimate-partner-violence-sexual-violence-and-stalking-among-men.html

Chang, S. C. (2017). EMDR therapy as affirmative care for transgender and gender nonconforming clients. In M. Nickerson (Ed.), *Cultural competence and healing culturally based trauma with EMDR therapy* (pp. 177–194). Springer Publishing Company.

Chang, S. C., Singh, A. A., & Dickey, L M. (2018). *A clinician's guide to gender-affirming care.* Context Press.

Chaplin, T. M. (2015). Gender and emotion expression: A developmental contextual perspective. *Emotion Review: Journal of the International Society for Research on Emotion, 7*(1), 14–21. https://doi.org/10.1177/1754073914544408

Clements-Nolle, K., Marx, R., & Katz, M. (2006). Attempted suicide among transgender persons. *Journal of Homosexuality, 51*(3), 53–69. https://doi.org/10.1300/J082v51n03_04

Connell, N., & Wilson, C. (1974). *Rape: The first sourcebook for women*. New American Library.

Creighton, S. (2001). Surgery for intersex. *Journal of the Royal Society of Medicine, 94*(5), 218–220. https://doi.org/10.1177/014107680109400505

DiMauro, J., & Renshaw, K. D. (2021). Trauma-related disclosure in sexual assault survivors' intimate relationships: Associations with PTSD, shame, and partners' responses. *Journal of Interpersonal Violence, 36*(3–4), NP1986–2004NP. https://doi.org/10.1177/0886260518756117

Edelman, E. A. (2011). "This area has been declared a prostitution free zone:" Discursive formations of space, the state, and trans sex worker bodies. *Journal of Homosexuality, 58*(6–7), 848–864. https://doi.org/10.1080/00918369.2011.581928

Fitzgibbons, R., & O'Leary, D. (2011). Sexual abuse of minors by Catholic clergy. *The Linacre Quarterly, 78*(3), 252–273. https://doi.org/10.1179/002436311803888276

Garnett, M. F., Spencer, M. R., & Weeks, J. D. (2023, November). *Suicide among adults age 55 and older, 2021* [NCHS Data Brief No. 483]. U.S. Department of Health & Human Services, National Center for Health Statistics, Centers for Disease Control and Prevention. https://www.cdc.gov/nchs/data/databriefs/db483.pdf

GLAAD. (2022, February 21). *GLAAD media reference guide* (11th ed.). https://glaad.org/reference

Herman, J. (1992). *Trauma and recovery*. Basic Books.

Jahoda, M. (1977). *Freud and the dilemmas of psychology* (p. 28). Hogarth Press.

Kennedy, A. C., & Prock, K. A. (2018). "I still feel like I am not normal": A review of the role of stigma and stigmatization among female survivors of child sexual abuse, sexual assault, and intimate partner violence. *Trauma, Violence, & Abuse, 19*(5), 512–527. https://doi.org/10.1177/1524838016673601

Kennedy-Root, A., & Denham, S. A. (2010). The role of gender in the socialization of emotion: Key concepts and critical issues. In A. Kennedy Root & S. Denham (Eds.), *New directions for child and adolescent development* (pp. 1–9, 128). Jossey-Bass.

Kenny, C., & Yang, G. (2021). *The global childcare workload from school and preschool closures during the COVID-19 pandemic*. The Center for Global Development. https://www.cgdev.org/sites/default/files/global-childcare-workload-from-school-closures-covid.pdf

Kimerling, R., Weitlauf, J. C., Iverson, K. M., Karpenko, J. A., & Jain, S. (2014). Gender issues in PTSD. In M. J. Friedman, T. M. Keane, & P. A. Resick (Eds.), *Handbook of PTSD: Science and practice* (2nd ed., pp. 313–330). The Guilford Press.

Masson, J. (1984). *The assault on truth*. Farrar, Staus & Giroux.

Nadal, K. L., Rivera, D. P., & Corpus, M. J. H. (2010). Sexual orientation and transgender microaggressions in everyday life: Experiences of lesbians, gays, bisexuals, and transgender individuals. In D. W. Sue (Ed.), *Microagressions and marginality: Manifestation, dynamics, and impact* (pp. 217–240). Wiley.

Nagata, J. M., Ganson, K. T., & Austin, S. B. (2020). Emerging trends in eating disorders among sexual and gender minorities. *Current Opinion in Psychiatry, 33*(6), 562–567. https://doi.org/10.1097/YCO.0000000000000645

National Institute of Mental Health. (2024, September). *Mental illness*. https://www.nimh.nih.gov/health/statistics/mental-illness

Ristock, J., Zoccole, A., & Passante, L. (2010). *Aboriginal Two-Spirit and LGBTQ migration, mobility, and health research project*. https://www.rainbowhealthontario.ca/resource-library/aboriginal-two-spirit-and-lgbtq-migration-mobility-and-health-research-project

Sagar-Ouriaghli, I., Godfrey, E., Bridge, L., Meade, L., & Brown, J. (2019). Improving mental health service utilization among men: A systematic review and synthesis of behavior change techniques within interventions targeting help-seeking. *American Journal of Men's Health, 13*(3), 1557988319857009. https://doi.org/10.1177/1557988319857009

Schauer, M., & Elbert, T. (2010). Dissociation following traumatic stress: Etiology and treatment. *Journal of Psychology, 218*(2), 109–127. https://doi.org/10.1027/0044-3409/a000018

Seidler, Z. E., Dawes, A. J., Rice, S. M., Oliffe, J. L., & Dhillon, H. M. (2016). The role of masculinity in men's help-seeking for depression: A systematic review. *Clinical Psychology Review, 49*, 106–118. https://doi.org/10.1016/j.cpr.2016.09.002

Senefeld, J. W., Lambelet, C. D., Johnson, P. W., Carter, R. E., Clayburn, A. J., & Joyner, M. J. (2020). Divergence in timing and magnitude of testosterone levels between male and female youths. *JAMA, 324*(1), 99–101. https://doi.org/10.1001/jama.2020.5655

Sharer, B., & Lukens, G. (2024, May 9). *Health coverage rates vary widely across—and within—racial and ethnic groups.* Center on Budget and Policy Priorities. https://www.cbpp.org/research/health/health-coverage-rates-vary-widely-across-and-within-racial-and-ethnic-groups

Shiner, B., Westgate, C. L., Harik, J. M., Watts, B. V., & Schnurr, P. P. (2017). Effect of patient-therapist gender match on psychotherapy retention among United States veterans with posttraumatic stress disorder. *Administration and Policy in Mental Health, 44*(5), 642–650. https://doi.org/10.1007/s10488-016-0761-2

Shlasko, D. & Hofius, K. (2017). *Trans allyship workbook: Building skills to support trans people in our lives.* Think Again Training.

Simmons, S., & Suárez, L. (2016). Substance abuse and trauma. *Child and Adolescent Psychiatric Clinics of North America, 25*(4), 723–734. https://doi.org/10.1016/j.chc.2016.05.006

Sullivan, C. L., & Brown, J. S. (2015). Masculinity, alexithymia, and fear of intimacy as predictors of UK men's attitudes towards seeking professional psychological help. *British Journal of Health Psychology, 20*(1), 194–211. https://doi.org/10.1111/bjhp.12089

Tolin, D. F., & Foa, E. B. (2006). Sex differences in trauma and posttraumatic stress disorder: A quantitative review of 25 years of research. *Psychological Bulletin, 132*(6), 959–992. https://doi.org/10.1037/0033-2909.132.6.959

University of California at Los Angeles Health. (2023, October 12). *Understanding undiagnosed autism in adult females.* https://www.uclahealth.org/news/article/understanding-undiagnosed-autism-adult-females

Villarroel, M. A., & Terlizzi, E. P. (2020, September). *Symptoms of depression among adults, United States, 2019* [NCHS Data Brief No. 379]. National Center for Health Statistics. https://www.cdc.gov/nchs/products/databriefs/db379.htm?utm_medium=email&utm_source=transaction

Wingfield, A. H. (2020). *Women are advancing in the workplace but women of color still lag behind.* Brookings Institute.

World Professional Association for Transgender Health. (2022). *Standards of care for the health of transsexual, transgender, and gender nonconforming people* (7th ed.). Author. https://www.wpath.org/publications/soc

CHAPTER 6

Sexual/Affectional Orientation and Relationship Status

Stephanie Baird

LEARNING OBJECTIVES

- Learn the definitions of heterosexual and LGBTQ+ sexual and affectional/romantic orientations and scales (including asexual and demisexual). A therapy case study example illustrates intersections of identity and sexual health concerns.
- Learn about heteronormative and romonormative societal pressure.
- Learn about the history of queer theory and its impact on identity.
- Learn about different relationship statuses (singlehood, monogamy, divorce, and consensual nonmonogamy/polyamory).
- Learn how affairs can impact relationships. A therapy case example demonstrates how eye movement desensitization and reprocessing (EMDR) therapy can treat the impact of affairs on sexual health.

SEXUAL AND AFFECTIONAL/ROMANTIC ORIENTATION

INTRODUCTION AND DEFINITIONS

Definitions and descriptions of *sexual* and *affectional/romantic orientation* continue to evolve as we blaze onward into the 21st century. Sexual orientation refers to how someone generally orients their predominant sexual attraction to other genders, in relation to their own gender.

However, sexual orientation is often about much more than sexual behavior. A former client once pointed out that when he came out as gay in his teens, he was mortified that people might imagine him engaging in sexual activity, upon hearing the label "gay." This particularly bothered him as he had no sexual experience yet, nor were his own sexual thoughts and fantasies developed. I am repeating this here as a reminder to understand that a person is much more than their sexual orientation or gender. As Walt Whitman (n.d.) famously wrote in his epic poem *Song of Myself*, "I contain multitudes."

As people, particularly the younger Generation Z and Generation Alpha, expand gender constructs and experiences, ideas of attraction are also expanding. We now know that orientation can include *both* sexual and affectional or romantic attractions. Affectional and romantic orientations relate more to the emotion-based closeness, attraction, and/or romantic, but nonsexual, interest experienced toward other. Romantic affection demonstrations might include physical gestures such as holding hands, cuddling, and/or kissing.

For example, someone might describe themselves as heterosexual and heteroromantic. Or they may describe themselves as bisexual (sexual attraction to more than one gender) *and* homoromantic (romantic/affectional attraction toward the same gender). Sexual and affectional orientation, like gender (gender is addressed in depth in Chapter 9), can remain consistent or change over one's lifetime. It is helpful to have welcoming language in your office or on your intake forms, allowing your clients to indicate pronouns, labels, and categories, if they wish.

Heterosexual/Heteronormativity/Heterosexism

Heterosexuality is generally defined as someone being attracted to someone from a different gender from their own. A more colloquial term is *straight*, and heterosexual stereotypes conjure images of masculine cismen holding hands with feminine ciswomen. Some people may use the term *heteroflexible* to describe an orientation of mostly attracted to a different gender from their own, but open to same or similar gender attraction. In mainstream media and in sociological and cultural research and critique, *heteronormativity* contributes to the privileging, centering, and emphasizing of representations portraying a cisman and ciswoman as the ideal sexual/romantic couple, most notable often centered in Disney and Hallmark channel films and series. Heterosexism takes this concept further and refers to discrimination or prejudice against nonheterosexual individuals or couples.

LGBTQIA2+

LGBTQIA2+ is a comprehensive anacronym that stands for **L**esbian, **G**ay, **B**isexual, **T**ransgender/nonconforming, **Q**ueer and/or **Q**uestioning, **I**ntersex, **A**sexual and/or **A**lly, **T**wo-Spirit, and other identities. These are defined further in the text that follows. Prior percentages of nonheterosexual identities have been estimated as 10% of the population. In a 2023 Gallup poll, ***one in five*** Gen Z adults (born between 1997 and 2012) identify as LGBTQ+ , with the majority of those nonheterosexuals identifying as bisexual (Jones, 2024). Pew Research Center (Brown, 2023) research found that 7% of surveyed U.S. adults identified as lesbian, gay, bisexual, or transgender in 2022.

Lesbian

Lesbian generally refers to ciswomen who are attracted to other ciswomen; additionally, some transwomen also identify as lesbian. Historically, particularly in the feminist movements of the 1970s through the 1990s, some lesbians might define themselves as *butch* (identifying with stereotypically masculine physical and/or personality characteristics), *femme* (identifying with stereotypically feminine physical and/or personality characteristics, or within a more "androgynous" [comprising both/and, or neither, masculine and feminine characteristics]) spectrum. Since the gender expansion explosion within the last decade, younger lesbians may not utilize these descriptors as much. They may instead discuss their identities in terms of *masculine of center* or *feminine of center.*

Gay/Men Who Have Sex With Men/Same Gender Loving Categories

Gay generally refers to male-identified individuals who are attracted to other male-identified individuals, although the term can more broadly refer to any individual attracted to a similar/same gender. Researchers since the 1990s have also identified a group called *men who have sex with men, males who have sex with males,* or *MSM.* These are (usually) cismen or cismale-identified who may answer "heterosexual" (among other identities) on questionnaires *and* engage in sexual activity with other male-identified individuals.

Similarly, for females, sometimes the term *women who have sex with women* (WSW) is used in gathering data. These terms were developed to solely capture the behavioral aspect of this group, originally for disease risk–based research.

Cleo Manago coined the term *same gender loving* in the early 1990s; it is often used in communities of color as a nonEurocentric–based term (compared to the White Eurocentric *gay* and *homosexual* terms). Some of our clients may choose this language to describe themselves.

Bisexual/Pansexual/Polysexual/Omnisexual

Bisexuality refers to people who recognize sexual attraction to more than one gender. Many bisexual folx understand there are more than two genders, and include those expanded possibilities in their personal definition. Folx may call themselves *pansexual/panromantic* ("gender-blind" attraction to others), *omnisexual* (sexual or romantic attraction toward all possible genders, with some possible gender preferences), or *polysexual/polyromatic* (attraction toward multiple genders).

Bisexuality (admittedly a binary term) has frequently been misunderstood as a "transition" or "fence-sitting" phase. However, many bisexual-identified folx claim this label as a lifelong identity. Bisexual activists continue to fight against biphobia, and often point out that for them, they prioritize getting to know a person, not what is "between their legs."

Boston-based Robyn Ochs is a bisexual activist who publishes and speaks widely. Ochs posted on Instagram, "If you are LGBTQ+, existing proudly and unapologetically in public is a form of activism. Surviving and thriving is a form of activism" (Ochs, 2021). She and other activists have also pointed out over the years that a bi/pan/omni identity does not mean one is attracted to everyone, just like a heterosexual ciswoman attracted to cismen gets to be picky about her "type" and is not attracted to *every* cisman. Nor does a bi/pan/omni identity always guarantee a Saturday night date.

Sexual Orientation Scales: Kinsey, Klein, Storms, Gender Unicorn

Kinsey and early sex researchers in the 1940s were the first to develop a sexual orientation scale called *The Kinsey Scale* (0 = *completely heterosexual attraction/behavior*, 6 = *completely homosexual attraction/behavior*). They discovered in their research of thousands of anonymous Americans that noticeable percentages of Americans reported gay (up to 37% of males) or lesbian experiences (based on questions about attractions, fantasies, and actual experiences), technically placing a surprisingly large group in the "bisexual" category at that time (Kinsey et al., 1948, 1953). However, how people choose to actually identify may be very different from their behavior.

Expanding on The Kinsey Scale to understand bisexuality and human nuance more accurately, other scales were later developed. *The Klein Sexual Orientation Grid*, developed in 1978 (F. Klein, 1993), asks about degree of sexual attraction, behaviors, fantasies, and emotional/social preference toward same and other genders, along with their own self-identification. The respondent uses a one to seven scale (from "another sex only" to "same sex only") to answer these questions about past, present, and ideal internal and external experiences.

Michael Storms's *Storms Sexuality Axis* (1980) plots eroticism on an *x/y* axis, respectively, and allows for the presence of asexuality and demisexuality (versus the prior scales). The *Erotic Attraction* dimension measures the degree of sexual attraction an individual experiences toward people of the same/similar sex and people of different sexes/genders. It acknowledges that individuals may experience varying levels of attraction toward both sexes simultaneously or at different times in their lives. *The Social Preference* dimension assesses an individual's preference for social interactions and emotional relationships with people of the same/similar or different sexes.

The *Gender Unicorn*, initially developed for youth, is a wonderful tool for looking at continuums of identity and attraction, which is helpful for all individuals (see **Figure 6.1**).

Available online are other visual representations called the Gender Galaxy and the Sexuality Galaxy, depicting many different sexual and romantic orientations and gender identities.

Asexual/Graysexual

Clients may also apply these descriptive terms to themselves or their partners: *asexual* (ACE; no experience of sexual attraction toward anyone, and may enjoy sexual experiences on their own) or *graysexual* (rarely experience attraction toward anyone). Yes, many factors can impact sexual interest (e.g., trauma history, relationship issues, mental health issues, communication, hormones, medications, medical conditions, parenting or work fatigue, negative sexual environment or lack thereof, and/or "sexual brakes" being fully pressed), AND a growing number of individuals, regardless of any of those factors, assert this term. An ACE or graysexual identity is legitimate and real, and often still stigmatized in a culture that prizes sexual activity as part of a romantic relationship.

Asexual clients may perceive clinicians' questioning about lack of sexual interest as pathologizing. If clients (whether ACE or not) express concern about a low or decreased sexual interest, then we need to ask for their full permission and consent to inquire about the possible aforementioned mitigating factors. We can also share information about asexuality or graysexuality, particularly if those are new terms to them. I have had asexual clients over the years state "asexual" at intake and

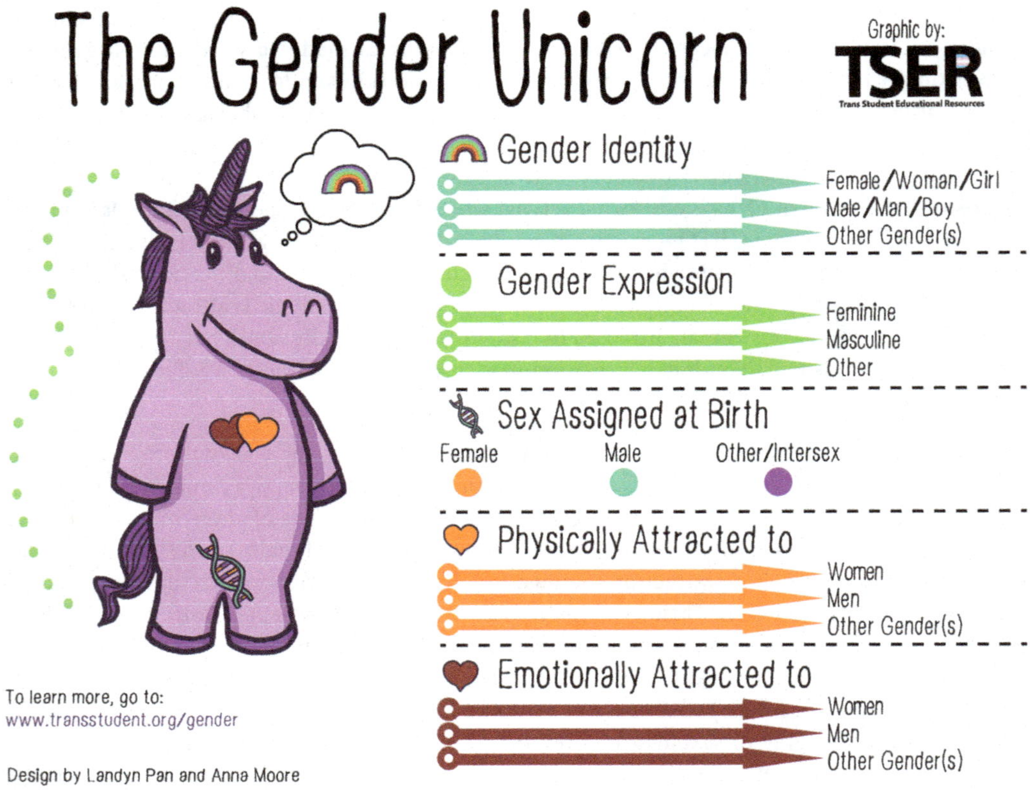

FIGURE 6.1. The Gender Unicorn

Source: Courtesy of Trans Student Educational Resources. (n.d.). *The gender unicorn*. https://transstudent.org/gender. Used under CC BY 4.0 (https://creativecommons.org/licenses/by/4.0).

remain asexual long after our trauma work was completed. By helping our clients discern whether they truly are experiencing a reduced sexual interest, or perhaps identify more with asexual or graysexual, we normalize and validate asexual and graysexual orientations.

Aromantic/Greyromantic

Someone identifying as *aromantic* (or "aro") experiences no romantic attraction to others, and has little or no desire to form a romantic relationship with anyone. An aro person may, however, have a sexual orientation where they experience sexual attraction and interest in other people. *Greyromantic* describes someone who identifies as rarely experiencing romantic feelings or interest toward others.

Demisexual

Another orientation clinicians might encounter more frequently is *demisexual* and/or *demi-romantic*. Demisexuals/-romantics experience sexual or romantic attraction AFTER they have developed a strong emotional connection with another person. Clients may not yet know this term, so it can be helpful to introduce it and normalize their experiences, which may be the opposite of what many mainstream movies and television shows portray (i.e., intense erotic attraction at first sight).

One of my colleagues, who identifies as demisexual, mentioned that she, as well as many of her demisexual friends, have all received comments from therapists that their demisexual orientation must be "due to unhealed sexual trauma or religious hangups." She reported that one of her good friends was "scared off of EMDR [eye movement desensitization and reprocessing] *this week*" (italics added for emphasis; personal communication, May 24, 2021) because her therapist made such a comment. As my colleague further explained her demisexuality, "I am not letting just anyone up in my energy and my emotions, and that feels like the most organic and honest thing I can do for myself. Sometimes I get jealous of my friends who can just 'hook up,' but alas, that is not me." Again, just like with a potentially asexual client, we must perform due diligence in following our clients' lead, asking their permission for any clarification as they disclose their experiences and identities, and not interject our own theories and assumptions.

Abrosexual

Abrosexual is a term to describe someone who notes changing sexual fluidity. For instance, they might identify with the term *lesbian*, and later feel attracted to people of all genders, and then a few days later feel little to no sexual attraction at all. Abrosexual people can experience fluctuations in terms of *the intensity of* their attraction. Identifying as abrosexual means someone is embracing the fact that their actual experiences and orientation change over time. The prefix "abro-" means "delicate" or "graceful."

Queer

Some people, especially Millennials and younger (in my clinical experience), reclaim and use the term *queer* to describe themselves, an umbrella term that can include living, loving, or identifying outside of binary expectations, in specific or multiple ways. A person will let you know if they use this term for themselves, so do not use this word unless they give you permission. Ideally they will feel comfortable to explain what "queer" means to them.

QUEER THEORY ***by Eve Ng, PhD*** *(Communication), PhD (Linguistics), Associate Professor and Associate Director of Graduate Studies, School of Media Arts and Studies Core Faculty, Women's, Gender, and Sexuality Studies Program, Ohio University, Athens, OH*

Introduction

Queer theory is sometimes distinguished from an earlier mode of "gay and lesbian studies," which had sought to catalog the diversity of human sexual experience across different cultural and historical contexts. Instead, although popular use of "queer" now encompasses a range of nonnormative sexual desires, practices, and identities, one of the most significant contributions of queer theorists has been fundamentally challenging assumptions about the categories of "sex", "gender", and "sexuality" themselves. Furthermore, queer theory interrogates knowledge production and theory-building more generally, where "queering" refers to processes of destabilizing assumed categories and conceptual foundations, including beyond the domains of sex/gender/sexuality. Finally, in critiquing heteronormativity and associated power structures, some queer theorists challenge common assumptions about what people should aspire to (such as "life, liberty, and the pursuit of happiness").

Rethinking "Sex", "Gender", and "Sexuality"

In many normative systems of sexuality in modern Western societies, not only are particular kinds of sexual orientation and sexual practices privileged (e.g., heterosexual, monogamous), but the system assumes multiple forms of fixedness and rigidity. Notably, an individual's biological sex is supposed to be determined at birth and unchanged through life, and their sexual orientation is assumed to be similarly fixed. The system is also structured by binary oppositions, for sex (male/female), gender identity (man/woman), and sexual orientation (heterosexual/homosexual). Feminist scholars have critiqued the system—which queer theorist Judith Butler termed the "heterosexual matrix"—for its failures to reflect actual lived experiences, for assuming that change is not possible, and for the ways that the privileged term in each binary dominates the subordinated terms.

At one level, individuals who most clearly fail to fit the heterosexual matrix expose its descriptive flaws. For example, as Fausto-Sterling (2000) discussed, intersex infants occur naturally, and yet modern Western medical practice has deemed them "abnormal" and in need of surgical interventions to make their bodies conform to the binary oppositions of the heterosexual matrix. Transgender and nonbinary people assert various gender identities different from what they were assigned at birth; moreover, the stigma, discrimination, and violence that trans/nonbinary individuals may experience also underscore the power relations of the matrix. Queer theorists such as Gayle Rubin have traced the history of "sexual minorities" and advocated for their academic and political recognition, to be viewed not as pathologic, deviant, or criminal, but as members of a human sexual diversity that includes different kinds of intimate relationships.

However, for scholars such as Butler, the more fundamental critique is that sex, gender, and sexuality are not identities (even a larger set of changeable identities) that individuals *are*, but rather, they are the result of a cumulative set of practices that individuals *do*. This is what Butler (1990) calls the "performative" and "iterative" character of sex/gender (and, by extension, sexuality); thus, "gender performativity" means that gender identity is the result of a series of repeated acts that many individuals in a society perform over and over again, such that there emerge generally recognized identities of "girl"/"woman" and "boy"/"man."

This goes beyond second-wave feminist critiques that gender identities are "socially constructed," which pointed out the problematic aspects of assuming that girls/women would or should be conventionally feminine and boys/men conventionally masculine, but left unexamined the assumption that the category of "gender" was a property of individuals. Rather, Butler's hugely influential retheorization of *gender as performative* argues that gendered (and sexual) practices are what produce individuals with gendered, sexed identities, rather than the other way around (i.e., rather than individuals expressing their gendered, sexed identities through their practices). This thesis is succinctly summarized as "there need not be a 'doer behind the deed,' but [rather] that the 'doer' is variably constructed in and through the deed" (Butler, 1990, p. 181).

Broader Challenges to Knowledge Production and Normativity

Butler's theory of performativity is linked to other critical reexaminations of commonly assumed building blocks for scholarly inquiry. Prior to queer theoretical approaches, there had already been challenges to the Enlightenment modes of "objective" scientific inquiry. This includes feminist standpoint theory, which argues that the sociopolitical location of human subjects, including scholars, crucially influences their perspectives, and the lived experiences of traditionally marginalized people is particularly important to reclaim.

However, the queering of knowledge production moves even further away from earlier epistemological approaches. For example, the phenomenon of an individual's "experience," besides having political importance, also serves as important data undergirding various social sciences, including psychology. Traditionally, historians have assumed that individuals exist *prior* to their experiences, and then are the subjects who have experiences. Instead, historian Joan Scott proposes that we must examine the larger contexts through which subject formation is possible at all, and consider how any person's experience is mediated through ideology and norms shaped by existing power structures. Otherwise, scholars risk "naturaliz[ing] categories such as man, woman, black, white, heterosexual, and homosexual" (Scott, 1991, p. 782).

Another important strand in queer theory's challenges to normative assumptions involves reconsidering and even embracing the "abject." If (hetero)normativity is about aiming to be a happy, productive (in both the economic and reproductive senses), and forward-looking member of society, then queer scholars have reevaluated the denigration or stigma associated with discomfort, sickness, death, and the lack of a future-oriented vision. In queer affect theory, Sara Ahmed has discussed particular forms of queer discomfort—such as feeling ill at ease when surrounded by straight people—as a kind of "not fitting" that is not necessarily negative or something to be avoided, but as a way of "*inhabiting norms differently*" (Ahmed, 2004, p. 155, emphasis in original).

Social theory has also given rise to the "temporal turn," with attention to the political implications of how time is conceptualized. At one level, queer scholars have underscored that the cycles of life/birth/death do not work the same for queer people as they do for those who conform to heteronormative trajectories. Additionally, a queer temporality approach extends to critiquing capitalism and its ideologies of success, which are entwined with heteronormative life cycles: education, graduation, work, promotion, capital accumulation to buy a house, starting a family, and so on. Perhaps most provocative are positions elaborated by scholars such as Lee Edelman, who celebrated the ways that queer people interrupt the replication of human generations and explicitly reject futures centered on the figure of the child, and Gregory Tomso, who reframed men who had unprotected sex with each other during the AIDS epidemic as epitomizing a queer "biopolitical resistance" to "coercive regimes of power" (Tomso, 2008, p. 276) associated with neoliberal capitalism, which seek to compel individuals to maintain maximum physical health and productivity.

Collectively, then, queer theory provides multiple avenues to rethink key categories pertaining to sexual identity and sexual practice, how social scientists pursue their research, and even what the goals of human life should or should not be.

HOMOPHOBIA AND DENOUNCING SEXUAL ORIENTATION CHANGE EFFORTS

It was only about 80 years ago that Kinsey brought homosexuality out in the open with his research, and only about 50 years ago (mid-1970s) that the *Diagnostic and Statistical Manual of Mental Disorders* (5th ed.; *DSM-5*; American Psychiatric Association, 2013) dropped homosexuality as a disorder. This was shortly after the 1969 Stonewall Riots which kicked off the modern LGBTQ movement, elucidated by interviews with participants in Jane Fleishman's 2020 book on the subject. Only 10 years ago, gay marriage in the United States was legalized (June 26, 2015). However, certain lawmakers continue to impede progress toward equality for all, and at present are particularly targeting transgender and gender-nonconforming individuals. Many individuals continue to harbor homophobic (fear and hatred of anything nonheterosexual) beliefs, attitudes, and violent behaviors. The second largest mass shooting by a single individual in U.S. history occurred in 2016 at a Florida gay nightclub, Pulse, killing 49 mostly Latinx individuals.

Sexual orientation change efforts (SOCE) involve any type of purported treatment or therapy intended to change someone's sexual orientation from lesbian, gay, bisexual/pansexual, etc. to heterosexual. Earlier terms for SOCE include "conversion" or "reparative" therapy.

The American Psychological Association issued a statement in 2009 condemning any kind of sexual orientation change efforts, noting the "longstanding consensus of the behavioral and social sciences and the health and mental health professions is that homosexuality per se is a normal and positive variation of human sexual orientation" (Anton, 2010, pp. 463–464).

The EMDR International Association (EMDRIA) also has a statement denouncing "conversion" or "reparative" therapy using EMDR therapy to "change" someone's orientation to heterosexual:

> EMDRIA™ recognizes the need and responsibility to address the use of EMDR therapy approaches in any SOCE that pathologizes sexual and gender minority (LGBTQIA+) persons and communities. EMDRIA™ does not believe that representations of sexual orientation and gender identity result from unresolved trauma. An individual's sexual orientation and gender identity are not matters of pathology. EMDRIA™ does not believe LGBTQIA+ individuals are in need of mental health treatment by virtue of their sexual orientation and gender identity. Therefore, the use of EMDR therapy in any SOCE program or other similar intervention is inappropriate and outside the norms and values of EMDRIA™. EMDRIA™ prohibits the use of EMDR therapy for this purpose by its Members, EMDR Certified Therapists™, EMDR Consultants™, Credit Providers, and EMDR Trainers™. (EMDRIA, n.d., Sexual Orientation Change Efforts)

Unfortunately, some conservative religious organizations have rebranded the word *conversion* in different and subtle ways, attempting to capture religious participants, particularly youth, who may be struggling with nonheterosexual desires and attractions. Research has shown SOCE to be particularly harmful to our vulnerable youth, leading to "depression, anxiety, drug use, homelessness, and suicide" (Human Rights Commission, n.d., para. 2).

As of April 2024, SOCE is outlawed in 26 states (all of New England), Washington D.C., and Puerto Rico, plus more than 100 municipalities. Many other national organizations have also publicly denounced SOCE, particularly citing the harm it has been shown to do to youth. These organizations include the American Psychiatric Association, American College of Physicians, American Academy of Pediatrics, American Counseling Association, Child Welfare League of America, and the National Education Association, among others.

We will certainly do harm if we attempt to use psychotherapeutic or clinical treatment (including EMDR therapy) to reduce or eliminate attractions and/or identities that have been eliminated from the *DSM*-5 (American Psychiatric Association, 2013) as a disorder since the mid-1970s (Marich, 2021), even if a client specifically requests therapy to eliminate LGBTQ thoughts and behaviors. Rather, we may find ourselves in the unique position to provide validation, affirmation, normalization, and psychoeducation of LGBTQIA+ identities (as well as basic information about systemic oppression) to our questioning clients. For some clients, this may be the first time they have ever broached the topic of nonheterosexual attractions with anyone. We do not want to mimic or exacerbate the external oppressions, frequent traumas, and *microaggressions* (discussed in more detail later in this chapter) that folx with these marginalized identities already encounter regularly, by complying with requests to "get rid of" this "problem." In fact, supportive psychotherapy (including EMDR therapy) can powerfully help *survivors* of SOCE programs (SOCE programs remain legal in nearly half of our states), potentially deprograming the negative and self-loathing self-image and increased shame perpetrated via SOCE.

Lastly, let us not forget that LGBTQIA+ individuals, especially those more visible in communities, tend to experience more direct violence, microaggressions, and negative targeting of their identities over their lifetime versus heterosexually identified folx.

John O'Brien (2017) has an informative and helpful chapter on "EMDR Therapy With Lesbian/Gay/Bisexual Clients" in Nickerson's book *Cultural Competence and Healing Culturally Based Trauma With EMDR Therapy*).

PREEMPTIVE RADICAL INCLUSION

CB Beal, sex educator, uses the term *preemptive radical inclusion* (PRI; Beal & Alves, 2018) to understand that whoever walks through our office door may have experienced erotic marginalization or engaged in erotically marginalized practices (nonheterosexual, nonmonogamy, kink, etc.). PRI also involves shifting away from penis-in-vagina sexual experiences, moving toward a shared language for sexual, intimate, and sensuous romantic practices, and is not orgasm focused. PRI means that "we ... position ourselves ... in the room, *to presuppose that everyone ... already, and always, [is] in the room* [and purposely] create experiences that preemptively involve them" (Beal, n.d., para. 10, emphasis in original). Rather than waiting for an individual to express their identity and need, we create experiences that *preemptively* involve them. Beal states that "PRI is a process, and justice and equity is the outcome" (Beal & Alves, 2018).

Case Study 6.1: Haley, Demisexual-Identified

Haley, an early thirties White ciswoman who worked as a middle school art teacher, sought EMDR therapy to work on posttraumatic stress disorder (PTSD) symptoms related to a sexual assault in high school. Haley had been able to ignore or shrug off these symptoms (specifically nightmares, avoidance, interfering thoughts, and exaggerated startle response) for many years. We surmised that the stability of her current relationship seemed to now provide a safe place for the symptoms to be recognized.

During the intake, Haley openly identified as demisexual and pansexual, and in a current monogamous relationship with a transwoman (male to female). Haley was very clear that she was happy with her demisexual identity, stating that over the years she learned that her sexual interest in a person begins *after* an emotional attraction develops. She related this about her current relationship, describing how sexual interest and attraction to her partner eventually grew from a slow courtship and increasing emotional connection. She noted greatly appreciating her partner's patience. However, now that PTSD symptoms were intruding in their sexual relationship, Haley was very motivated to address the past trauma so that she and her partner might resume formerly pleasurable and desired sexual activity. I also provided information about sexual brakes and accelerators during these initial sessions, and we conceptualized that the prior trauma was now fully pushing on her sexual brakes, eliminating any interest in sex.

Additionally, during medical history gathering, Haley disclosed she had recently sought medical help due to menstruation issues. An exam revealed that she possessed two uteruses. She reported feeling incredibly distressed by this information, and like a "freak." Lastly, Haley also noted growing up in Alabama in a fundamentalist Baptist household where any nonmarried sexually active and/or nonheterosexual identity was considered "blasphemous" and grounds for "going to hell." Although she no longer identified as Baptist, she noted some lingering internalized homophobia and erotophobia.

Sorting through her background, we determined there were many EMDR targets beyond the presenting high school sexual assault. Our EMDR target list included:

- Several preteen targets of noticing same-gender attraction, yet feeling incredibly shameful (we processed the shame).
- Occasions when she asked her pastor and parents roundabout and vague questions about sexual orientation, and being harshly rebuked and censored.
- The original reason for referral—the high school sexual assault (this occurred right after a football game where she was a cheerleader).
- Some early college dating experiences with cismen that involved nonconsensual actions perpetrated by them.
- Shame regarding these initial sexual experiences due to her nonconsent as well as the heavy "no sex" messaging in her family of origin and early religious environment.
- Two initial same-gender dating experiences in her mid-twenties where her partners moved faster sexually than she wanted.
- Shame around not being out as pansexual to her family of origin, and worry about eventually being outed.
- Haley's recent medical examinations where she learned of her particular anatomical configuration—both the doctor's insensitivity in relating and explaining the information, and her own medical concerns of potential fertility issues.

Thankfully, as mentioned before, Haley had a very supportive relationship, stable job, and positive community of friends and coworkers. We were able to proceed through the EMDR targets without much trouble, getting through the timeline over the course of a few months. Her negative cognitions (NCs) for the EMDR targets related to sexual identity and biological anatomy tended to be either "there is something wrong with me" or "I'm abnormal." For the sexual assaults, her NCs were "I'm not strong, I'm vulnerable, it's my fault."

Haley's positive cognitions (PCs) related to sexual identity targets and biological anatomy included "I'm worthy of being my authentic self," "I am normal," and "I'm fine as I am." PCs for her sexual assault experiences included "I'm strong/capable, I'm safe," and "It's not my fault." For emotions during EMDR therapy phase 3 assessment and phase 4 desensitization, she often reported shame followed by anger and grief. Physically, these emotions generally presented as tightness in her chest or throat. As the targets processed, she would report a loosening of the tightness, particularly as she found her voice during processing, often speaking aloud things she wished she had said during the various events. Once the targets were fully processed, Haley noted a return of interest in sexual activity with her partner, and an even fuller enjoyment of their sexual interactions than before.

We also completed several future templates, which included (a) making complaints to the doctor's office of the initial handling of her anatomical difference, (b) confidently coming out to her parents as pansexual and involved with a transgender person, (c) capably handling running into the more recent assailants that continue to live in the same region, and (d) expressing some new sexual fantasies to her partner.

RELATIONSHIP STATUS

Every client seeking therapy will have a relationship status, whether single, celibate, partnered, cohabitating, married, in a polyamorous relationship, divorced, widowed, and so on. It is helpful to have an understanding of these statuses and possible strengths and issues each can bring to therapy and sexual health.

SINGLEHOOD

We encounter clients who are single, whether by choice or circumstance. Some may be proud of their singlehood and may have chosen some form of abstinence or celibacy for particular reasons (i.e., religious/spiritual; healing from trauma; and/or increasing focus on academic, professional, creative, athletic, or other pursuits). Others may wish to be dating or in a relationship and may express some shame or feel they are single due to some sense of unworthiness or unattractiveness. It can be beneficial to spend some time unraveling their attitudes on relationships and singlehood, as there may (or may not) be clinical material related to negative beliefs they may hold.

INVOLUNTARY CELIBATES (INCELS)

Incels refer to a subset of individuals (mostly cisgendered males) who feel they are "involuntarily celibate" due to an inability to find a sexual or romantic (generally cisfemale) partner. Incels have been visible in online forums since the 1990s, and often communicate misogynist beliefs, blaming (cis)women for their lack of success in dating. Some perpetrators of mass shootings have claimed allegiance to incel ideologies. Researchers correlate issues such as online radicalization, isolation, untreated mental health problems, and changing gender dynamics and continued misogyny with the rise of incels. Efforts to address these issues often focus on promoting healthy relationships, addressing toxic masculinity, and combating online extremism.

CASUAL DATING/HOOK-UP CULTURE

Many "single" people may be sexually or romantically active to varying degrees; they may enjoy casual dating, one-night stands, or brief courtships (facilitated by the ease of proximity dating apps like "Tinder" and "Grinder"). Although these people may be at any age in life, they are particularly prevelant in their early twenties as they simultaneously pursue self-discovery goals including academic and/or professional interests. Older people who have left a marriage or long-time partner, or who have been widowed, may also spend some time enjoying casual, no-commitment dating. In my own clinical practice, I have observed many divorced or widowed ciswomen thoroughly enjoy casual dating, refusing to commit or marry a new long-term partner and often preferring to live alone.

ROMONORMATIVITY

In her article "Rom-Com Without Romonormativity, Gays Without Homonormativity: Examining the People Like Us Web Series," Eve Ng (Associate Professor of Media, Women's, Gender, and Sexuality Studies at Ohio University) coined the term *romonormative* to describe privileging "monogamous romantic relationships," a phenomenon that also often involves "downplay[ing] same-sex eroticism" (Ng, 2020, Abstract). Finally, we have a word for all the Disney-forced monogamous romance plots (not to mention the all-too-common heteronormativity of mainstream media).

Unfortunately, many single individuals do experience pressure from well-meaning relatives and friends to date, find someone, settle down, get into a relationship, and ultimately get married. These friends and relatives may be worried their single friend will get lonely, or be in need of a helper at some point (particularly as they age). However, it always remains a personal choice whether to pursue companionship versus be only responsible for oneself, and that choice should be respected by others. We therapists can certainly inquire of our clients about their current feelings regarding being single, should it become appropriate, and ideally take the lead from them as to whether this needs more exploration, or if this is simply their preferred and/or default relationship status.

MONOGAMY

Many of our Westernized clients will experience monogamy (one person committed sexually and/or romantically to one other person) as their relationship status at some point in their lives. Many clients might identify as serial monogamists (having one monogamous relationship after the other) or fervently desire a committed long-term or life-long monogamous relationship. However, a surprising number of clients may report experiences and preferences that do not meet that definition, despite the heavy societal pressure toward relationships and monogamy. Some people are also more recently identifying as *monogamish*—mostly monogamous with some occasional open relationship elements.

The United States has a powerful $60 billion a year wedding industry, further enforcing the monogamous relationship as the highest pinnacle of romantic (or interpersonal) achievement. Many fortunes ride on the fairytale notion of two people falling in love, committing, then getting married. However, the marriage rate in the United States is 6.5 per 1,000 people, dropping considerably since the 1990s. Zimmer (2013) explains that only 17% of human cultures across the world are strictly lifetime monogamous—many cultures embrace some flexibility regarding sexual and emotional relationships such as serial monogamy, polygamy, secret dual monogamous relationships, and so on. In the United States, reports from the Pew Research Center reveal that only "half of Americans ages 18 and older were married in 2017 ... down 8 percentage points since 1990" (Geiger & Livingston, 2019, #1).

While marriage rates are declining (potentially due to folks waiting till later ages, more economic independence for ciswomen, and/or lack of access and high expense for some), cohabitation rates have steadily increased. Divorce rates have dropped overall 18% between 2008 and 2016, according to a recent study on divorce by sociologist Philip N. Cohen (2019), yet are on the rise among Baby Boomers and older individuals (Geiger & Livingston, 2019).

CONSENSUAL NONMONOGAMY/POLYAMORY

Monogamy, marriage, and divorce are not the only options for sexual and/or romantic relationships. While monogamy has been the Western puritanical default assumption of what humans should aspire to, more and more folx, especially Millennials and Generation Z, are also exploring and articulating nonmonogamous orientations, defining and ascribing to *open* relationships, *consensual nonmonogamy* (CNM), *ethical nonmonogamy* (ENM), and/or *polyamory*—being intimate with more than one person at a time.

CNM is often defined broadly as being sexually involved with two or more people and can include things like negotiated one-night-stands. Any kind of CNM involves the knowledge and consent of all partners involved (Tallon-Hicks, 2010). ENM, another term in use, tends to emphasize a more ethical framework of honesty, communication, respect, and transparency.

Polyamory tends to be defined as ongoing emotional and/or sexual relationships with more than one partner. *Fluid-bonded* is another term clients may use to describe their relationships. Individuals in the defined fluid-bonded group may feel comfortable, after negative sexually transmitted infection (STI) testing results, being sexually intimate with the other individuals in that bonded group without using safer sex barriers such as condoms or dental dams.

A favorite illustrated book, *How to Have Feminist Sex* (Perry, 2019), has a wonderful section on the history of nonmonogamy. She essentially notes that many other cultures and similar species (chimps and bonobos) do not have an overriding monogamous expectation. She mentions several human peoples from nonWestern cultures that have these ideas: any child in that group could potentially have any number of fathers (Naskapi tribe, Canada), and therefore all children are loved and cared for, and every woman is possibly a little bit pregnant by more than one man (some Amazon tribes). Some tribes have a built-in agreement in romantic relationships about not getting too jealous of other lovers (the Canela in Brazil) and making sure no one is neglected (the Siriono in Bolivia). There are folks on many fronts (academic, sociological, civilian, artistic) challenging the Western monogamy paradigm.

Many CNM clients are well-informed and utilize the ethical ideals of honesty, communication, and transparency as detailed in these books: *The Ethical Slut* (Easton & Hardy, 2009), *Opening Up* (Taormino, 2008), and Polysecure (Fern, 2020), among others. Other clients may be new to CNM and in exploration mode, having had learning experiences worthy of therapy. According to various research investigations ranging from 2,000 to 8,000 participants, anywhere from 4% to 20% identified some type of nonmonogamous practice.

It is also helpful to know that some folks may identify as *relationship anarchists*, that is, people who do not prioritize any type of relationship or partner.

Polycules and Polyships

Folks who practice CNM or polyamory might mention being part of a *polycule* (the entire network of folks romantically or sexually interconnected to each other) within one group or polyship (the specific connections and/or relationships within members of a polycule). Members may also mention their *metamour. A metamour* is a partner who has an intimate relationship with a second partner—their partner's partner. For example, Jim is involved with Andre. Andre is also involved with Ruth, but Ruth is not involved with Jim. Ruth is Jim's metamour.

Some clients may also describe themselves as existing within an *alternative family structure* (a structure that diverges from the traditional nuclear family structure of two parents and their children). Polyamorous familes, communal families, blended, adoptive, extended, and single-parent families all fall under this umbrella term.

Compersion

Folks in poly relationships might report feeling *compersion*, the opposite of jealousy. Compersion means feeling happy and delighted that an intimate partner had a wonderful sexual experience with another person. Compersion can also exist alongside jealousy (Tallon-Hicks, 2010). Joli Hamilton, sex educator/activist, has a TEDx Talk on "Compersion—The Opposite of Jealousy" (TED, 2020). However, some of our openly CNM clients, just like our monogamous clients, may struggle with jealousy at times, adding unwanted jealousy to their list of themes and events to therapeutically process. We can also ask our clients about any positive and negative experiences with CNM. This can help ascertain more general positive resourcing and/or potentially difficult clinical content to examine and process.

New Relationship Energy

Both monogamous and CNM clients might mention and/or experience *new relationship energy* (NRE). This often occurs at the beginning of a new relationship, when giddiness, excitement, and endorphins for the new partner are high. CNM clients may notice that NRE with a new partner may cross over into current long-term relationships, infusing the more established relationships with zest as well. Conversely, unskillfully navigated NRE (i.e., spending all one's free time with the new partner) can sometimes result in long-term partners feeling neglected and jealous. Experienced polyamorists anticipate, accept, and plan for NRE. Community wisdom advises folks to put off making major decisions during NRE, and to make extra effort to do special things for the current partner(s) (Sheff, 2019).

Alternative Family Structures Approach

Sennott (2011) developed a comprehensive framework *alternative family structures approach* (AFSA) through which to view therapeutic modalities (e.g., cognitive behavioral therapy [CBT], dialectical behavior therapy [DBT], group, family therapy) in the provision of care to nontraditional romantic and familial configurations. This CNM/poly/open relationship affirming lens has an 8-session structured assessment and treatment planning components, with the goal of understanding what is bringing the family structure into therapy. Please consult the text *Sex Therapy With Erotically Marginalized Clients* (Constantinides et al., 2019) for greater detail in utilizing this feminist and transfeminist approach.

INFIDELITY

Infidelity can occur in both monogamous and CNM relationships. One-third of a group of 2000 surveyed American adults reported cheating in a monogamous relationship either physically, emotionally, or in both categories (Domitru, 2022). If two people have committed exclusively to each other, then the experience and discovery of a sexual, romantic, or emotional affair, whether via the internet or in person, can be gut-wrenching for all involved.

Conversely, infidelity can occur in open relationships when one person violates the terms of the consensual nonmonogamy (e.g., seeing a new sexual/romantic interest yet not informing their partners; not using a condom when the agreement included universal condom use; spending the night at a partner's house when that was not an agreed option). It is important for clients in relationships to check in regularly with each other about what constitutes cheating for them, especially with the opportunities and possibilities made available by technology of emotional to cyber affairs.

It is helpful to understand some of the dynamics that may be encountered for clients who have discovered their partner's affair, or have been the one to conduct the affair. While there are many esteemed and respected books published on navigating and recovering from affairs (see resources in Chapter 13), what follows here is some basic information to provide a small foundation for your clinical practice.

The intense betrayal and devastating havoc inflicted by this type of up-close and personal behavior is sometimes the very first reason why a person finds themselves in a therapist's office. Many of my own clients have benefited from receiving EMDR therapy, which is normally a therapy reserved for treating trauma, in helping them heal from the fallout, which indicates how severely an affair can impact someone.

There are several different types of affairs. The go-to image that comes to mind is something *physical* of a sexual nature happening between people who are committed to other partners. These are the images of coworkers making out or engaging in sexual activity with each other in their cars during their lunch break or on business trips, then returning to their married or monogamous domestic partners at night, no one the wiser.

Emotional affairs are another category. A relatively recently identified category, this addition speaks to the progress of civilization into more nuanced territory. One can argue that movies and books of yesteryear (particularly before the internet) made a clear distinction of what constituted a true affair. In this earlier 20th century media (such as in *M*A*S*H*), an affair only happened if something physical occurred between the two people. If lips got within one centimeter, but never kissed, then the people could, and would likely, deny being part of an affair.

However, now, in our collective progress into further attending to and understanding emotional relationships (especially among Generation X and Millennials, in my opinion), we understand that emotional intimacy with someone other than one's proclaimed sexual and/or romantic partner might be cause for concern. In other words, baring one's soul to one's "work-spouse" day in and day out may eventually supplant the emotional bond with one's actual spouse, if not careful with boundaries. Our modern need for our primary relationship to meet all our needs (best friend, lover, coparent, support person, hobby partner) may also have helped contribute to this more recent phenomenon.

Digital living and communicating has also provided us with a third type of infidelity: the *digital* affair. This is an interesting category because nothing physical may ever occur between the two individuals, including never even hearing each other's voices, yet now they are charged with committing a digital affair due to content they wrote or shared with each other.

I have had a few clients in recent years express great distress over discovering a partner's steamy Facebook or reddit messages with a random person or a previous acquaintance, to the point that we targeted these disturbances with EMDR therapy.

Some additional types of affairs include (a) one-night stands, (b) distraction affairs (using the affair to distract from a professional or health problem), (c) the "double-life" affair (essentially developing a full emotional, sexual, and physical relationship with another person, perhaps even having another family with them), and (d) out-of-control sexual behaviors (someone who feels compelled and has persistent urges to sexually interact with other people, over and over). The out-of-control person may frequent strip bars, sex workers, or internet sex and not consider any of this behavior cheating (especially if they state that no emotions are involved).

Many affairs simply end and do not result in new marriages between the two people cheating together.

Because of the many possible affair types and nuances now available, it is important for stated monogamous partners to discuss the parameters of their monogamy from time to time—like an annual relationship definition and evaluation. Often two people can have very different ideas of what monogamy entails, so clear communication is essential to avoid the tears that can spring unspoken assumptions. In fact, ongoing research shows that cisgender men and women are not in full agreement of what constitutes cheating behavior in any category—from sharing intimate thoughts with another person (40% of men compared to 52% of women consider this cheating) to physical sex acts (90% of men to 96% women; Dumitru, 2022).

Ester Perel, couples sex and relationship guru, has a lot to say about affairs and modern monogamy. I often point my clients to her classic books *Mating in Captivity: Unlocking Erotic Intelligence* (2006/2017a) and *The State of Affairs: Rethinking Infidelity* (2017b), as well as her 2015 TED Talk *Rethinking Infidelity: A Talk for Anyone Who Has Ever Loved.* In her TED Talk, Perel explicitly states that the definition of cheating keeps expanding and is quite variable depending on whom you speak to (some consider staying active on dating apps, once committed, an act of cheating). Due to this variability, global estimates range from 26% to 75% of folks cheating in monogamous relationships. Additionally, she notes that not only would nearly all of us decry our partners lying about an affair, we ourselves would also lie "if we were having" an affair (Perel, 2015, 4:08).

Perel likes this definition of affairs: a relationship that includes (a) secrecy, (b) "emotional connection to one degree or the other," and (c) "sexual alchemy." She states that infidelity is "a violation of trust, a crisis of identity" (Perel, 2015, 7:02) and that "[a]ffairs in the digital age are death by a thousand cuts" (Perel, 2015, 8:12). Even people in open relationships might have a secretive affair.

To help explain why people commit affairs, Perel says affairs are "an expression of longing and lost ... yearning for emotional connection, for novelty, for freedom, for autonomy, for sexual intensity, a wish to recapture lost parts of ourselves or an attempt to bring back lost vitality" (2015, 10:58) or find an "antidote to death" (2015, 13:21).

Interestingly, Perel finds that the majority of couples remain together after the affair. The advantage to this reconciliation is that the one being cheated on "no longer has to uphold the status quo that may have not been working for them either" (Perel, 2015, 15:40). It goes without saying that trust needs to be regained. This involves the "perpetrator acknowledge[ing] their wrongdoing [and taking the responsibility to] hold vigil for the relationship" (Perel, 2015, 13:34). It is the transgressor that needs to check in about the affair.

The victim also needs to find ways to live without learning "the sordid details" (Perel, 2015, 17:50). I have found this last detail especially true for my clients, as specific images described to them of the affair can burn a vivid imprint in their imagination. EMDR therapy has been particularly helpful to eliminate this disturbance regarding the vivid image they conjured. Additionally, although most cheaters instinctively do NOT want to share specifics or gory details of the affair, they can unfortunately be swayed by their partner's beseeching entreaties.

Couples therapy can help people navigate this tricky terrain, and so can trauma-focused treatment. A couples therapist can help the victim investigate questions around meaning (i.e., *what were you getting out of the affair that this relationship wasn't giving you*?). Perel ultimately notes that affairs are a two-sided coin with "hurt and betrayal on one side and growth and discovery on the other" (2015, 20:29).

Jealousy, break-ups, divorces, and infidelity, whether from short-term, long-term, monogamous, married, or CNM relationships, can provide a wealth of clinical content to explore.

Case Study 6.2: Kai, Infidelity and Low Sexual Interest

Kai is a late-forties, heterosexual, Southeast Asian cisman, working as an anesthesiologist. He is married and in a consensual nonmonogamous (open) marriage. He sought EMDR therapy after discovering his wife's (similar age, working professional, White) affair with a much younger man. Although they had a CNM relationship, Emily had chosen to keep this new partner, a younger cisman, from him.

After Kai learned of the affair, some time prior to entering therapy, he spent many hours pressing Emily for details (which she gave) and listening to her apologies and renewed professions of loyalty, love, and commitment to him as her primary and fully informed partner. Kai searched the internet and found images of the man. Armed with details of their affair, plus a visual of the person, Kai conjured unshakable mental images of the sexual details of the affair. Kai noted previously enjoying compersion for Emily and her other lovers (and enjoying her compersion for him). His goal for treatment was to find a way to forgive her, be comfortable and trust her again, and stay married (they had children together and Emily stated over and over that she wanted to stay married to him and was willing to do anything).

We were able to develop a timeline of the events now corroborated as cheating moments (i.e., when Kai was away at a conference or working late) and populate them with the mental images he formed. Other targets also included the events surrounding the disclosure and early conversations about the affair. Kai's NCs over the course of many targets included: "I'm abandoned, unimportant, not worthy, a loser, tricked/betrayed, second rate," and so on. His PCs included: "I'm important, I have power, choices, I'm desired, able to trust and move on." He reported emotions of betrayal, anger, disgust, grief, and sadness, and experienced the associated disturbance as tightness in his chest.

Once we worked through most of these EMDR targets, Kai spoke of wanting to be able to enjoy some affection from his wife. We were able to develop and install EMDR future templates of effectively "enjoying being touched by her." This was his explicit goal, as he adamantly wanted to remain married, despite having trouble regaining full trust for her. These EMDR future templates helped him to begin enjoying touch with Emily again.

As we wrapped up individual EMDR therapy, Kai and Emily entered couples therapy. Kai acknowledged that their marriage health was not yet fully restored. However, he felt optimistic about their marriage moving forward, resolving the lingering notes of betrayal and recently identified off-balance dynamics of their relationship (Emily felt he made more of the decisions and rules, contributing to some of her unhappiness).

PERSONAL AND CLINICAL CONSIDERATIONS

If you feel comfortable identifying in any of the categories described in this chapter (queer, gay, poly, bisexual, demisexual, as an asexual person ["ACE"], etc.) in your practice information, this may help certain clients who might feel invisible find their way to you, thereby benefiting from your psychotherapy and sexual health psychoeducation to address stigmatization, microaggressions, and/or traumas resulting from erotic marginalization (Sennott, 2020). Additionally, if you hang rainbow flags or check off in your profile that you serve LGBTQIA+ clients, make sure you are fully comfortable treating folx from these categories (Marich, 2021).

MICROAGGRESSIONS

Microaggressions are "subtle insults that are delivered through dismissive looks gestures, and tones (verbal, nonverbal and over visual) that are often directed toward people of color" (Sue & Constantine, 2007, p. 137) and can also be experienced by other marginalized populations such as LGBTQIA+ individuals. Microaggressions can be intentional or unintentional; they communicate a negative or derogatory stereotype, belief, or assumption and dehumanize or belittle the receiver. Many of our clients from these erotically marginalized communities may report experiencing any number of microaggressions, which are potentially worthy of addressing in therapy.

Additionally, heterosexism (cultural victimization of LGBTQIA+ individuals) and heteronormativity (privileging of heterosexual relationships) can be seen as a form of abuse that oppresses LGBTQIA+ individuals (Neisen, 1993).

It is quite possible that a client may perceive and share that their therapist (possibly you) or another treatment provider has enacted a microaggression toward themselves during the therapeutic process. The *CPR model* (Manser et al., 2018) can help you and your client move gracefully through this potential pitfall through the following steps: (a) "***C***alm yourself" (breathe, don't get defensive), (b) "***P***ractice humility" (be accountable; focus on the harm, not your intent; prioritize the impact on the other person), and (c) "***R***epair" (center the relationship, ask what you can do to repair).

POLYSEMICITY

Polysemicity refers to how one word or idea can have multiple meanings or be expressed in very different ways. In other words, another person's experiences may not mimic or duplicate one's own experience, even if we both perform the exact same behavior (M. Klein, 2010). Everyone has different and unique experiences, so a Black lesbian client in her early twenties may not behave and/or have many similar experiences to another Black lesbian client or clinician in her early twenties, late fifties, or at age 75. Understanding that our clients may have different definitions and experiences of sexuality and gender, even those that appear to identify the same as we do, is helpful to remember. Another helpful catchphrase to keep in mind as we broaden our sexual health knowledge is "don't yuck my yum"—every person is entitled to their own preferences and interests regarding consenting adult sexual activities.

NINE PRINCIPLES OF CLINICAL SUPPORT

Constantinides et al. (2019) have written the highly informative and valuable book *Sex Therapy With Erotically Marginalized Clients: Nine Principles of Clinical Support* detailing principles to consider when working with people from marginalized groups. Marginalized groups include folks who have a nonheterosexual identity (i.e., identifying as lesbian, bisexual, gay, etc.), a non-monogamous orientation (i.e., folks who practice polyamory), and/or noncisgender identity (i.e., transgender or nonbinary person). Their comprehensive and groundreaking book also has many in-depth case examples of working with marginalized folks, illustrating the use of these nine principles to enhance the therapeutic process. Briefly, the nine principles are:

1. *"Maintain transparency and name systemic/individual oppressions."*—"Therapists have the potential, and responsibility, to see and name power dynamics related to erotic marginalization both inside and outside the therapy room."
2. *"Challenge binary thinking and its constrictions."*—Binary thinking "creates a framework of seeing the world that limits possibilities ... and creates distance and separateness."
3. *"Support willingness to experience the anxiety of uncertainty."*—Although clients come to therapy seeking answers and solutions, it is critical to be able to sit in "the murky grey area without answers."
4. *"Practice a relational and dialogic approach" (not "expert").*—As a therapist, bring an open and collaborative mind-set and curiosity, remain aware of power differentials, and invite clients to explore their intersecting identities.
5. *"Emphasize the client's own words, knowledge, and narratives."*—Center the client's own descriptions and experiences.
6. *"Locate oneself and respond to client's meta-communication"* (notice nonverbal cues).—Practicing preemptive radical inclusion (assuming that every client may be erotically marginalized in some way) "is a way of de-centering the therapist's own experience in order to make space for their clients."
7. *"Support participation of family and network."*—"Supporting participation of family and/or communities in clinical work helps clients create a space in which they feel good about themselves."
8. *"Practice active allyship."*—"Participate in the creation of a network for clients, and see oneself as an active participant in the social support, emotional scaffolding, and the larger network of affirming provider care."
9. *"Build a community of colleagues."*—It is vital "to have safe spaces both personally and professionally to get support, supervision, affirmation, and be understood without extensive explanation or scrutiny."

Keeping as many of these principles in mind as you work with your clients, especially those experiencing marginalization, oppression, or any of the existing isms or phobias, will help you provide invaluable support for them.

SUMMARY

Sexual and affectional/romantic attraction and orientation can be important parts of our clients' relational identities and can remain stable, or change, throughout their lifetimes. Sexual and affectional orientations encompass a wide range of healthy and normal human experiences including attraction to other genders, similar genders, many or all genders, or little to no attraction to anyone.. A very short list of the enumerable descriptors clients might utilize include: heterosexual, gay, lesbian, same gender loving, bisexual, pansexual, omnisexual, demisexual, graysexual, asexual, abrosexual, and/or queer. It is helpful to know and remember that homosexuality was removed from the *DSM* over 50 years ago (in 1973), based on the psychological, sociological, scientific, and cultural consensus that "homosexuality per se is a normal and positive variation of human sexual orientation" (Anton, 2010, p. 464).

Bisexuality, pansexuality, and/or omnisexuality are often misunderstood as transitional or fence-sitting identities, when in actuality a surprisingly large number of individuals have had experiences and attractions to similar and different genders. Clients may also identify as asexual (very little or no sexual interest) and/or demisexual (sexual attraction grows once an emotional connection is established). Both of these are valid and do not need to be seen as a result of trauma or pathologized as a hyposexual disorder. A brief history of queer theory and its impact on sexual and gender identity is also explored.

The American Psychological Association, EMDRIA, and many other national organizations (plus 26 states) have formal statements and/or laws denouncing any kind of SOCE. Unfortunately, SOCE is legally allowed in some states, despite research showing the harm it often causes to people subjected to it (especially youth). We must never use, condone, or be complicit in any kind of SOCE therapy; in fact, our clients who have experienced SOCE may likely need trauma-informed therapy (i.e., EMDR therapy) to process and ameliorate the trauma from harmful and deleterious SOCE experiences.

PRI, an ongoing justice-oriented process, presupposes that any or all of our clients may possess marginalized (erotically or otherwise) experiences and/or identities. We must perform due diligence in understanding each unique client, their experiences, and attractions.

Our clients may be single (by choice or default), committed to one person, married, or in a CNM relationship. Our society puts incredible pressure on people to comply with heteronormativity and romonormativity. Validating and affirming singlehood, types of open relationships, or other nonmonogamous relationship structures is an essential practice of supportive therapy. Compersion can occur in open relationships and is when one partner derives happiness from their partner's enjoyment of a separate romantic or sexual relationship. However, jealousy can occur in any type of relationship. Infidelity can result in responses of grief, shock, betrayal, loss, trauma, and so on. Any and all emotional and psychological responses can be supported and processed through individual and/or couples therapy, potentially strengthening and uplifting the relationship to a better place.

DISCUSSION QUESTIONS

- Discuss sexual versus romantic/affectional orientations, as well as potential combinations a client might disclose in therapy.
- Discuss some of the ways folks identifying as LGBTQIA+ might experience marginalization and/or homophobic behaviors.
- Provide an example of a microaggression a client may report, and detail how the CPR method might help process the situation.
- What are some reasons why an infidelity might occur, even in a nonmonogamous relationship? How might the infidelity impact all involved (i.e., the involved partner, the noninvolved partner, and the third party?)

LEARNING ACTIVITIES

CourseConnect

To access self-assessment questions and interactive, competency-based learning activities for this chapter, visit www.springerpub.com/courseconnect. See inside front cover and tear-out card for CourseConnect details.

ADDITIONAL RESOURCES

Additional resources are online and available at www.springerpub.com/courseconnect.

REFERENCES

Ahmed, S. (2004). *The cultural politics of emotion*. Edinburgh University Press.

American Psychiatric Association. (2013). *Diagnostic and statistical manual of mental disorders* (5th ed.). https://doi.org/10.1176/appi.books.9780890425596

Anton, B. S. (2010). Proceedings of the American Psychological Association for the legislative year 2009: Minutes of the annual meeting of the Council of Representatives and minutes of the meetings of the Board of Directors. *American Psychologist, 65*, 385–475. https://doi.org/10.1037/a0019553

Beal, C. B. (n.d.). *Preemptive radical inclusion*. Justice and Peace Consulting. Retrieved May 13, 2025, from https://justiceandpeaceconsulting.com/preemptive-radical-inclusion

Beal, C. B., & Alves, C. L. (2018, March). *OWL facilitator training for young adult, adult, and older adult levels*. New England Region UUA.

Brown, A. (2023, June 23). *Five key findings about LGBTQ+ Americans*. Pew Research Center. https://pewrsr.ch/430nOXY

Butler, J. (1990). *Gender trouble: Feminism and the subversion of identity*. Routledge.

Cohen, P. N. (2019, January 1). The coming divorce decline. *Socius, 5*. https://doi.org/10.1177/2378023119873497

Constantinides, D. M., Sennott, S. L., & Chandler, D. (2019). *Sex therapy with erotically marginalized clients: Nine principles of clinical support*. Routledge.

Domitru, Oana (2022, October 4). *How many Americans have cheated on their partners in monogamous relationships?* YouGov. https://today.yougov.com/society/articles/43605-how-many-americans-have-cheated-their-partner-poll

Easton, D., & Hardy, J. (2009). *The ethical slut: A practical guide to polyamory, open relationships, and other adventures*. Celestial Arts.

EMDR International Association. (n.d.). *EMDR International Association policies*. https://www.emdria.org/about-emdria/emdr-international-association-policies. Reprinted with permission from the EMDR International Association Professional Code of Conduct.

Fausto-Sterling, A. (2000). *Sexing the body: Gender politics and the construction of sexuality*. Basic Books.

Fern, J. (2020). *Polysecure: Attachment, trauma, and consensual nonmonogamy*. Thornapple Press.

Fleishman, J. (2020). *The stonewall generation: LGBTQ elders on sex, activism, and aging*. Skinner House Books.

Geiger, A. W., & Livingston, G. (2019, February 13). *8 facts about love and marriage in America*. Pew Research Center. https://www.pewresearch.org/fact-tank/2019/02/13/8-facts-about-love-and-marriage

Human Rights Commission. (n.d.). *The lies and dangers of efforts to change sexual orientation or gender identity*. Author. Retrieved September 17, 2021, from https://www.hrc.org/resources/the-lies-and-dangers-of-reparative-therapy

Jones, J. M. (2024, March 13). LGBTQ+ identification in U.S. now at 7.6%. *Gallup News*. https://news.gallup.com/poll/611864/lgbtq-identification.aspx

Kinsey, A., Charles, P., Wardell, B., & Martin, C. E. (1948). *Sexual behavior in the human male*. W.B. Saunders.

Kinsey, A. C., Pomeroy, W., Baxter, M., Clyde E., & Gebhard, P. H. (1953). *Sexual behavior in the human female*. W.B. Saunders.

Klein, F. (1993). *The bisexual option*. Taylor & Francis.

Klein, M. (2010, April). *When sex gets complicated: Pornography, kink, cybersex, and other clinical challenges*. American Association of Sexuality Educators, Counselors and Therapists.

Manser, K., Campbell, J., & Criniti, A. (2018). CPR model. training@accessmatters.org

Marich, J. (2021, June 13). *EMDR therapy and LGBTQ+ experiences* [Webinar]. The Institute for Creative Mindfulness. https://icm.thinkific.com/courses/emdr-therapy-lgbtq-experiences-webinar-replay

Neisen, J. H. (1993). Healing from cultural victimization: Recovery from shame due to heterosexism. *Journal of Gay and Lesbian Mental Health, 2*(1), 49–63. https://doi.org/10.1300/J236v02n01_04

Ng, E. (2020). Rom-com without romonormativity, gays without homonormativity: Examining the 'People Like Us' web series. *New Review of Film and Television Studies, 18*(1), 83–100. https://doi.org/10.1080/17400309.2019.1664057

O'Brien, J. M. (2017). EMDR therapy with lesbian/gay/bisexual clients. In M. Nickerson (Ed.), *Cultural competence and healing culturally based trauma with EMDR therapy: Innovative strategies and protocols* (pp. 195–208). Springer Publishing Company.

Ochs, R. [@robynochs]. (2021, May 4). If you are LGBTQ+, existing proudly and unapologetically in public is a form of activism. Surviving and thriving is a [Post]. Instagram. https://www.instagram.com/p/COdqJalMkFH/?igsh=ZXBzcnFhNnBjemVw

Perel, E. (2015, March). *Rethinking infidelity ... a talk for anyone who has ever loved* [Video]. TED Conferences. https://www.ted.com/talks/esther_perel_rethinking_infidelity_a_talk_for_anyone_who_has_ever_loved/transcript

Perel, E. (2017a). *Mating in captivity: Unlocking erotic intelligence.* HarperCollins. (Original work published 2006)

Perel, E. (2017b). *The state of affairs: Rethinking infidelity.* HarperCollins.

Perry, F. (2019). *How to have feminist sex: A fairly graphic guide.* Penguin Random House.

Scott, J. W. (1991). The evidence of experience. *Critical Inquiry, 17*(4), 773–797. https://doi.org/10.1086/448612

Sennott, S. (2011). Gender disorder as gender oppression: A tranfeminist approach to rethinking the pathologization of gender non-conformity. *Women and Therapy, 34*(1–2), 93–113. https://doi.org/10.1080/02703149.2010.532683

Sennott, S. (2020, May). *Sex therapy with erotically marginalized clients: Nine principles of clinical support.* [Workshop]. Smith College School for Social Work.

Sheff, E. (2019, October). New relationship energy: What it is & how to deal with it. *Psychology Today.* https://www.psychologytoday.com/us/blog/the-polyamorists-next-door/201910/new-relationship-energy-what-it-is-how-deal-it

Storms, M. D. (1980). Theories of sexual orientation. *Journal of Personality and Social Psychology, 38*(5), 783–792. https://doi.org/10.1037/0022-3514.38.5.783

Sue, D. W., & Constantine, M. G. (2007). Racial microaggressions as instigators of difficult dialogues on race: Implications for student affairs educators and students. *College Student Affairs Journal, 26*(2), 136–143. https://files.eric.ed.gov/fulltext/EJ899387.pdf

Tallon-Hicks, Y. (2010, June). *Polyamory for professionals.* [Workshop].

Taormino, T. (2008). *Opening up: A guide to creating and sustaining open relationships.* Cleis Press.

TED. (2020, January 27). *Compersion—The opposite of jealousy | Hamilton, Joli* [Video]. YouTube. https://www.youtube.com/watch?v=bIojP4MnTwg&t=11s

Tomso, G. (2008). Viral sex and the politics of life. *South Atlantic Quarterly, 107*(2), 265–285. https://doi.org/10.1215/00382876-2007-066

Whitman, W. (n.d.). *Song of myself, 51.* https://poets.org/poem/song-myself-51

Zimmer, C. (2013, August 2). Monogamy and human evolution. *New York Times.* https://www.nytimes.com/2013/08/02/science/monogamys-boost-to-human-evolution.html

II

Treatment

CHAPTER 7

Sex Therapy Frameworks

Wendy Stock and Stephanie Baird

LEARNING OBJECTIVES

- Learn about modern sex therapy frameworks, including the *new view of women's sexual problems.*
- Learn about common sexual problems reported in sex therapy.
- Learn about persistent sexual myths and corrective psychoeducation.
- Learn about conditions for good, great, and magnificent sex.
- Learn about basic sex therapy treatment strategies such as sensate focus, Kegels, and mindfulness.
- Learn how to use the *Sexual History Questionnaire* to obtain client sexual health information.

INTRODUCTION TO SEX THERAPY FRAMEWORKS

HISTORICAL UNDERSTANDINGS OF THE BASIS OF SEXUAL PROBLEMS

How culture constructs sexuality profoundly impacts our understanding of sexual health and how we define sexual problems. It guides and often narrows what we look for as we assess individuals seeking treatment, and what areas we may overlook. Culturally determined conceptions of sexuality, if we are unaware of their limitations, potentially impede our ability to offer the most effective treatment to our therapy clients. As clinicians, it is incumbent on us to be aware of cultural lenses, and to select the best components from the range of different models of sexuality, building upon existing models with critical awareness. The field of sex therapy has undergone an exciting evolution as it has matured to encompass broader models that better describe sexuality across different populations and social contexts.

For many decades, the prevailing dominant cultural model of human sexuality was based on a model that narrowly defines sexual functioning as an unvarying progression of physiological responses, and failure to experience this progression as sexual dysfunction and therefore mental illness. These traditional approaches developed with a heteronormative focus, holding the ability to "achieve" penis-vagina sexual intercourse as the main criterion of healthy sexual functioning.

MASTERS AND JOHNSON

Early approaches to sex therapy were based on a model of sexual arousal by Masters and Johnson (1966) that proposed a four-stage model of sexual arousal: excitement, plateau, orgasm, and resolution. Masters and Johnson's work provided invaluable information about the human physiology of sexual arousal, including the role of the clitoris in female orgasm, which was previously largely overlooked. Their work provided the basis to contest the dominant and inaccurate view that women should always orgasm during penetrative sex, and that the inability to do so was a form of pathology. Unfortunately, in emphasizing sexual physiology, this model lent itself to medicalized approaches to solving sexual problems, to the exclusion of relational factors and social context.

To their credit, Masters et al. (1979) revised their treatment model to incorporate a relational view, defining the couple, rather than the individual, as the appropriate focus of therapy. However, as Perelman (2014) notes, couples-based sex therapy was seen as a short-term, problem-focused, and directive approach that often overlooked the context of overall relationship dynamics, power issues, and the social context in which sexual problems emerged.

KAPLAN

Later, Helen Singer Kaplan (1979) proposed a three-stage model, adding a desire phase to arousal and orgasm. The addition of a desire phase encouraged consideration of physical and psychological factors that may affect desire for sex (Magon et al., 2012). Kaplan integrated behavioral techniques alongside some of the psychodynamic approaches. Kaplan's approach paid specific attention to the way in which clients approached therapy and sought to understand the unconscious factors that inhibit change.

MEDICAL MODELS

Medical models for treatment of sexual issues are predicated in the assumption that the sexual symptoms have a biological etiology, and that biological interventions can be of some assistance in treating sexual concerns. The emphasis on a medical contribution emerged after the 1970s, in response to the emphasis on applying a psychodynamic perspective to sex problems and a response to greater popularity in drug options for treatment, as well as more reimbursement for medical issues over psychological issues (Tiefer, 1996).

BEHAVIORAL MODELS Kat Hertlein

Behavioral models include those that mainly focus on behavior; however, they can also include cognitions. Cognitive behavioral therapy (CBT) is one of the most empirically validated treatments for sexual dysfunction, and has been demonstrated as effective in treating hypoactive sexual desire disorder, orgasm issues, anxiety, body image issues, and many others (Stephenson et al., 2013). Techniques in behavioral therapies include skills training, directed masturbation training, and conditioning techniques to associate arousal and orgasm with certain stages of sexual cycles and stimuli.

CRITIQUES OF HISTORICAL SEX THERAPY MODELS

The current diagnostic nomenclature for sexual dysfunctions (*Diagnostic and Statistical Manual of Mental Disorders* [5th ed.; *DSM-5*, American Psychiatric Association [APA], 2013) is based on these earlier models of sexual functioning (desire, arousal, and orgasm), and adds a category for sexual pain disorders. Although these linear stage-based models may be descriptive for some individuals, they have been criticized for failing to account for the social and relational context in which sexual problems occur. This lack of context has vast implications for the treatment of sexual problems. Several alternative approaches are discussed that provide contextual, multifaceted analyses of causes of sexual problems, and suggest effective directions to address them.

MOVING TOWARD INTEGRATIVE MODELS

Schnarch Approach

The Schnarch approach was based on the work on Murray Bowen and the concept of differentiation. Schnarch theorized that differences in expressions of love, affection, and intimacy can underscore and impact the partners' sexual satisfaction. Schnarch's work teaches partners to understand how one's level of differentiation impacts their communication with their partner, and helps couples to be able to grow together. Those who have higher levels of differentiation feel more grounded in who they are and can permit people to be close to them and be vulnerable to others; those with lower levels of differentiation are unable to connect as well with others because they are not secure in themselves. Schnarch argues that engagement in sexually fulfilling relationships requires that people operate from a grounded place with an established sense of self to engage relationships (Schnarch & Regas, 2012).

Biopsychosocial Model

The biopsychosocial model proposes a view of etiology that allows room for a complex interplay of emotions, thoughts, and conditions that contribute to the development and maintenance of sexual problems. This allows therapists to not solely focus on one factor exclusively. Perelman (2024) uses an example of how cancer treatment also may have negative side effects on one's sex life. In this way, the treatment has to incorporate an appreciation for both biology and psychology in treatment. For example, other conditions such as depression and anxiety can also impact the presence of a sexual dysfunction (Perelman, 2024).

Intersystems Approach

A specific type of biopsychosocial approach is called the intersystems approach. Developed by Weeks and Gambescia (Hertlein et al., 2019), the intersystems model puts forth five different domains under which sexual dysfunctions might emerge: individual biological, individual psychological, couple/dyadic issues, family of origin, and cultural. Like the biopsychosocial model, any of these elements can disturb the perception of satisfaction with the sexual relationship or also suggest the presence of any of the other dysfunctions. For example, partners may have a high level of conflict or power imbalance, which will create issues in their sexual relationship; however, the way that they have learned to talk to one another, and the way that they have learned about power, might be from their family of origin. Therapists who operated out of the intersystems approach can bring attention to each of these areas and develop a treatment plan consistent with the etiology of the symptoms: issues that stem from one's family of origin are addressed through a family of origin lens; issues that stem from a psychological issue are addressed psychologically, and so on.

Feminist Reconceptualization of Sexual Problems

Feminist sex therapy has led the field in recognition of the limitations of a biologically based approach to human sexuality. Tiefer (1988) critiqued sexual examples from the dysfunction nomenclature as omitting empirically based information on what people socialized as women ("women" in this historical context refers to individuals with clitorises and vulvas) consider important in their sexual lives, including intimacy, negotiation, and communication. Tiefer recommended that feminist-informed sex therapy include "corrective genital physiology education, assertiveness training, body image reclamation, and masturbation education" (1996, p. 53). Naomi McCormick (1994), another feminist sex therapist, recommended that therapists treat individuals and couples for deficits in tenderness, poor communication, sexual selfishness, disinterest in oral sex, and unwillingness to cuddle.

A feminist approach to sex therapy uses existing scientific knowledge about biology, medical approaches, and empirically validated treatment techniques while adding the following ingredients: recognition and willingness to intervene to address gender inequality, power differentials in relationships, valuing emotional and subjective aspects of sexuality, recognition that traditional sex roles underlie sexual problems, and awareness of the role of sexual coercion, abuse, and trauma in causing sexual problems. Finally, awareness of the relational context of sexual dysfunction is inherent in a feminist approach to sex therapy.

Rosemary Basson (2002) introduced a circular model of the female sexual response cycle that emphasizes subjective experience. An important tenet in Basson's model is that a person's sexual response can be ignited at any phase in the cycle, and that not all sexual encounters begin with spontaneous sexual desire. Her model emphasizes that the relational context of the sexual encounter greatly influences motivations to have sex, and the ultimate outcome of a sexual interaction.

The New View of Women's Sexual Problems

The most prominent and organized challenge to the dominant paradigm of sexual dysfunction comes from the new view of women's sexual problems, a collaboration of feminist academics, researchers, scholars, clinicians, and activists. Incorporating Basson's (2002) model and extending far beyond, sexual disorders (including but not limited to those people with clitorises) defined by the field of psychiatry as mental illness can alternatively be understood as problems tied to lack of information, lack of access to healthcare, powerlessness, relational issues, or the result of violent trauma. Sexual problems are seen as arising within a broader framework of cultural and relational factors. The competent clinician should take a history inclusive of all these issues.

A new view of women's sexual problems offers a blueprint for a comprehensive assessment with inherent implications for treatment, depending on the information obtained. The utility of this model for assessment and intervention will become apparent in the following section, which addresses the prevalence, frequency, and treatment of common sexual dysfunctions (Kaschak & Tiefer, 2002).

The "new view" considers four main categories of causes of sexual problems (Kaschak & Tiefer, 2002):

I. Sexual Problems Due to Socio-cultural, Political, or Economic Factors

A. Ignorance and anxiety due to inadequate sex education, lack of access to health services, or other social constraints
1. Lack of vocabulary to describe subjective or physical experience
2. Lack of information about human sexual biology and life-stage changes
3. Lack of information about how gender roles influence … sexual expectations, beliefs, and behaviors
4. Inadequate access to information and services for contraception and abortion, [sexually transmitted infection (STI)] prevention and treatment, sexual trauma, and domestic violence

B. Sexual avoidance or distress due to perceived inability to meet cultural norms regarding correct or ideal sexuality, including:
1. Anxiety or shame about one's body, sexual attractiveness, or sexual responses
2. Confusion or shame about one's sexual orientation or identity, or about sexual fantasies and desires

C. Inhibitions due to conflict between the sexual norms of one's subculture or culture of origin and those of the dominant culture

D. Lack of interest, fatigue, or lack of time due to family and work obligations

II. Sexual Problems Relating to Partner and Relationship

A. Inhibition, avoidance, or distress arising from betrayal, dislike, or fear of partner[;] partner's abuse of couple's unequal power[;] or arising from partner's negative patterns of communication

B. Discrepancies in desire for sexual activity or in preferences for various sexual activities

C. Ignorance or inhibition about communicating preferences or initiating, pacing, or shaping sexual activities

D. Loss of sexual interest and reciprocity as a result of conflicts over commonplace issues such as money, schedules, or relatives, or resulting from traumatic experiences, e.g., infertility or death of a child

E. Inhibitions in arousal or spontaneity due to partner's health status or sexual problems

III. Sexual Problems Due to Psychological Factors

A. Sexual aversion, mistrust, or inhibition of sexual pleasure due to:
1. Past experiences of physical, sexual, or emotional abuse
2. General personality problems with attachment, rejection, co-operation, or entitlement
3. Depression or anxiety

B. Sexual inhibition due to fear of sexual acts or of their possible consequences, e.g., pain during intercourse, pregnancy, sexually transmitted disease, loss of partner, loss of reputation.

IV. **Sexual Problems Due to Medical Factors** Pain or lack of physical response during sexual activity despite a supportive and safe interpersonal situation, adequate sexual knowledge, and positive sexual attitudes. Such problems can arise from:
   A. Numerous local or systemic medical conditions affecting neurological, neurovascular, circulatory, endocrine or other systems of the body
   B. Pregnancy, [STIs], or other sex-related conditions
   C. Side effects of many drugs, medications, or medical treatments
   D. Iatrogenic conditions

COMMON SEXUAL PROBLEMS REPORTED IN SEX THERAPY

A large demographically representative study (Laumann et al., 1999) in the United States found that 43% of women and 31% of men reported at least one sexual dysfunction.

Among subjects identified as women:
- 33% lacked interest in sex
- 24% were unable to orgasm
- 14% experienced pain during sex
- 21% reported trouble lubricating

Among subjects identified as men:
- 16% lacked interest in sex
- 8% were unable to orgasm
- 29% orgasmed too early
- 10% had trouble maintaining or achieving an erection

CORRECTIVE SEXUAL EDUCATION: DEBUNKING SEXUAL MYTHS AND PROVIDING INFORMATION

Tiefer (1996) referred to the need for "corrective sexual education" in addressing sexual problems. Sex therapy almost invariably requires a psychoeducational component, sometimes during the assessment phase and sometimes as treatment progresses. The myths discussed in the following are commonly held, and astoundingly impervious to the availability of more accurate information provided by science and readily accessible online. Providing accurate information can have a profound impact on presenting symptoms, and at times can ameliorate them, as described in the examples. Space prevents a thorough debunking of each myth.

COMMON AND PERSISTENT SEXUAL MYTHS

General Cultural Myths

- People should be able to read their partner's physical signals during sex without any verbal communication.
- Pornography accurately portrays sex.

Myths About Female Sexuality

- All people with vaginas should be able to orgasm through penetrative sex.
- Misunderstanding the significance of vaginal lubrication: It is commonly believed that the presence or absence of vaginal lubrication is an accurate indicator of female sexual arousal.
- Sex is only good if you have an orgasm.
- Douching is necessary to keep the vagina clean.
- Painful sex is normal.

Myths About Male Sexuality (As Identified by Bernie Zilbergeld's *Male Sexuality* [1992])

- People with penises should not have certain feelings (e.g., vulnerability, sadness).
- In sex, as elsewhere, it is performance that counts.

- The man must take charge of and orchestrate sex.
- The man is always ready and always wants to have sex.
- All physical contact must lead to sex.
- Sex equals intercourse.
- Sex requires an erection.
- Sexual intercourse is always a linear progression on increasing excitement terminated only by orgasm.
- Sex is natural and spontaneous.

Case Study 7.1: Alexis, Lubrication Is Not a Valid Measure of Sexual Arousal

Alexis, a cisgender woman, is being seen in treatment for lack of sexual desire with her cisgender male fiancé. Relationship issues had already been successfully addressed (i.e., equalizing relative contribution to household chores). With further assessment, it became apparent that Alexis has a healthy interest in sex, and masturbates on average three times weekly. However, she often makes excuses to avoid having sex with her partner, although she does experience pleasure and orgasm when she "gets past the initial part," as she put it. What became apparent was that both partners were relying on the state of her vaginal lubrication to determine how and when to initiate intercourse. As Masters and Johnson (1970) suggest, vaginal lubrication is not a dependable measure of sexual arousal or desire

On some occasions, Alexis was profusely lubricated but was not feeling ready for penetrative sex. Both partners assumed that she was, and what resulted was sometimes painful cramping when the penis hit the cervix in her essentially unaroused vaginal barrel (not elongated with the uterus being pulled back and out of the way). An unaroused vaginal barrel is about 3 inches in depth; an aroused vaginal barrel is approximately 6 inches in depth. Lubrication is not a good independent measure of female arousal, yet it is often used as such. Alexis did not feel empowered to ask to slow things down, as she assumed that she was aroused, even if not subjectively aware of it.

On other occasions, Alexis was feeling aroused but wasn't lubricated at all. Her partner kept stimulating her very dry vaginal tissues manually—the fragile mucous membrane was easily abraded with extended rubbing and friction. This became so irritating physically and experientially that Alexis would sometimes preempt further stimulation by initiating intercourse, which caused further irritation that sometimes became painful.

This example is included here because this scenario is encountered frequently in sex therapy. Sharing the following information proved quite helpful in Alexis's treatment: Vaginas may lubricate more, less, or not at all during different phases of their menstrual cycle, when using oral contraception, or when using certain medications (antihistamines dry out *all* mucous membranes; diuretics can have the same effect). Lubrication is a misleading measure of sexual arousal. When in doubt, the female partner should be asked and should be encouraged to trust her subjective sense of her body. When sex is desired, lubrication can be applied *proactively*—it makes stimulation feel more pleasurable and less irritating from the onset and does not need to imply a lack of responsivity in the female partner, nor a lack of skill in the other partner (frequent misapprehensions in this situation).

Another myth at play in Alexis's case was the belief that it is normal for sex to sometimes hurt, accepting this as a precondition for having sex. This led to her avoiding sex completely, or initiating painful intercourse to "get it over with." This case also illustrates the relevance of the new view of women's sexual problems model (described earlier) in identifying multiple factors that may apply to ciswomen's sexual problems: inadequate sex education, lack of vocabulary to describe subjective or physical experience, lack of information about human sexual biology, anxiety about one's sexual responses, lack of time and energy due to family and work obligations, ignorance or inhibition about communicating sexual preferences or pacing of sexual activity, and loss of interest over conflicts regarding commonplace issues.

CORRECTIVE SEXUAL EDUCATION: SEXUAL ANATOMY AND PHYSIOLOGY

Understanding one's own sexual response and having the means to verbalize preferences are often greatly facilitated by sharing materials on sexual anatomy and physiology with sex therapy clients. The illustrations provided by Suzann Gage in *A New View of a Woman's Body* (Federation of Feminist Women's Health Centers, 1981) dramatically increase accurate and empowering education. Chapter 3 of her book, titled "The Clitoris: A Feminist Perspective," redefines the clitoris as a much more substantial sexual organ that includes a complex of connected erectile tissue underlying the skin, in contrast to the popular understanding of the clitoris as only the head of the clitoris (see **Figures 7.1 and 7.2**). This chapter contains illuminating illustrations of a nonaroused and aroused clitoris, comparing these to the equivalent in the penis, with striking similarity. Sharing these illustrations with accompanying explanation often paves the way for better communication in couples of any gender combination. When clients see that their sexual arousal is physiologically real, it often results in a radical change within them as they feel more entitled to pursue their own sexual pleasure.

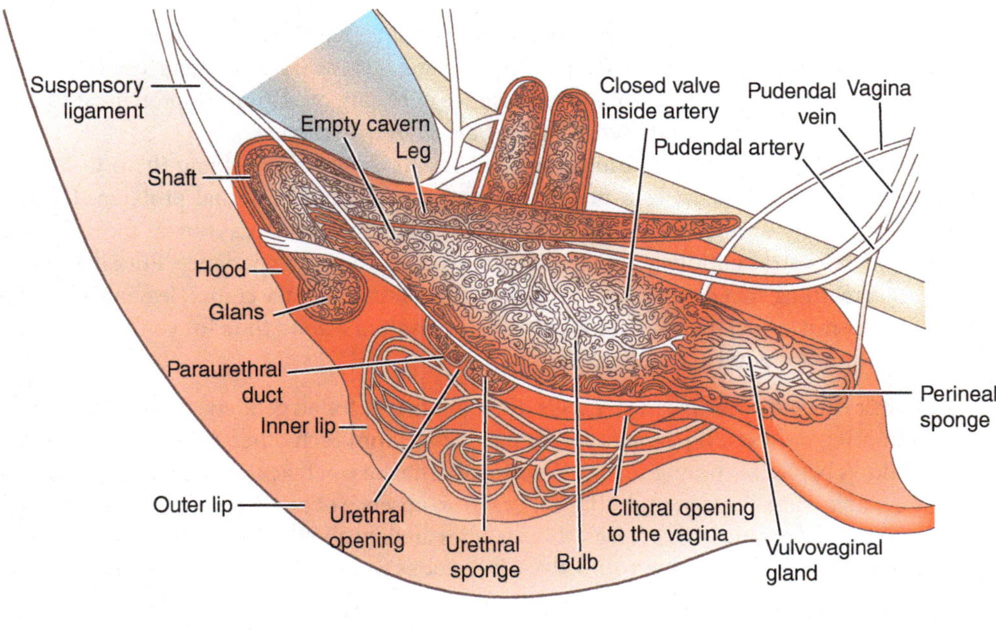

FIGURE 7.1. Cross-Section of the Nonerect Clitoris

Source: Adapted from Federation of Feminist Women's Health Centers. (1981). *A new view of a woman's body*. Feminist Health Press.

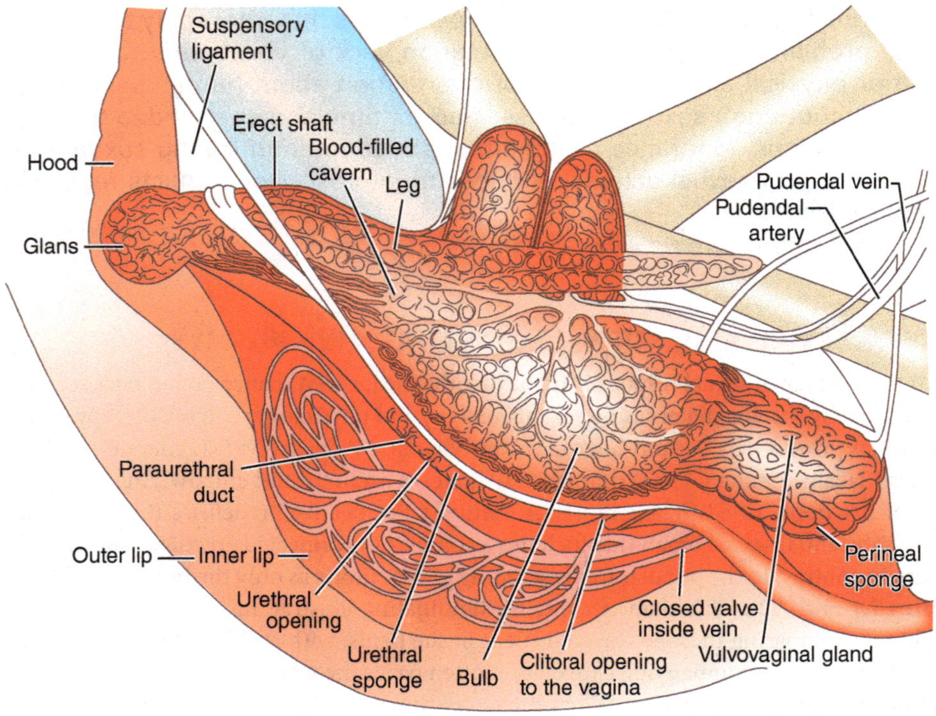

FIGURE 7.2. Cross-Section of the Clitoris During Sexual Arousal

Source: Adapted from Federation of Feminist Women's Health Centers. (1981). *A new view of a woman's body.* Feminist Health Press.

CONDITIONS FOR GOOD AND GREAT SEX

Dr. Bernie Zilbergeld, in his book *The New Male Sexuality* (1992), suggests that knowing our conditions for good and great sex is essential to optimizing our sexual enjoyment. The converse is also true: When people are unaware of the importance of having conditions or prerequisites, they are at risk for disappointment, and even sexual problems or dysfunctions.

Introducing the concept of conditions for good sex to clients, and helping them to identify their own conditions, is crucial as a prelude to treating any kind of sexual problem. On this, Zilbergeld writes: "In a sexual situation, a condition is anything that makes you more relaxed, more comfortable, more confident, more excited, more open to your experience. Put differently, a condition is something that clears your nervous system of unnecessary clutter, leaving it open to receive and transmit sexual messages in ways that will result in a good time for you" (1992, p. 89) General conditions for good sex include:

1. Feeling intimate with your partner. This is often important for all genders, despite stereotypes of men wanting only sex. If partners are feeling distant from each other, they may need to talk about feelings before becoming sexual. Emotional distance can take the heart out of sex.
2. Feeling sexually capable. Generally, this relates to an absence of anxieties about sexual performance. For people with penises, this includes anxiety about becoming erect or ejaculating too soon. For people with vulvas, it includes worry about painful intercourse or lack of orgasm. For everyone, it includes concern about whether one is a good enough lover.
3. Feeling trust. Both partners may need to know they are emotionally safe with their partner. They need to feel confident that they will not be judged, ridiculed, or talked about.
4. Feeling aroused. A person does not need to be sexual unless they are sexually aroused or excited; simply because one's partner wants to be sexual does not mean that you must.

5. Feeling physically and mentally alert. This condition requires a person not to feel particularly tired, ill, stressed, or preoccupied. It requires minimal influence of excessive alcohol or drugs.
6. Feeling positive about the environment and situation. A person may need privacy, to be in a place where they feel protected from intrusion. Each needs to feel that the other is sexually interested and wants to be sexually involved.

Zilbergeld continues to suggest conditions for **great** sex:

1. Accurate information about sexuality, especially your own and your partner's
2. An orientation toward sex based on pleasure, such as arousal, fun, love, and lust, rather than performance and orgasm
3. Being involved in a kind of relationship that allows each person's sexuality to flourish
4. An ability to communicate verbally and nonverbally about sex, feelings, and relationships
5. Being equally assertive and sensitive about your own sexual needs and those of your partner
6. Accepting, understanding, and appreciating differences between partners sexually

Case Study 7.2: Maddie, Advocating for Her Conditions for Good Sex

Maddie rarely turned down her partner's initiations for sex, but she reported frequently being distracted by self-consciousness and unable to respond fully during sexual interactions. Some of her distracted thinking was about having had a hard day at work, and not having had time to unwind. Easily addressed in therapy, Maddie now felt comfortable taking more time to unwind. More prominent were Maddie's worries about her body (perspiration, vaginal odor), especially when her partner engaged in oral sex. Maddie shared that she specifically worried excessively about her vaginal odor, although her partner had been reassuring and engaged, even when they had sex after Maddie's gym workout. She felt that she should not insist on taking a shower first, because her partner didn't seem to mind. Reinforcing Maddie's right to have her own conditions for comfort, and therefore respond sexually, allowed her to speak up about these conditions. Maddie became more engaged, present, and comfortable, enjoying her sexual encounters more fully.

CONDITIONS FOR MAGNIFICENT SEX

Kleinplatz and Menard have spent decades researching the components of good, great, and magnificent sex. In their seminal work, *Magnificent Sex: Lessons From Extraordinary Lovers* (2020), they interviewed 75 individuals who self-identified as having experienced "great, remarkable, wonderful, and memorable sex," asking in-depth questions in order to discover the commonalities within the reports and descriptions. They also interviewed 20 sex therapists on their perspectives on what extraordinary sex is. From these qualitative interviews, Kleinplatz and Menard (2020) identified eight common components of magnificent sex:

1. *Complete mindfulness* (i.e., "being completely present in the moment, embodied, focused, and absorbed"). They noted that this quality was often the first and most prominent aspect mentioned in the interviews. Some also described it similarly to a state of "flow." If we consider the idea of sexual brakes and accelerators, then this would also correspond with all brakes being off (no awareness of laundry on the floor, emails waiting in the inbox, just being fully present and absorbed in the sexual activity).
2. Fully *"in sync" connection/merger/alignment with partner*, often described by respondents as "electricity, energy, and/or conductivity" between partners.
3. "*Deep sexual and erotic intimacy* ... characterized by deep feelings of mutual respect and trust for their partners," with no mention of any particular sexual activity.

4. "*Extraordinary communication and deep empathy*," including ease, openness, and receptivity with verbal communication, nonverbal communication, and a focus on kissing as a communication method. This aspect is in glaring contrast to many erotophobic messages humans receive in their sexual development of NOT openly discussing sexual interest and pleasure, NOT asking for needs and boundaries, and simply "tolerating" unpleasant interactions.
5. "*Genuine, authentic, transparent*," uninhibited (i.e., unselfconsciously sharing one's deepest fantasies, fears, and wishes).
6. "Vulnerability and surrender" (i.e., "letting go ... being swept away, going with the flow" and even a "loss of conscious thought."
7. *Exploration, safe risk taking, and fun* (i.e., playing, pushing, and expanding boundaries; incorporating fun, humor, and lightness; experimenting; and being comfortable with making mistakes and recovering from them (in opposition to a focus on technique).
8. "*Transcendence and transformation*" (i.e., a "combination of heightened states—mental, emotional, physical, relational, and spiritual")

These eight qualities starkly contrast the ubiquitous negative erotophobic messaging we receive (or lack of any kind of messaging, whether negative, neutral, or positive). In fact, the majority of the respondents mentioned having to unlearn societal expectations and stereotypes around sex.

TREATMENT OF COMMON SEXUAL DIFFICULTIES

THE WILLINGNESS MODEL

The willingness model, created by Joanne Loulan, a lesbian sex therapist, provides a useful way to help couples with decreased frequency of sex or low desire. Loulan (1984), based on her observations of lesbian couples' sexuality, developed a new model of sexual response that contained a new component—willingness. This model reflects the fact that for many ciswomen, desire does not always occur spontaneously. However, if individuals decide that they are willing and interested in engaging in sexual activity—despite lacking desire—they may find that desire occurs as they become physically aroused and experience pleasure.

True willingness requires consent; it is not an excuse for sexual coercion. The guidance to couples utilizing this technique is for the low desire partner to be willing to engage in physical affection and sexual touching to explore whether their desire can be "kindled." If the flames of arousal catch on, then the couple can proceed to have a sexual encounter, however this is defined. If no "kindling" occurs, the partners do not need to proceed. The higher desire partner must be willing to accept frustration if this happens.

The willingness model is helpful for people who know they enjoy having sex with a partner, but are too tired, depressed, or stressed to want to initiate sex—they "want to want" sex.

It gives permission to say to one's partner, "I'm not really in the mood, but I might be if we start to fool around," and then see what happens.

SENSATE FOCUS, THE FOUNDATION OF SEX THERAPY INTERVENTIONS

The brilliance of the sensate focus technique, developed by Masters and Johnson (Linschoten et al., 2016), fulfills both a diagnostic function and also a therapeutic intervention that allows improvement of communication deficits in couples. Utilizing this technique before addressing a specific presented sexual dysfunction is crucial in laying a groundwork of constructive communication and sensual, nondemand touching. This method often serves to alleviate some of the contributing factors of performance pressure and poor communication patterns.

In the beginning stages of sensate focus, couples are encouraged to touch each other's bodies and feel for sexual sensations but refrain from touching breasts or genitals or engaging in intercourse or direct genital touching. The exercises work to build gradual desire for full genital sexual involvement. As the couple becomes more skilled at giving and receiving verbal feedback and being present in the moment, they are then encouraged to touch breasts and external genitals, and then eventually to include intercourse, penetrative, or orgasmic sexual activity.

The primary benefits of this approach are:

Introducing sensual touching and deeper connection: In our culture, sex often becomes narrowly focused on genitals, and the rest of the body is ignored. The sensate focus exercise helps to remind us to reintroduce sensual touching as a pleasurable end, as well as a practice that can help awaken us to a deeper and more gratifying sexual experience with our partners. The exercises work to build gradual desire for full genital sexual involvement. As the couple becomes more skilled at giving and receiving verbal feedback and being present in the moment (may take several sessions), they are then encouraged to touch breasts and external genitals, and then eventually to include intercourse or penetrative sexual activity.

Communication deficits assessed and improved: The ubiquitous myth that verbal communication should not be needed during sexual interactions is a major factor in sexual dissatisfaction and sexual dysfunctions. Many individuals believe that providing feedback during sex is unromantic and takes away from the desired mood. Individuals socialized as women often fear being too "bossy" in bed, fearing disapproval from their partners should they speak up. In many cases, "a miss is as good as a mile" in not receiving the precise touching that is needed to orgasm. A partner's deep sigh can be interpreted as the partner being highly aroused, when in reality it can be a sigh of frustration and disappointment when the sexual touching is not working. With sensate focus exercises, partners learn to communicate first with each other about nongenital touch preferences, knowing that these may change over the course of the encounter. Hence, ongoing communication in real time can be learned first with nongenital touch, and then gradually extended to the ability to provide supportive, gentle feedback about the exact level of touch that will work for the recipient.

Diagnostic function: Sensate focus also provides crucial diagnostic information to the therapist, a window in therapy to explore and develop methods of working with barriers to intimacy, rather than trying to ignore or "bypass" negative feelings. Ignoring one's feelings and pretending to feel comfortable prevents true intimacy. Therefore, it is productive for clients to be as aware as possible of *all* of their feelings while doing this exercise. Clients provide access to information that is crucial to their treatment, and which is otherwise inaccessible to the therapist.

Goals of Sensate Focus as Presented to Clients

- To learn ways to touch each other in a sensual, pleasing manner, not dependent on an expectation or demand for sexual arousal or sexual "performance" for oneself or for one's partner
- To practice communicating to your partner your preferences in being touched, in a direct, clear, and constructive manner
- To fully recognize any barriers to physical and emotional intimacy

Sensate Focus Exercise Instructions

Timing/scheduling: Collaboratively schedule 1 hour for each sensate focus session. Sex and sex therapy homework often take a back seat to most other activities, including the laundry. Scheduling time for a sex therapy date is the best way to ensure that it will happen, and is a valuable approach after therapy is over to maintain changes that you have/will make. Try to space these sessions during the week, rather than trying to squeeze them in under pressure on the day before your next therapy appointment.

Setting/environment: The partner who initiates the session is responsible for creating a comfortable environment—setting the room temperature, establishing lighting, providing a beverage, and so on. You are encouraged to try using massage lotion (almond oil or commercial massage lotion) in consultation with your partner. Some people prefer the feel of talcum powder or cornstarch powder, rather than liquid emollients. You may wish to use a large towel to protect your sheets (Stock, n.d.).

Make certain that your cell phones are off and that you will not be interrupted. If you share your home with others, you may choose to let them know that you are spending an hour of "we" time. This is also excellent role-modeling behavior for maintaining a healthy couple relationship.

Take turns (alternating who gets to go first and last) with one partner being the "giver" and the other the "receiver" for 30 minutes each. Make sure that you allow your partner to touch the front and back of your body during your turn as receiver. Although you may experience sexual arousal at times during the sensate focus exercise, sexual arousal is not the goal of this exercise, and it is not intended as a prelude to sexual engagement.

During your turn as receiver, you are only responsible for relaxing and focusing on your sensations, and telling your partner, at the time, three things that feel good about how they are touching you. You also need to tell your partner at least one thing that doesn't feel good, but phrased in terms of what you would like them to do to make it feel better (please move your touching up/down, right/left, harder/softer, to a different location, etc.).

During your turn as giver, try touching your partner in different ways. Breasts and genitals are "off-limits." Use different parts of your hands; different pressures; long, short, circular stroking; and so forth. Do pay attention to your partner's verbal feedback. Also, try to be aware of how you feel in the giver role. Remember that no one is a mind reader, and that it is your partner's responsibility to verbally guide you if they want something different from what you are doing.

KEGELS

Many folks have heard of learning and practicing Kegel exercises to improve continence and decrease postchildbirth vaginal wall slackness. Clients should make sure they have accurate information and instructions. I myself (S. Baird) suffered from reduced continence, 7 years after giving birth vaginally. My own pelvic floor physical therapist, Stacy Troy, MS, PT, noted that most people learn and perform Kegels inaccurately, and emphasized the importance of learning and practicing Kegel exercises correctly.

Buehler's (2022) book on sex for mental health professionals includes several pleasure-enhancing techniques. Early in the book she shares "Kegels for Everyone" as a way for people with clitorises and vaginas to develop a "greater awareness of sexual sensation and arousal, as well as improved capacity for orgasm" (p. 35). Kegels can also "improve [the] quality of [penis] erection and increase ejaculatory timing" (p. 35). Kegels involve tightening and relaxing pelvic floor muscles, often identified initially by stopping the "flow of urine" for folks with vaginas, or trying to stop gas from leaving the body, for folks with penises.

The proper exercise involves pulling up and squeezing the pelvic floor muscles for both short and longer periods. It does *not* involve practicing stopping urine midstream (although, as previously mentioned, that can be helpful to *initially* identify these muscles) nor does it involve squeezing your abdomen or butt cheeks together. The Mayo Clinic website (Mayo Clinic Staff, 2022) has a very helpful and accurate guide to performing Kegel exercises (www.mayoclinic.org/healthy-lifestyle/womens-health/in-depth/kegel-exercises/art-20045283).

"Slow Kegels" (also good for mindfulness) involve tensing the muscle group for 3 seconds, then fully relaxing for 3 seconds. Typically one performs about 10 of these squeezes for a full set, about five times a day. It is important to consult with a pelvic floor physical therapist or expert and vetted websites to ensure proper instruction. If done improperly (for instance, too much tightening, not enough relaxation), then you can make "the muscle too tight" (Buehler, 2022, p. 35).

MINDFULNESS

Buehler (2022) and Ogden (2018) both mention the importance of breath and mindfulness in both getting in touch with and increasing pleasure. Buehler offers advice for the client to first pay attention to their breath (taking slightly slower breaths), then add in more focus (helping the mind follow the body), then finally link the mind and body. Once this is established, clients can tune into "what [they] are feeling and experiencing [which] can increase arousal, emotional connection, and pleasure" (Buehler, 2022, p. 197). Clients can say to themselves, "'Breathing in, I am aware of my [sexual] body.'… 'Breathing out, I am aware of my [sexual] body'" (Buehler, 2022, p. 197). This practice can be particularly helpful during sex with another partner to help remain calm and present. Ogden discusses the neuroscience behind how "consciously regulating our own breathing (can) strengthen the neuro networks that will change our automatic breathing rhythm to support excitement, arousal, and other sex-positive attributes" (2018, p. 35)

PLEASURE

We would be remiss if we did not devote a section on the role of *pleasure* in contributing to positive sexuality, sexual health, and overall sexual functioning.

Many educators, researchers, and writers such as Debbie Herbenick (*Because It Feels Good: A Woman's Guide to Sexual Pleasure and Satisfaction,* 2009), Betty Dodson, and adrienne marie brown *(Pleasure Activism,* 2019*),* among many others, have thankfully added a focus on pleasure in their work over the last couple of decades. Sex counselor and long-time midwife Evelyn Resh, in her book *Women, Sex, Power & Pleasure* (2013), points out how a lack of pleasure overall in women's lives (she is mainly referring to ciswomen) is often correlated with overall dissatisfaction and unhappiness. In her introduction, she names her thesis of how, although countless books and articles discuss how to increase happiness, very few specifically mention the importance of "pleasure, sensuality, and sexuality" within this context as an essential ingredient.

Resh herself discusses her own solution for dealing with times when her own sexual energy is nonexistent: she returns to her belief that "pleasure begets pleasure and that in order to increase [her] pleasure quotient [she] needs to feel powerful" (2013, p. 5). For her, this equation to regain sexual interest/energy means "emotional wellness equals powerful living equals increased interest and access to all pleasures, including sex" (2013, p. 5). If she is not feeling emotionally sturdy, then she works on increasing that sturdiness and well-being.

Resh notes that for the women who state that they could care less if they ever have sex again (despite deeply loving their partners, and feeling attraction to them), she surmises the low energy is often related to trouble with one or more of what she considers the six markers of emotional well-being ("*self-confidence* and *self-esteem, health-seeking behaviors, spiritual satisfaction, creativity, resilience,* and *compassion*" [emphasis added; 2013, p. 6]). In other words, most likely one (or many) sexual brakes have been engaged for some time, to the exclusion of remembering or being in touch with sexual accelerators. Nagoski famously repeats in her books and TED Talks that "pleasure is the measure"—people are most likely to seek out (and continue to seek out) sexual activity and interaction if it feels good.

Resh further reinforces the need to keep pleasure front and center in her chapter on menopause: "when hormones decline, which all … naturally do with aging, a conscious hedonism—a genuine willingness to try new things and a good sense of humor—should take their place and is more than capable of compensating for changes in biology" (2013, p. 117).

Resh also describes something she coined *sensual atrophy syndrome* (SAS) as a marked estrangement from life's pleasures. This also ties into Emily Nagoski's discussion of Kate Manne's *human giver syndrome* from Nagoski's book on burnout (2019): a system in which one caste of people (*givers*) are expected to offer their time, attention, affection, and bodies willingly to another class of people: the *human beings.*

Constantinides et al. (2019) adapted information from Timmers et al.'s (1976) non-goal directed sexual experience to develop a *circle of sexual pleasure* to "help clients expand their own sexual possibilities and desires" (p. 52; see Figure 7.3). With client sexual pleasure in the center of the circle, different lines shoot outward, like spokes in a wheel, where clients can write the answers to these questions: "I like to _____; it feels good when _____; I get turned on when _____" (p. 51). "Each spoke is one activity or behavior that the client finds sexually arousing or pleasurable" (p. 52) and can range from connecting to sensual/erotic to sexual behaviors.

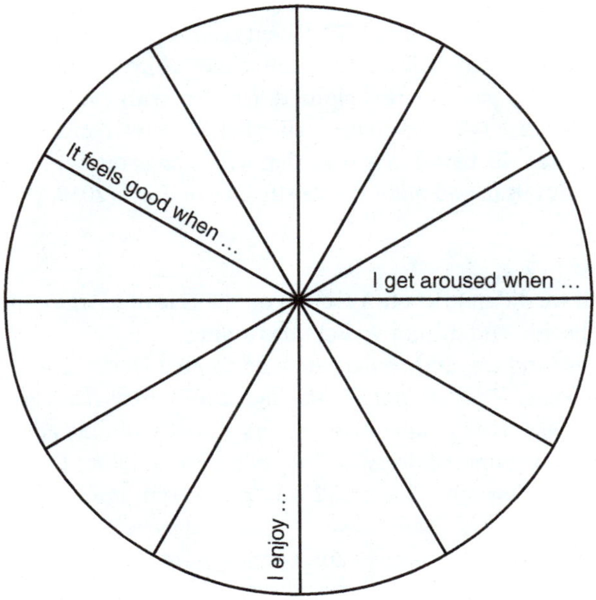

FIGURE 7.3. Circles of Pleasure

RESOURCE: STRENGTHENING A CONFIDENT AND JOYFUL SEXUAL SELF

INTRODUCTION

Emily Nagoski's helpful TED Talk, "Confidence and Joy Are the Keys to a Great Sex Life" (TED, 2016), inspired the development of this resource. This resource is also influenced by the development needs meeting strategy (DNMS) healing circle (Schmidt, 2009) and eye movement desensitization and reprocessing (EMDR) future templates (Leeds, 2016; Shapiro, 2018), and is designed to be a slightly more boundaried and potentially less explicit version of the future template Sabitha Pillai-Friedman provides within her sexual dysfunction EMDR protocol (2009).

The goal of this resource is to provide your clients with another opportunity to recognize and experience a positive sexual moment. Many humans in general, especially clients with trauma histories, do not spend much time prioritizing or focusing on their sexual health and pleasure. Experiencing this resource is a chance to slow down and allow one's neural networks to bathe in positive associations (whether from memory or fantasy).

If your client is unable to identify a positive sexual moment, that is okay; they can initially identify a positive moment from another area of life. Go through the resource two or three times, each time assisting your client in identifying something more closely approximating sexual content. Remember, this resource is appropriate for clients who actively wish to enhance a positive and joyful sexual self. If your client is not interested, do not proceed.

This resource is best facilitated toward the end of EMDR therapy when the client has reported a reduction in posttraumatic stress disorder (PTSD) symptoms and/or negative triggers to sexual material. However, any client who is relatively stable and interested in increasing a positive relationship with their sexuality may benefit from this resource. Ideally, your client is expressing a wish to gain more confidence or get more in touch with their sexual needs. Hold off on this resource if your client is actively dissociating, continues to show trouble self-regulating, or is unable to stay in the window of affective tolerance.

Good bilateral stimulation (BLS) options include the Butterfly Hug tapping, theratappers, and audio. These options allow the client to close their eyes and absorb into the experience. It is helpful to reiterate therapist/client boundaries before doing this resource. Remind the client that they are in charge of their body and can ask for a time out, report only what is comfortable, take as much distance physically as is allowable, or even move further from the video screen if this is through telehealth (but instruct them to keep their camera on).

Provide your client with the accompanying "Strengthening a Confident and Joyful Sexual Self" client worksheet ahead of time, instructing your client to follow the directions in the Preface daily between appointments. If your client has difficulty identifying and writing down their positive physical attributes, or seeing the "door to their sexual self," then more processing regarding body image and/or sexually related targets may be needed.

Anecdotally, some people who have experienced this resource reported the positive cognition automatically popping into their mind during sex. One person noted having an orgasm less than 2 minutes after the appearance of her positive cognition.

CLINICIAN SCRIPT

Based on Emily Nagoski's 2016 TED Talk "Confidence and Joy Are the Keys to a Great Sex Life"

- If difficulties arise with the event, choose another event.
- Reiterate sexual boundaries.

Preface

(Read slowly one to two sessions before planning to use the script.)

"Confidence is knowing what is true about your body. Joy is loving what is true about your body" (TED, 2016; 10:11). Some things that can help body confidence: (a) Every day look at yourself in the mirror and write down everything you like **OR** (b) for 2 minutes a day enter a calm mind-set, see the door that opens to your authentic sexual self. Shine a beacon of kindness and compassion through the door.

The Script

I. Think of a time when you had a completely positive sexual encounter (with yourself or someone else), when many or all of the skills that follow were applied. If no such encounter exists yet, think of a moment in your sexual or affectionate fantasy life, or a different moment when you felt particularly confident (perhaps with work, sports/athletics, movement, or a creative activity like art or music), or something positive you've seen or read that embodies the following skills or aspects.

When you felt many or most of these:

1. present and grounded;
2. affirmed and consenting;
3. open to new, different, and positive ways of sexually interacting;
4. in touch with your needs;
5. able to express your needs clearly;
6. in touch with pleasant physical sensations and/or smells;
7. deserving of giving and/or receiving pleasure;
8. confident;
9. desiring to share this energy in some form (i.e., journaling, art, telling an appropriate friend or therapist, or transforming this energy into other domains); and
10. perhaps spiritually connected or in "flow."

II. Have you identified a **moment from your life**, either a physical moment, or from your mind?

What emotions are you noticing for yourself? ______________________ (looking for a positive emotion)

What physical sensations go along with this moment? ______________________

Do you have an image or simple word or phrase to represent this? ______

What is a positive cognition (PC) thought we can put with this image? ______
(i.e., I'm worthy of pleasure. I'm safe as I pursue pleasure. I enjoy connection. I radiate joy.)

How true is this PC feeling right now on a scale from 1 to 7 (1 is "false," 7 is "true")? ______
Hold the PC ______ with the image/name ______.
Apply BLS (slow alternating tapping).

How true is the PC now from 1 to 7? ____ (Continue to apply BLS sets until the PC gets to a 6 or 7.)

III. Now let's go through each skill I mentioned in the beginning. I'll have you hold the positive thought with the moment and each skill. We will let each skill get strengthened, moving on to the next when you signal me. If a problem arises, let me know.

Now think of ______ (event/moment/image/name), ______ PC, notice any positive body sensation, and focus on feeling ...

1. present and grounded;
2. affirmed and consenting;
3. open to new, different, and positive ways of sexually interacting;
4. in touch with your needs;
5. able to express your needs clearly;
6. in touch with pleasant physical sensations;
7. deserving of giving and/or receiving pleasure;
8. confident;
9. desiring to share this energy in some form (i.e., journaling, art, telling an appropriate friend or therapist, or transforming this energy into other domains); and
10. perhaps spiritually connected or in "flow."

Check in with your PC ...

IV. Now imagine a desired **future** encounter, whether with yourself or someone else. Take a moment to develop the setting, determine activities, and so on. How true is the PC ______ as you imagine this scenario? (Install to a 7 using BLS sets. Once the PC is at a 7, use slower BLS and have your client take some deeper, slower breaths, staying with the scenario for half a minute or so, breathing in the positive words and sensations.)

V. *Optional:* Ask the client for a challenge that may arise in the desired future encounter.

When you think of this future encounter, are there any possible challenges that come to mind that may interfere with full enjoyment? ______

Notice and eliminate any negative physical disturbances, or strengthen any positive physical sensations with BLS.

Install the PC to a 7.

Case Study 7.3: Eliza, Strengthening Her Confident and Joyful Sexual Self

Eliza, a late-30s cisgender bicultural African American and Colombian (one parent was an immigrant from Colombia) married lesbian, had worked through all her prior EMDR targets (two were related to sexual assaults, three were related to family of origin denying her sexual orientation) and was now working on improving the quantity and quality of sexual interaction with her wife mainly through psychoeducation (both were completing *The Come as You Are Workbook* [Nagoski, 2019]). Physical boundaries between the therapist and client were reiterated. Eliza understood we could stop the resource at any time, and that she could report only what she felt comfortable articulating.

Eliza was able to note some positive physical features for herself on the days between our appointments. She also reported using her calm place (a beach in Maine) to enter in a calm mind-set and shine a beacon of kindness and compassion through it. As this was telehealth, the client worksheet had been emailed ahead of time. Eliza had printed it out and was ready to complete it as we progressed.

Eliza identified a positive sexual moment from a few years ago when she and her wife Chris were traveling. At one particular hotel in Georgia they experienced a great deal of sexual satisfaction and intense erotic connection, both very much feeling alive, free, and in flow. Eliza, very appropriately, did not go into detail, but affirmed that this was a positive sexual experience and chose to call it "Georgia hotel." The PC she chose to use was "I can capably and confidently enjoy giving and receiving pleasure." The PC started at a 5, and was able to increase to a 6.5 after two BLS rounds. She reported feeling confident and happy, noting that her sternum felt expansive and that she had butterflies in her stomach. We then combined the cue phrase ("Georgia hotel"), the PC ("I can capably and confidently enjoy giving and receiving pleasure"), and the 10 positive qualities. Eliza affirmed that each item strengthened, and reported that her PC was now at a 7.

For her future encounter, Eliza imagined a sexual encounter with Chris on a road trip at an upcoming hotel in New Hampshire. She reported easily being able to imagine details, sensations, and positive emotions. Her PC remained at a 7. As for a potential challenge, she wondered how this scenario would transpire if her wife was not interested in sex once they arrived at the hotel. We spent a few moments discussing various strategies, including conversations ahead of time to help set the tone and mood, and courting behavior Eliza might apply. We recognized that her wife often swims more in the "responsive desire" domain. As long as Chris consented to Eliza initiating courtship behaviors, there was a high chance Chris would be interested in engaging in sexual activity. Eliza reported initially feeling some tension in her sternum as we sorted through this challenge. After the strategizing, we applied BLS. Eliza noted that the tension dissipated almost immediately and that once again she felt "good" butterflies in her stomach. Her PC of "I can capably and confidently enjoy giving and receiving pleasure" was once again at a 7.

Two weeks later, Eliza reported that she and her wife indeed enjoyed a wonderful sexual experience in New Hampshire, and even continued with increased sexual activity after returning home. They continued to work on communication and awareness regarding sexual needs, feeling positive about their mutual increase in interest and concern.

SEXUAL HISTORY QUESTIONNAIRE

Jassy Casella Timberlake's multipage, open-ended *The Sexual History Questionnaire* (2019), included at the end of this chapter, is one very comprehensive tool to use with any individual, regardless of genital configuration, to help determine difficulties and pleasures. The clinician ideally asks these questions verbally to clients, or can send home sections of the questionnaire if the client seems well regulated and motivated to answer on their own. If administered verbally, it could take one to several sessions. The information gathered may generate both positive associations with their sexuality and sexual life experiences (perhaps leading to strengthening some resources), as well as potential topics for further exploration, discussion, and processing.

SUMMARY

Humans can experience many pleasures, and many difficulties, with sexual activity. The sex therapy field continues to evolve, taking into account the diverse experiences across gender, physical, cultural, spiritual, and familial background, and so on. Since Masters and Johnson, and other early researchers, many other sexologists have expanded views of sexual functioning beyond medically based origins. Schnarch, for instance, theorizes that greater differentiation of partners' identity supports increased sexual satisfaction. Intersystems theory promotes understanding of sexual difficulties from a multiprong approach. The new view of women's sexual problems is another comprehensive approach assessing factors impacting all genders, including lack of information, access, interest, energy, or time; erotophobic attitudes; and so on.

The Sexual History Questionnaire (Timberlake, 2019) is one tool to help obtain a comprehensive client sexual health history.

Sensate focus is an enduring important and helpful tool that sex therapists often prescribe to help clients increase awareness of sensation and communication with their partner. Many other resources exist to help individuals increase their capacity for sexual pleasure, including Kegels, breathing, mindfulness, creating a sexy context (whether in one's mind or environment), good communication with oneself and partner(s), and nondemand sensual time. Taking care of one's physical body can also improve sexual response and pleasure.

There are many conditions which help create good, great, and/or magnificent sex for all genders. It is helpful to know what they are for oneself, and communicate needs to others.

A new resource, "Strengthening a Confident and Joyful Sexual Self," provides your clients with another opportunity to access, recognize, and experience a positive sexual moment (whether from their life or imagination). This resource is a chance to slow down and allow one's neural networks to bathe in positive associations.

DISCUSSION QUESTIONS

- How have modern sex therapy frameworks evolved to encompass broader models that better describe sexuality across different populations and social contexts?
- What are the limitations of the traditional approaches to sex therapy that were based on a model of sexual arousal by Masters and Johnson and how have later models addressed these limitations?
- In what ways do culturally determined conceptions of sexuality impact our understanding of sexual health and the treatment of sexual problems in therapy?

LEARNING ACTIVITIES

CourseConnect

To access self-assessment questions and interactive, competency-based learning activities for this chapter, visit www.springerpub.com/courseconnect. See inside front cover and tear-out card for CourseConnect details.

ADDITIONAL RESOURCES

Additional resources are online and available at www.springerpub.com/courseconnect.

REFERENCES

American Psychiatric Association. (2013). *Diagnostic and statistical manual of mental disorders* (5th ed.). https://doi.org/10.1176/appi.books.9780890425596

Basson, R. (2002). Women's sexual desire—Disordered or misunderstood? *Journal of Sex Marital Therapy, 28*(Suppl. 1), 17–28. https://doi.org/10.1080/00926230252851168

brown, a. m. (2019). *Pleasure activism: The politics of feeling good.* AK Press.

Buehler, S. (2022). *What every mental health professional needs to know about sex* (3rd ed.). Springer Publishing Company.

Constantinides, D. M., Sennott, S. L., & Chandler, D. (2019). *Sex therapy with erotically marginalized clients: Nine principles of clinical support.* Routledge.

Federation of Feminist Women's Health Centers. (1981). *A new view of a woman's body: A fully illustrated guide* (Illustrated by S. Gage).

Herbenick, D. (2009). *Because it feels good: A woman's guide to sexual pleasure and satisfaction.* Author.

Hertlein, K. M., Gambescia, N., & Weeks, G. R. (Eds.). (2019). *Systemic sex therapy* (3rd ed.). Routledge.

Kaplan, H. (1979). *Disorders of sexual desire.* Brunner/Mazel.

Kaschak, E., & Tiefer, L. (Eds.). (2002). *A new view of women's sexual problems.* Haworth Press [manifesto on pp. 1–8, also available online: http://www.newviewcampaign.org/manifesto3.asp].

Kleinplatz, P., & Menard, A. (2020) *Magnificent sex: Lessons from extraordinary lovers.* Routledge.

Laumann, E., Paik, A., & Rosen, R. C. (1999). Sexual dysfunction in the United States: Prevalence and predictors. *JAMA: Journal of the American Medical Association, 281*(6), 537–544. https://doi.org/10.1001/jama.281.6.537

Leeds, A. (2016). *A guide to the standard EMDR therapy protocols for clinicians, supervisors, and consultants* (2nd ed.). Springer Publishing.

Linschoten, M., Weiner, L., & Avery-Clark, C. (2016). Sensate focus: A critical literature review. *Sexual and Relationship Therapy, 31*(2), 230–247. https://doi.org/10.1080/14681994.2015.1127909

Loulan, J. (1984). *Lesbian sex.* Spinsters Ink.

Magon, N., Chauhan, M., Malik, S., & Shah, D. (2012). Sexuality in midlife: Where the passion goes? *Journal of Mid-lLfe Health, 3*(2), 61–65. https://doi.org/10.4103/0976-7800.104452

Masters, W., & Johnson, V. (1966). *Human sexual response.* Little, Brown.

Masters, W., & Johnson, V. (1970). *Human sexual inadequacy.* Little, Brown.

Masters, W., Johnson, A., & Kolodny, L. (1979). *Textbook of sexual medicine.* Little, Brown.

Mayo Clinic Staff. (2022). *Kegel exercises: A how-to guide for women.* Retrieved August 24, 2024, from https://www.mayoclinic.org/healthy-lifestyle/womens-health/in-depth/kegel-exercises/art-20045283

McCormick, N. B. (1994). *Sexual salvation: Affirming women's sexual rights and pleasures.* Praeger.

Nagoski, E. (2019). *The come as you are workbook: A practical guide to the science of sex.* Simon & Schuster.

Nagoski, E., & Nagoski, A. (2019). *Burnout: The secret to unlocking the stress cycle.* Random House.

Ogden, G. (2018). *Expanding the practice of sex therapy: The neuro update edition* (2nd ed.). Routledge.

Perelman, M. (2014). The history of sexual medicine. In D. L. Tolman & L. M. Diamond (Eds.), *APA handbook of sexuality and psychology: Vol. 2. Contextual approaches* (pp. 137–179). American Psychological Association.

Perelman, M. (2024). Reframing the bio-psychosocial model. For sexual medicine. *Journal of Sexual Medicine, 21*(Suppl. 1), qdae001.341. https://doi.org/10.1093/jsxmed/qdae001.341

Pillai-Friedman, S. (2009). Sexual dysfunction EMDR protocol. In M. Luber (Ed.), *Eye movement desensitization and reprocessing (EMDR) scripted protocols: Special populations* (pp. 151–166). Springer Publishing Company.

Resh, E. (2013). *Women, sex, power & pleasure.* Hay House.

Schmidt, S. J. (2009). *The developmental needs meeting strategy: An ego state therapy for healing adults with childhood trauma and attachment wounds.* DNMS Institute.

Shapiro, F. (2018). *Eye movement desensitization and reprocessing (EMDR) therapy, third edition: Basic principles, protocols, and procedures.* Guilford Press.

Schnarch, D., & Regas, S. (2012). The crucible differentiation scale: Assessing differentiation in human relationships. *Journal of Marital and Family Therapy, 38*(4), 639–652. https://doi.org/10.1111/j.1752-0606.2011.00259.x

Stephenson, K. R., Rellini, A. H., & Meston, C. M. (2013). Relationship satisfaction as a predictor of treatment response during cognitive behavioral sex therapy. *Archives of Sexual Behavior, 42*(1), 143–152. https://doi.org/10.1007/s10508-012-9961-3

Stock, W. (n.d.). *Sensate focus instructions* (unpublished handout).

TED. (2016, February 12). *Confidence and joy are the keys to a great sex life | Emily Nagoski* [Video]. YouTube. https://www.youtube.com/watch?v=HILY0wWBlBM

Tiefer, L. (1988). A feminist perspective on sexology and sexuality. In M. Gergen (Ed.), *Feminist thought and the structure of knowledge* (pp. 16–26). NYU Press.

Tiefer, L. (1996). Toward a feminist sex therapy. *Women & Therapy, 19*(4), 53–64. https://doi.org/10.1300/J015v19n04_07

Timberlake, J. C. (2019). *The sexual history questionnaire.* New England Sex Therapy.

Timmers, R. L., Sinclair, L. G., & James, J. R. (1976). Treating goal-directed intimacy. *Social Work, 21*(5), 401–402. https://doi.org/10.1093/sw/21.5.401

Zilbergeld, B. (1992). *The new male sexuality: The truth about men, sex, and pleasure.* Bantam Books.

SUPPLEMENTAL MATERIALS FOR CLINICIANS AND CLIENTS

For PDF versions of this material, access the "Downloads" feature on Course Connect (www.springerpub.com/courseconnect).

Sexual History Questionnaire

By Jassy Casella Timberlake

New England SexTherapy, LLC

newenglandsextherapy.com

Client Name:

Date(s) of Administration:

CURRENT CONCERN

What prompted you to come at this point for therapy?

Who initiated seeking therapy?

Have you seen therapists previously? What were your experiences with these professionals?

DESIRED OUTCOME

What is your primary goal for our work together?

If therapy is successful, what will you be able to do that you are unable to do now?

How will this change anything in your current life, relationship, personality, or partner's personality?

What significance does the problem have with respect to your own sexual functioning? How does the problem affect your partner's sexual functioning?

HISTORY OF CONCERN

When did the problem first occur? What was happening in your life at that time?

(If there is more than one problem, or both/all partners have a problem): Which problem do you recall as having developed first?

Is there any situation in which the problem improves?

When does the problem occur? Is there anything that makes it worse?

SEXUAL HISTORY

Contact with other children:

As a child, did you engage in sexual play or exploration with other children? Describe where and how you did this.

How often did you do this?

Who initiated these games? What role(s) did you play?

How did you feel about doing this?

Were you ever caught doing this? What happened?

What was your major source for information about sex?

In what ways has your religion and family background influenced your attitudes toward sex? Were you allowed to ask questions?

What was the age of your first sexual feeling (in whatever way you define that)?

MASTURBATION

At what age did you first experiment with masturbation? How old were you when you first masturbated? Where were you and what did you do?

With what frequency did you masturbate in your teens?

How did you learn about masturbation?

How did you feel about masturbation?

What techniques have you used for masturbation?

How often do you currently masturbate?

Are you able to talk with your partner about self-pleasuring/masturbation?

UNWELCOME SEXUAL CONTACT/ABUSIVE BEHAVIORS

As a child, did anyone ever touch you, or make you touch them, in a way that made you uncomfortable either at the time or looking back on it now?

Did anyone ever make sexual comments to you or comment on your body in a way that made you uncomfortable, then or now?

Did you have any sexual contact with adolescents or adults? Were you forced or coerced to have sex against your will?

Did you ever sexually touch other children your own age in a way that was upsetting to them at the time? Were you aware that what you were doing might be upsetting?

What words or label do you use to describe these experiences?

Did you ever tell anyone else about any of these experiences? What happened when you did?

Was there ever hitting, biting, pushing, shoving, slapping, or other physical aggression toward you, siblings, or a parent in your home? Could you describe this?

Were there any upsetting experiences related to sex as a child that we have not discussed? If so, could you describe them?

PUBERTY AND ADOLESCENCE (AGES 10–20)

Body changes for adolescents assigned female at birth:

When did you first notice your breasts beginning to develop? Were you the first person to notice? How did it come to your attention?

Did you experience breast development earlier, later, or about the same as most of your friends?

How did you feel about your developing breasts? How did others react?

Did you have erotic dreams as an adolescent? If yes, was there a theme to them? When did you begin to menstruate? Describe the circumstances when it first occurred.

Had you been taught about menstruation in advance? By whom?

Was this information shared with one or more family members? With whom?

Was it discussed among your friends? What were your feelings about the possibility of beginning to menstruate? Were you earlier, later, or about the same as most of your friends?

Did you develop a regular menstrual cycle? How long did this take? Have you had any menstrual difficulties?

Have you had sex during your period, or during the period of a partner who menstruates? How do you feel about this?

How did you feel when you first learned that some people have nocturnal emissions ("wet dreams")?

Body changes for adolescents assigned male at birth:

How old were you when your voice began to change? How did you feel about it? How long did it take to settle into your adult range?

How old were you when you had your first nocturnal emission ("wet dream")? How did you react? Had you been taught about these in advance? By whom?

Was this information shared with one or more family members? With whom? Did you take steps to conceal the evidence of your wet dreams?

Did you have any problems with the developments of puberty?

How did you feel when you first learned that some people have menstrual periods?

Have you ever had sex with someone who menstruates while they were having their period?

How do you feel about this idea?

Body changes for all:

How and when did your body change during puberty?

How did you feel about these changes?

Were these changes what you expected or hoped for?

How did you feel about your height, weight, hair, skin?

How are your feelings about your body connected to your race, ethnicity, culture, and so on? Did you engage in attempts to change or control your weight while you were growing up?

How did you feel about this? How was your family involved in noticing, commenting on, or trying to control your weight?

Did the body changes you experienced during adolescence bring up any concerns for you about your gender identity or gender presentation?

ADOLESCENT DATING BEHAVIOR

How would you describe your junior/senior high school social life? Were most of your friends male, female, or other genders?

At what age did you start to notice the sexual development of your peers? How did you feel about it?

At what age did you start to date? In groups? On single dates? Did you date same sex partners, different sex partners, or a variety? Did your parents allow dating or did you have to take steps to conceal it?

How did you feel about the dating behavior of your peers?

Did you date many different people or did you usually have a steady relationship with one person at a time? How old were you when you had your first steady relationship? How old was your partner, and what was their gender?

How did your social life change when you left home or went to college?

ADOLESCENT GENDER JOURNEY

How did your sense of your gender change, stabilize, or evolve during adolescence?

Did you talk to anyone about the thoughts and feelings you were having about your gender? How did they respond?

How did you cope with any negative or confused feelings you had about your gender during this time? Did you seek any medical or counseling support? What was that experience like?

Did your behaviors and gender presentation during adolescence match with the expectations those around you had for someone of the gender assigned to you? If yes, what was that like for you? If no, what was that like for you?

Were you ever targeted for harassment or violence because of your gender or gender presentation in adolescence?

Did anyone ever suggest that the adults in your life should try to change or affirm your gender presentation and/or gender identity? What happened?

FOR SEXUAL AND GENDER MINORITY CLIENTS

At what age did you first begin to identify yourself as potentially "different" in terms of your sexuality or gender?

At what age did you become aware of others who might be like you?

At what age did you acknowledge that you might be [your sexual orientation], or [your gender]? At what age did you decide to tell someone else? Whom did you choose to tell first? How did they respond? What was that like for you?

Can you talk about what the process of coming out to yourself and others was like during adolescence? Who knew and who did not know?

How did your close friends respond if and when they knew?

How did people in your school environment respond if and when they knew? Were you ever the victim of intimidation or violence at school? Who could you talk to about this?

Who else was supportive of you during this time?

How was your family life affected by your sexual or gender identity?

Were you able to date and engage in sexual activity with partners of your preferred gender(s)?

How were you able to express your sexual or gender identity at this time? What was it like to live in your community as a sexual or gender minority?

What else should I know about your experiences with sexuality and gender as an adolescent?

ADULT GENDER JOURNEY

How has your sense of your gender changed, stabilized, or evolved during adulthood?

Have you talked to anyone about the thoughts and feelings you were having about your gender? How did they respond?

How have you coped with any negative or confused feelings you have/had about your gender during adulthood? Did you seek any medical or counseling support? What was that experience like?

Have your behaviors and gender presentation during adulthood matched with the expectations those around you had for someone of the gender assigned to you? If yes, what was that like for you? If no, what was that like for you?

Have you ever been targeted for harassment or violence because of your gender or gender presentation in adulthood?

Did anyone ever suggest that you should try to change or affirm your gender presentation and/or gender identity? What happened?

At this time, do you have any desire to change anything about your lived gender identity or your gender presentation? What, if anything, do you think you might do about that?

UNWELCOME SEXUAL CONTACT/ABUSIVE BEHAVIORS

As an adolescent, did anyone ever touch you, or make you touch them, in a way that made you uncomfortable either at the time or looking back on it now?

Did anyone ever make sexual comments to you or comment on your body in a way that made you uncomfortable, then or now?

Did you have any sexual contact that you did not want at the time?

Were you forced or coerced to have sex against your will?

Did you ever feel taken advantage of sexually?

Did you ever sexually touch other adolescents in a way which was upsetting to them at the time?

Were you aware that what you were doing might be upsetting?

What words or labels do you use to describe these experiences?

Did you ever tell anyone else about any of these experiences? What happened when you did?

Was there ever hitting, biting, pushing, shoving, slapping, or other physical aggression toward you from an intimate partner? Could you describe this?

Were there any upsetting experiences related to sex as an adolescent that we have not discussed? If so, could you describe them?

ADULTHOOD (AGE 20 TO PRESENT)

Current attitudes toward sex:

How would you describe your attitude toward sex and your own sexuality at present?

What specific aspects of sex are enjoyable to you?

What aspects do you dislike or find unpleasant?

Is there anything about your current sexual life that causes you to feel guilty or distressed? What are your beliefs about the purpose of sex?

How important is sexual pleasure?

How important is procreation?

What is the importance of sex in your life?

What is your current attitude toward each of the following:

- Your genitals, your partner's(') genitals
- Menstruation
- Vaginal secretions
- Semen
- Masturbation
- Fellatio ("blowjobs")
- Cunnilingus ("eating pussy")
- Foreplay
- Penetrative sex
- Anal penetration or intercourse
- Sexual fantasy
- Adult films/pornography
- Erotic literature
- Sex toys
- Nudity
- Bondage and discipline, dominance and submission, sadism, and masochism

FANTASY

Have your fantasies changed significantly over the course of your adult life? How frequently do you engage in sexual fantasy currently?

What kinds of fantasies are most frequent for you at this time?

Are you comfortable with the content of your fantasies?

Who can you share your sexual fantasies with?

MENOPAUSE

Type of hormone supplement used, if any: ___________

For how long? Was it prescribed or over the counter?

What are any concerns you may have about being pre-/peri-/postmenopausal?

ORGASM

What have been your experiences with orgasm?

Alone?

With a partner?

Would time seem wasted without an orgasm with a partner?

BODY IMAGE

How did and how do you feel about your body? Please talk about how you felt as a child, growing up, as a young adult, and now.

How would you *like* to feel about your body?

Does the way you feel about your body impact your enjoyment of sex?

PAINFUL SEX

Have you ever experienced pain during sex play?

If yes, please describe the nature of that pain.

What have you done to address this issue?

HISTORY OF SEXUAL EXPERIENCES AND RELATIONSHIPS

Describe the history of your sexual relationships. Talk about the number of partners, what sexual activities you have experienced, and the issues and conflicts that have emerged for you in intimate relationships. If you have had a "type" please describe that type:

IF CURRENTLY PARTNERED

How many emotional partners do you have? How many sexual partners? How do you define the boundaries of your current relationship(s)?

What label(s) do you use to describe the relationship(s)?

If you are in a current relationship, how often do you and your partner(s) have affectionate nonsexual contact? Is that enough for you? For your partner(s)?

How attractive do you think you are on a scale of 1 to 10? _____

How attracted are you to your partner(s) on a scale of 1 to 10? _____

How attracted do you think your partner(s) is/are to you?

How do you feel about your own body?

If you are in a relationship, how do you feel about your partner(s)' body(ies)? How do you imagine your partner(s) feel(s) about your body?

How are these feelings communicated?

Are you ever criticized or shamed by a partner about your body?

Does anyone in your life try to control how your body looks?

How comfortable are you with your sexual orientation?

Have you ever thought you might like to have a relationship or sexual contact with someone of another gender?

Have you discussed this with anyone?

Is it something you have seriously considered acting on?

Have any of your partners experienced such feelings?

How has this affected the relationship?

How much conflict is there in your relationship(s)? How well do you each deal with conflict?

What kinds of stressors are you experiencing currently in your lives that might affect your sexual or emotional relationship(s)?

If you are currently in a long-standing relationship, how has sex changed over the course of the relationship?

Why do you think it has changed?

How do you and your partner(s) feel about this?

If you are currently in a long-standing relationship, have you ever been sexually involved with another person outside of the boundaries of the relationship(s)?

How many times? For how long?

How did you feel about this?

Did your partner(s) know about the outside relationship?

What effect has this activity had on your relationship(s)?

What was the purpose or meaning of the outside sexual activity?

Has/have your partner(s) ever been sexually involved with another person outside the boundaries of the relationship?

Did you know about it at the time? How did you feel about this?

What effect has this activity had on your relationship(s)?

What was the purpose or meaning of the outside sexual activity?

Describe any feelings you may have about having sexual contact with your present or possible sexual partner(s).

Describe your present sexual interactions, such as penetrative sex or masturbation, turn ons, your present pattern for sexual pleasure, frequency of sexual interactions, your current number of partners, and so on. (Do partners cuddle, hug, spoon, kiss hello/goodbye. Who initiates what kinds of touch?)

Do you feel you most often "give your best" when having sex with your partner(s)?

Are you proud of the way you express your feelings toward your partner(s) at this time? If not, what's missing in your opinion?

Do you WANT your partner(s) during sex or just "want sex"?

Do you WANT to be aroused and involved sexually?

What would you like from an ideal sexual partner, or your current partner? What would you be willing to give to such a partner?

Do you tell your partner what pleases you most sexually? What displeases you?

What do you want most in the way of attitude, behaviors, and so on from your partner that they do not provide you now?

What attitudes or behaviors do you receive from your partner that you value the most?

What attracts, excites, and stimulates you sexually? Describe the situation you find most desirable and stimulating for being sexual?

What trait, behavior, or habit does your partner have which tends to diminish your sexual feeling for them?

Are you interested in sexual practices that include power and pain play, that is, dominance/submission/bondage?

Do you look at pornography? If so, with what frequency? Do you use pornography to masturbate? What kinds of pornography do you enjoy?

Specific sexual acts:

Do you or your partner have sex with more than one person at a time? If yes, do you usually do so together, or separately?

Do you ever use sex toys during your sexual activity? What kind, and how do you use them? How often?

Do you read erotic or pornographic books or magazines, or watch adult erotic or pornographic videos?

How often?

Is/are your partner(s) aware of this? How do they feel about it?

Do you ever share these materials with your partner(s)?

Do you visit adult websites? How often?

What activities do you engage in online?

Is/are your partner(s) aware of this?

How do they feel about it?

How do you feel about your partner's(') use of erotic or pornographic materials or adult websites?

Do you or your partner(s) ever prefer to dress in certain clothing (such as clothing of another gender or costumes) or materials (such as rubber or leather) for the purposes of sexual enhancement?

Who else knows about this?

How does this affect the relationship?

Do you engage in activities that you would describe as "kinky"? What activities? Describe them. How often do you engage in them (bondage and discipline, dominance and submission, sadism, and masochism)?

How do you feel about this activity?

Is/are your partner(s) aware of this? How do they feel about it?

Do they engage in these activities with you?

Have you ever engaged in sexual activities for money, including exotic dancing, posing for photos, engaging in sexual acts, working a phone sex line, engaging in online sexual activities?

For how long? How often?

Describe what activities you engaged in.

How do you feel about this activity?

Is your partner aware of this? How do they feel about it?

Have you ever paid money for sexual activities or services, including hiring an escort, hiring a sex worker or prostitute, "erotic massage with release," purchasing subscriptions to adult websites, phone sex lines, paying for bondage and discipline, dominance and submission, sadism and masochism activities?

How often? How do you feel about this activity?

Is your partner aware of this? How do they feel about it?

Are there other specific activities I have not asked about that are an important part of your sexual life?

ALCOHOL/SUBSTANCE USE

How often and how much do you (and does your partner) drink/use?

Do either you or your partner smoke? How much?

Do you use recreational drugs? What kinds, how much, and how often? Have you ever had a blackout or memory loss while drinking/using?

SEXUAL HEALTH

Are you currently seeing a body worker (e.g., chiropractor, acupuncturist, phsyical therapist)?

If yes, please describe the nature of your physical discomfort:

Do you have any preexisting medical conditions that may affect your sexuality (e.g., diabetes, hypertension, heart disease)? Are you currently taking any prescribed medications (such as for hypertension, diabetes, depression, anxiety, or cardiovascular disease)? If yes, list: ____________________

What medications or drugs, including over the counter drugs and herbal supplements, do you use?

How has HIV/AIDS or other sexually transmitted infections impacted your sexual activity?

Do you know about safer sex practices? To what extent do you engage in safer sex? Why or why not?

Have you or your partner(s) ever experienced an unwanted pregnancy? What happened?

How was the decision made about what to do?

How do you feel about that?

Do you have any worries or concerns about your sexual health and well-being as an adult?

Who can you go to for information or feedback?

Do you have any disabilities or other physical or mental conditions that affect your ability to function sexually?

Do you require assistance from a partner or caregiver in order to participate in sexual activity with yourself or a partner?

Are you able to get assistance when you need it?

Do you have sufficient privacy and adaptive equipment for the sexual activities you want to engage in?

Are you noticing any effects of aging on your body and your sexual activity?

Any other information

Describe anything else related to your past or present experiences. Include anything that may be important for me to know, so that I may assist you in reaching your sexual goals.

Strengthening a Confident and Joyful Sexual Self

By Stephanie Baird, LMHC

(adapted and inspired by Emily Nagoski's TED Talk "Confidence and Joy Are the Keys to a Great Sex Life")

Preface: "Confidence is knowing what is true about your body. Joy is loving what is true about your body." Some things that can help body confidence: (a) Every day, look at yourself in the mirror and write down everything you like. (b) For 2 minutes a day, enter your calm place, and see the door that opens to your authentic sexual self. Shine a beacon of kindness and compassion through the door.

I. **List of desired qualities in a positive experience (ideally sexual, but can be affectional, work-related, sensual, athletic, creative, etc.):**

1. present and grounded;
2. affirmed and consenting;
3. open to new, different, and positive ways of sexually interacting;
4. in touch with your needs;
5. able to express your needs clearly;
6. in touch with pleasant physical sensations and/or smells;
7. deserving of giving and/or receiving pleasure;
8. confident;
9. desiring to share this energy in some form (i.e., journaling, art, telling an appropriate friend or therapist, or transforming this energy into other domains); and
10. perhaps spiritually connected or in "flow."

II. Identify a completely positive (sensual/erotic, if possible) **moment from your life**, either a physical moment, from your imagination, or something you've seen or read. **STOP here for now.**

Think of an image, word, or symbol to represent this (write or draw in this box):

What emotion are you noticing ___________ and where/how is that emotion in the body_______ ?

What positive cognition (PC) can we put with this image? ____________________ (i.e., I'm worthy of pleasure. I'm safe as I pursue pleasure. I enjoy connection. I radiate joy.)

Hold the cue word with the PC:

Cue word:	+	PC:

How true is the PC from 1 to 7? ____.

III. Now think of ______________ (cue word), your PC ______________________________, notice any positive body sensation, and focus on ... (a few of the previously listed 10 qualities), with slow BLS.

IV. Now imagine a desired **future** encounter, whether with yourself or someone else. Take a moment to develop the setting, determine activities, and so on.

____

How true is the PC ______________ as you imagine this scenario? Add BLS until completely true.

CHAPTER 8

Vulvar, Vaginal, and Pelvic Sexual Dysfunctions, Disorders, and Treatment

Wendy Stock, Katherine Hertlein, and Stephanie Baird

LEARNING OBJECTIVES

- Learn about vulva- and vaginal-related sexual disorders as well as a variety of treatment strategies related to desire disorders and arousal disorders.
- Learn about vulva- and vaginal-related orgasm disorders (preorgasmic, situationally orgasmic).
- Learn about the persistent orgasm gap and corrective psychoeducation.
- Learn about vulva- and vaginal-related genito-pelvic pain penetration disorder (e.g., vaginismus, dyspaurenia), as well as other pain disorders and difficulties (e.g., sex headaches).

INTRODUCTION

Several models of sexual arousal have been developed to address the diversity through which people incorporate cognitive, social, and biological factors in the process of arousal (Basson, 2002; Walen & Roth, 1987). There is also literature that suggests that people are different in their propensity toward arousal: that is, some people are more prone to be aroused than others. The work of Michael Perelman and Andrew Goldstein (Lipshultz et al., 2016) highlights the complex interplay of what contributes to arousal and what detracts from it. Perelman's (2018) approach is known as the sexual tipping point. This approach helps individuals and partners determine what factors turn each person on, what factors turn each person off, and how to organize those factors so that one can have satisfying sexual experiences.

Sexual dysfunctions are embedded in social and relational contexts, including those with a history of sexual trauma. The following diagnostic and treatment strategies and protocols must be understood and implemented with the requirement of having already conducted the broader, contextual assessment practices described earlier in this text. The focus in the following is primarily on treatment techniques, predicated on completion of a thorough assessment. Using these methods presupposes that treatment of other conditions has occurred (e.g., unprocessed sexual trauma, severe depression) that could interfere with treatment of sexual problems.

Additionally, while many of the titles of these disorders are gendered, it is understood that transgender individuals that possess relevant anatomy and genitalia (e.g., a transmale who possesses a clitoris), or intersex folks with different combinations, may also experience these issues.

(MALE) HYPOACTIVE SEXUAL DESIRE DISORDER

DIAGNOSIS AND DESCRIPTION

Sexual desire, often referred to (inaccurately) as *sex drive* or *libido*, includes interest in sexual stimuli, wishing for sexual activity, planning for sexual activity, or feeling frustrated when sexual activity does not occur. Many clinicians are using the words *desire* or *sexual interest*, as these words indicate a more temporal state, rather than a permanent or "innate" trait suggested by "drive."

The *Diagnostic and Statistical Manual of Mental Disorders* (5th ed.; *DSM-5;* American Psychiatric Association [APA], 2013) defines Male Hypoactive Sexual Desire Disorder (HSDD) as persistent or recurrently deficient sexual or erotic thoughts, fantasies, and desire for sexual activity that has persisted for a minimum of 6 months and causes significant distress to the person experiencing these symptoms.

The *DSM-5* has controversially combined desire and arousal diagnoses for people with vaginas and termed them Female Sexual Arousal and Interest Disorders. To clarify, the *DSM-5* term that was used in previous versions of the *DSM*, Hypoactive Sexual Desire Disorder (which included all genders), now only refers to desire disorders for people with penises (now termed Male Hypoactive Desire Disorder; APA, 2013). It has been argued that this amalgamation of these two diagnoses is not supported by empirical findings (Althof et al., 2017). For purposes of this chapter, desire and arousal disorders will be considered separately.

Many people reporting low desire function quite well sexually by all objective criteria, yet they have no subjective experience of sexual desire. Individuals presenting for treatment of low sexual desire can be characterized as "wanting to want" sex. Low desire can be either global or situational. Some clients have sexual desire but do not want to sexually engage with their partner, yet still masturbate regularly. Others do not experience any sexual urges, reporting few or no sexual thoughts or fantasies. Still others may identify as asexual or greysexual, and may simply need permission to embrace this identity.

Biological/Psychopharmacological Factors

Many factors can influence a lower desire and *must* be addressed before implementing specific techniques designed to increase sexual desire. Some factors include hormonal influences (e.g., age-related/postmenopausal decrease in estrogen or testosterone, lower level of testosterone, elevated prolactin during nursing that can dramatically decrease desire), medication side effects (such as effects from selective serotonin reuptake inhibitors [SSRIs] and serotonin-norepinephrine reuptake inhibitors [SNRIs]), medical conditions or treatments, and/or substance abuse.

Individual Factors

Individual factors not included in the category of biological factors include history of trauma and psychological functioning. For example, a history of untreated trauma or abuse can result in the client having intrusive thoughts or "flashbacks" at any point in the sexual response cycle, including arousal, engagement in sexual activity, and during reflection after the sexual activity. On the other hand, the impact of one's mood and mood disorders such as depression or anxiety on sexual desire can result in varied impact on desire, with depression and anxiety being related to less desire in some cases and being related to more desire in other cases (Bittoni & Kiesner, 2022).

Relational Factors

Societal, conjoint, and cultural background can play a role in decreased desire (sexual norms often socialize women to believe that desiring sex is wrong or sinful, resulting in guilt and shame). Relationship conflict and/or poor or absent communication can also impede desire and interest. In addition, relationship factors impact sexual desire and affect willingness to participate in sex. The prevalence rate of low sexual desire in ciswomen is high, reaching 43% (Kingsberg & Rezaee, 2013). Desire is often embedded in a relational context, and it is important to attend to the underlying motivational forces that trigger it. For example, having children and being in a longer relationship are often associated with lower levels of desire. Differentiation of self is another factor related to desire, with the presumption that partners who are well-differentiated can emotionally regulate, handle conflict better, and provide protection in the relationship against desire problems (Ferreira et al., 2016).

TREATMENT AND INTERVENTION STRATEGIES

For all of the treatment methods that follow, it can be helpful to consider the dual control model of sexual interest, that is, helping the client identify their sexual inhibition system (brakes) and sexual excitation system brakes (accelerators). Once the client can identify brakes getting in the way of potential sexual interest, the treatment strategies that follow may help to reduce or eliminate any specific situational or low-level chronic brakes (e.g., overwork, ongoing stress, prior interfering traumatic material, relational conflict). Additionally, while it may be relatively easy to pinpoint circumstances blocking sexual interest, it may be more difficult for some clients to identify potential sexual accelerators. They may need permission to engage in fantasy and solo exploration to help identify interest-generating context and material (i.e., what they consider a "sexy context").

Cognitive Behavioral Therapy Treatment Strategies and Tools

Cognitive behavioral therapy (CBT) treatment for clients with low sexual desire generally focus on a "priming" effect of increasing the frequency of sexual thoughts, fantasies, and awareness of sexual stimuli via a desire diary, desire checklist, priming the pump (seek out erotic material), fantasy time-outs during the day, scheduling sex, and so on. Additionally, most recent writing about sex emphasizes the importance of experiencing and centering pleasure as a way to continue to increase interest in pleasurable activities: "pleasure is the measure" (and pleasure begets more pleasure).

Relational Factors in Creating/Increasing Sexual Desire/Interest

Sexual desire is often embedded in a relational context, and it is important to attend to the underlying motivational forces that trigger it. Basson's (2002) nonlinear model of sexual response, discussed in Chapter 3, is circular, rather than the traditional linear model of sexual response. Her model incorporates the need for intimacy, and acknowledges that desire can be responsive or spontaneous, and may occur either before or after arousal.

Prekatsounaki et al. (2019), in a survey of 662 heterosexual cisgender women, identified three specific factors for ciswomen that corelate with a greater likelihood of increased sexual desire for a partner: *intimacy*, *celebrated otherness*, and *object-of-desire affirmation*. Increased levels of all three factors within the relationship were associated with the subject having more sexual desire for their partner. These results lend support to Basson's nonlinear model of sexual arousal.

Intimacy refers to feelings of closeness, deep involvement, and affection for the partner that create the conditions for desire because of emotional connection. Couples/relationship therapy can address increasing the quality of communication and emotional intimacy.

Celebrated otherness refers to the sense of personal autonomy in a relationship, of perceiving your partner as different and exciting, in contrast to the experience of fusion or enmeshment. Therapy (individual and couples/relationship) can address issues of overenmeshment and promote differentiation in the relationship. Differentiation can include helping clients develop and increase alone time and space, individual interests and friendships, and their relationship with themselves, as that has often become submerged in the primary relationship and family systems. This issue is particularly common among people socialized as women, who continue to assume more responsibility in the caretaking of family members and management of the household, regardless of outside employment.

Object-of-desire affirmation, the confirmation that someone feels they are viewed as attractive and desirable by their partner, was found to be the most significant factor determining desire for people with vulvas. Clinical implications following from this research would include addressing body image issues and encouraging verbal expression of interest and appreciation of the attractiveness of one's partner.

Systemic Treatment Strategies and Tools

Systemic treatment refers to the types of interventions that focus on the multiple systems. In the case of HSDD, treatments can be implemented across biological systems such as the incorporation of hormone replacement therapy and increasing testosterone levels (Gambescia et al., 2021). Cognitive work can focus on maladaptive schemas and learning to redirect one's focus away from arousal. Relational strategies include communication training, relationship skill-building, and conflict resolution (Meana & Steiner, 2014).

Eye Movement Desensitization and Reprocessing Therapy Treatment Strategies and Tools

As eye movement desensitization and reprocessing (EMDR) therapy follows a similar eight-phase protocol to process distressing, disturbing, or traumatic events and/or symptoms, more detail will be provided toward the end of this chapter. For EMDR therapy specific to low desire, targets regarding sexual desire shame, erotophobic beliefs and messages, prior history of trauma or abuse, and relationship conflict, anxiety, or stress may help reduce blocks to sexual desire.

FEMALE SEXUAL AROUSAL DISORDER

DIAGNOSIS AND DESCRIPTION

Female sexual arousal disorder (FSAD; considered separately from male hypoactive sexual desire here) is described as absent or reduced sexual excitement or pleasure in most sexual encounters, absent or reduced internal or external "sexual cues," and absent or reduced genital or nongenital sensations during sexual activity in all or mostly all sexual encounters. These symptoms must cause clinically significant distress for the person experiencing these symptoms, and have persisted for a minimum of 6 months.

FSAD has some unique features that differ from male HSDD. Sometimes FSAD co-occurs with reduced or absent sexual desire, but in other cases it exists as a separate entity. For example, a client may report that they are quite interested in having a sexual interaction, or that they attempted to masturbate, but that despite sufficient stimulation there was diminished or no genital arousal response. This can be frustrating for the individual who is interested and willing to become aroused.

Biological/Psychopharmacological Factors

In general, accepted models of understanding desire in cisgender women suggest developmental, individual, and relationship factors influence one another (McCabe, 2016). Meston and Stanton (2017) reviewed existing research on FSAD, summarized here. Biological contributing factors to FSAD overlap with those that can also contribute to female HSDD: medical health, hormones, and medications. Other specific medical/biological conditions include hypothalamic-pituitary axis dysfunction, surgical/medical castration, menopause, chronic oral contraceptive use, premature ovarian failure, drug and alcohol use, and cigarette smoking.

Individual Factors

Individual psychological factors such as stress, difficult or unsatisfying relationships, comorbid mental illness, history of sexual abuse, and negative body image can impact arousal (Meston & Stanton, 2017). Memory can also impact desire (Ricky et al., 2019). Research cites that for women, forgetting or neglecting their own self-identity differentiation is associated with decreased desire, which then affects sexual frequency (Costa et al., 2018).

Another important factor in arousal is the degree to which one is stimulated. A common issue (especially for ciswomen) is that they may not be adequately stimulated cognitively, emotionally, physically, and so on. Several models of arousal—for all genders—highlight the importance of cognition in arousal (e.g., Walen & Roth, 1987).

Symptoms of dissociation (likely related to prior sexual trauma) may result in feeling cut off or experiencing numbness of the genitals. Trauma and erotophic society and culture can also contribute to a feeling of disgust for one's genitals, potentially related to a lack of sensation.

Relational Factors

Inhibitors of sexual arousal can include fear of negative consequences for sexual activity (e.g., bad reputation, pregnancy) or feeling used by a sexual partner. Basson's (2002) nonlinear model of sexual response (discussed earlier) incorporates the need for intimacy, acknowledges that desire can be responsive or spontaneous, and notes that desire may occur either before or after arousal. Cisgender women's perceptions of their partners' responses affirmed a link between ciswomen's relationship satisfaction and (reduced) anxiety and their partners' responses (Rosen et al., 2020).

TREATMENT AND INTERVENTION STRATEGIES

Similar to hypoactive desire difficulties, for all of the treatment methods that follow regarding arousal difficulties, it can be helpful to consider the dual control model of sexual interest, that is, helping the client identify their sexual inhibition system (brakes) and sexual excitation system brakes (accelerators).

Psychoeducation

Implications for the treatment of FSAD include attention to psychological and historical factors that may impact the ability to be aroused. The factors mentioned within the discussion of HSDD would be applicable for treatment of arousal deficits in women as well. Help the client assess whether they are receiving effective and sufficient stimulation to allow their bodies to become sexually aroused. Genital self-exploration, self-touch and partner-touch psychoeducation and practice, as well as sensate focus exercises, are often helpful.

Medical Intervention and Treatments

In the instance of decreased or no lubrication, proactively applying lubrication to the external inner labia and clitoral area at the beginning of sexual activity can make a dramatic difference in the experience of pleasurable sensation from touch. Topical lubricants do not in themselves create sexual arousal, but instead may facilitate and optimize the possibility of experiencing arousal. Lubrication can be very helpful for postmenopausal clients who may generate less lubrication and experience atrophy of vaginal tissues and epithelial density (rendering the vaginal tissue more subject to abrasion and microscopic tears).

Hormonal (off-label use of the testosterone patch, estrogen treatment) and nonhormonal therapies (the antidepressant bupropion) have been used to treat both reduced desire and arousal in clients (reviewed by Meston & Stanton, 2017). Comparable drugs to the PDE5 inhibitors (Viagra, Cialis, Levitra) can increase vaginal engorgement and vaginal blood flow, but not increase subjective sexual arousal.

Cognitive Behavioral Therapy Treatment Strategies and Tools

As with treatment of low desire, psychological treatments for FSAD include psychoeducation about factors that can inhibit desire, partners' interventions (e.g., scheduling time for physical and emotional intimacy), communication training, cognitive restructuring of dysfunctional beliefs (e.g., a good sexual experience does not always end with an orgasm), sexual fantasy training, and sensate focus exercises. Participants can learn to be present and respond to their partner without worry about meeting performance criteria, goal orientation, or having to mind-read their partner's wishes. Treatment may also include identifying distracting, negative thoughts and learning to let go of these during sexual activity. These might include myths and misconceptions about sex, negative emotions, performance anxiety, and body image concerns. Cognitive restructuring can help people identify their fears and dysfunctional beliefs.

Systemic Treatment Strategies and Tools

Systemic treatment strategies involve addressing the integration of factors that contribute to the arousal issue. Systemic therapists must do a comprehensive assessment identifying potential factors such as medications and/or medical conditions, relationship issues, societal/cultural factors, as well as family messages that may contribute to the arousal difficulties. This means treatment might involve individual therapy, sex therapy, couples/relationship therapy, and coordination with physicians. It can mean teaching skills, psychoeducation on pleasurable and arousing conditions, communication skill building, cognitive therapy, and many other types of treatment.

Eye Movement Desensitization and Reprocessing Therapy Treatment Strategies and Tools

As EMDR therapy follows a standard eight-phase protocol to process distressing, disturbing, or traumatic events and/or symptoms, more detail will be provided toward the end of this chapter. For EMDR therapy specific to lack of physical arousal, targets regarding sexual and/or genital shame or disgust, erotophobic beliefs and messages, negative thoughts, prior history of trauma or abuse, dissociation, sexual anxiety, performance anxiety, body image concerns, and fears and anxiety about communicating sexual needs may help reduce blocks to experiencing arousal and sensation in the genitals.

ORGASM DISORDERS

FEMALE ORGASMIC DISORDER

Female orgasmic disorder is the inability for a person with a vulva to reach orgasm during sexual stimulation. As defined in the *DSM-5* (2013), Female Orgasmic Disorder is characterized by difficulty experiencing orgasm and/or markedly reduced intensity of orgasmic sensations and must cause clinically significant distress or interpersonal difficulty for the person experiencing the symptoms to be diagnosed. There is wide variation in the type and intensity of stimulation that elicits orgasm in people with vulvas as well as the subjective experiences of orgasm. Female orgasmic disorder may be lifelong or acquired, as well as generalized (occurring in all situations) or situational (occurring in select situations). An example of the situational type of the disorder is a woman who has orgasms through masturbation but not during partnered sexual activity.

Primary Female Orgasmic Disorder

Diagnosis and Description (Complete Absence of Orgasm)

People with primary female orgasmic disorder have not previously experienced orgasm in any situation. Generally no medical conditions are associated with this lifelong absence of orgasm. A thorough assessment should include early learning history about sexuality, presence of sexual trauma, cultural or religious influences that may have contributed, and lack of information about sex, among many other factors that may emerge as influential. This dysfunction can be due to a learning deficit, and some therapists, including this writer (W. Stock), characterize these clients as *preorgasmic* rather than anorgasmic.

Treatment Strategies

Directed Masturbation and Masturbation Strategies

The most effective treatment to date for preorgasmic clients to experience their first orgasm is a program of directed masturbation developed by LoPiccolo and Lobitz (1972). Masturbation has been shown to be the most probable method of producing an orgasm, as well as producing the most intense orgasm (Masters & Johnson, 1966). Learning to masturbate provides accurate proprioceptive feedback, enabling identification of effective sexually arousing stimulation techniques for the person.

The masturbation program developed by LoPiccolo and Lobitz (1972) is based on a sexual skills learning model and is an adjunct to a behavioral, time-limited treatment program. This can be offered to an individual client, or can involve all sexual participants.

The directed masturbation components include self-exploration, body awareness, effective self-stimulation training, and the use of *orgasm triggers* (Heiman et al., 1976; LoPiccolo &

Lobitz, 1972). This program involves nine steps, progressing from education on basic sexual physiology and anatomy, visual and tactile self-exploration, directed masturbation, development of sexual fantasy and imagery, sensate focus individually and with a partner, and eventually sharing effective techniques of masturbation with the partner. Clitoral stimulation is encouraged to facilitate orgasm during intercourse. Although vaginal/vulva/clitoral orgasm during intercourse should not be stressed as a goal for all partners, as this is not always a realistic expectation, concurrent clitoral stimulation may maximize this occurrence, if so desired by someone in treatment.

Self-help books are often used as adjuncts to treatment. *Becoming Orgasmic* (Heiman et al., 1976) was the original book developed for this treatment program. Other books such as *Becoming Cliterate: Why Orgasm Equality Matters and How To Get It* (Mintz, 2018), *Come As You Are* (Nagoski, 2015), and *Sex for One: The Joy of Self-Loving* (Dodson, 1996) are also very helpful for clients.

Secondary Female Orgasmic Disorder

Diagnosis and Description

A second type of orgasmic dysfunction, which perhaps includes an even larger group than those who have not yet experienced an orgasm, involves situational or secondary orgasmic dysfunction. Masters and Johnson (1970) used the term *secondary orgasmic dysfunction* to include (a) anyone who was previously able to achieve orgasm from some means of stimulation but who is currently rarely orgasmic, and to describe (b) anyone who is currently able to attain orgasm only in response to restricted types of stimulation.

The latter category is sometimes seen in clients who have only learned to orgasm with the use of a vibrator, and want to learn how to have orgasms with other forms of stimulation. The label of *secondary anorgasmia* has also been applied to clients with a wide range of sexual functioning, including those who experience orgasm only with strong interfemoral pressure or while lying face-down in bed.

Treatment Strategies for Both Primary and Secondary Orgasmic Disorders

Psychoeducation

For dependence on vibratory stimulation, the client can go "cold turkey" from using the vibrator, as the intense stimulation provided by vibrators exceeds what is possible from self or partner stimulation. The period of withdrawal is thought to help the brain "reset" to being able to experience less intense stimulation as pleasurable. During this period of withdrawal, employing the directed masturbation treatment program described previously can help the client begin to discover other ways of touching themselves that can be effective, as their nervous system learns to tune in to less intense stimulation.

The treatment for clients who are dependent on only one form of stimulation to orgasm and who want to broaden their repertoire of effective stimulation can follow this procedure as well. It is common that masturbation in positions that allow for greater ease of partner access may feel awkward or unnatural at first, but most clients are able to learn new patterns of arousal.

Many people with vulvas require clitoral stimulation to reach orgasm, and many do not receive adequate clitoral stimulation to reach orgasm in their sexual relationships, as discussed earlier in this chapter and throughout this entire book. Inadequate or ineffective stimulation is a rule-out prior to diagnosing female orgasmic disorder. Only a relatively small number of people with vaginas report that they consistently experience orgasm during intercourse, although due to cultural mythology, many people continue to feel inadequate about this. Some clients with vulvas still present for treatment of orgasmic dysfunction under the misapprehension that there is something wrong with them as they do not orgasm consistently or at all during penetrative vaginal sexual intercourse.

Psychoeducational intervention is appropriate for these clients, and sometimes for their partners, if under the same misapprehension. Patients may define unrealistic goals (e.g., orgasm during intercourse without clitoral stimulation) for treatment. Enabling someone to experience orgasm through some means of partner stimulation, if they have only yet experienced orgasm through masturbation, is perhaps a more realistic goal to adopt. Psychoeducation can help normalize clitoral orgasms.

If interpersonal or significant contextual factors, such as severe relationship distress, intimate partner violence, or other significant stressors, are present, then a diagnosis of female orgasmic disorder would not be made.

Treatment of secondary female orgasmic dysfunction may include sensate focus exercises as described previously, with an emphasis on effective, direct, and real-time communication between partners to ensure that the client is able to direct their partner to provide the most effective stimulation. Utilizing the hand-over-hand method is helpful in having the partner rest their hand lightly over the client's hand as they stimulate oneself, allowing their partner to learn more effectively the degree of pressure, pacing, and timing that the client needs.

Deemphasizing goal orientation regarding wanting to have an orgasm in every sexual encounter has been stressed in the sex therapy literature. However, ciswomen as a group have long undersold themselves in many heterosexual relationships by not insisting on adequate stimulation and not putting their sexual pleasure on equal standing with that of their partners. For this reason, the instruction to deemphasize having orgasms may need to be tempered with the encouragement to feel entitled to the fullest measure of sexual pleasure and satisfaction that is desired by these clients.

Medical Intervention and Treatments

Because secondary sexual dysfunctions such as anorgasmia are often created and maintained by a context of poor sexual interaction, clinicians generally do not overtly treat the secondary sexual dysfunctions (IsHak et al., 2010). In some cases, problems with orgasm are the result of substance use. Ceasing using the substance may relieve the anorgasmia. In addition, when the anorgasmia is the result of other medications to treat psychological disorders such as a client taking antipsychotics, antiepileptics, or medications for mood disorders, medication treatment can include lamotrigine, yohimbine, or alpha-1 agonists such as imipramine or ephedrine (Naghibi & Hosseini, 2023; Nguyen et al., 2023).

In fact, it is well known that taking antidepressants in particular can cause sexual problems (lack of interest in sex, numb genitals, orgasms that do not feel pleasurable) in as much as half of people (of all genders) prescribed these medications (Montejo et al., 2001). A recent *New York Times* article (Ghorayshi, 2023) details these reported side effects, including the potential lifelong impact of any course length of antidepressants, and the growing concern by patients, doctors, researchers, and regulating organizations regarding the impact of antidepressant treatment on the sexuality and sexual functioning of increasingly younger patients (teens and young adult).

Systemic Treatment Strategies and Tools

Systemic treatments for orgasmic disorder may be more helpful than some of the pharmacological interventions. Directed masturbation is an important treatment component. Engaging in individual work to increase comfort with masturbation, or increasing partner support for masturbation through couples therapy, may be necessary in order to encourage and facilitate directed masturbation. In addition, because poor communication is a contributing factor to orgasm problems, improved communication may help. Partners can be directed to engage in I-statements, "sofa" sessions (where the partners discuss what they enjoy during physically intimate activities), attenuation exercises, or other opportunities to generate the emotional connection through communication.

Case Study 8.1: Anya

Anya is a 45-year-old marketing manager who grew up Catholic and was married to a cisgender man for 10 years before she came out as lesbian to her husband. After they processed their amicable divorce, Anya spent 5 years married to Samantha and is now reporting having difficulty achieving orgasm through clitoral stimulation when it involves her partner, a method that was previously successful. She relies increasingly on a vibrator and laying face down in bed to reach orgasm, leading to decreased sexual satisfaction and a sense of inadequacy. Symptoms include anxiety about her sexual performance, pressure to perform, and frustration with her limited responsiveness to stimulation that does not include her vibrator. Anya perceives her partner Samantha to be frustrated that she cannot reach orgasm unless the vibrator is also in the bedroom, even though they had a satisfying time in the bedroom up until this point

Anya's year-long reliance on a vibrator for orgasm and decreased sexual desire are indicative of secondary orgasmic disorder. Secondary orgasmic disorder can be effectively addressed through a comprehensive treatment plan, promoting positive sexual health and a fulfilling relationship. Therapy can help address her anxieties, performance pressure, and negative beliefs about her sexuality and lead to significant improvements like reduced anxiety, increased sexual agency, enhanced communication and intimacy with her partner through sensate focus exercises, decreased reliance on the vibrator, the ability to achieve orgasm through various methods, and increased sexual satisfaction and overall well-being. Continued therapy sessions can aim to solidify progress and equip Anya and her partner to address any future sexual concerns, fostering a sense of empowerment and improved sexual health.

Eye Movement Desensitization and Reprocessing Therapy Treatment Strategies and Tools

As EMDR therapy follows a standard eight-phase protocol to process distressing, disturbing, or traumatic events and/or symptoms, more detail will be provided toward the end of this chapter. For EMDR therapy specific to lack of orgasm or trouble orgasming consistently, targets regarding sexual and/or genital shame or disgust, erotophobic beliefs and messages, negative thoughts, prior history of trauma or abuse, dissociation, sexual anxiety, performance anxiety, body image concerns, and fears and anxiety about communicating sexual needs may help increase and generalize orgasm potential.

GENDERED ORGASM GAP

The large gap in orgasm frequency between ciswomen and cismen in heterosexual sexual activity provides a good illustration of the influence of relational factors on sexual problems. Laumann et al. (1999) reported that, while 75% of heterosexual cisgender men reported having orgasms from partnered sex on a regular basis, only about 29% of cisgender women reported the same. Recent research of approximately 25,000 participants confirms this continued gap, with men reporting orgasm rates during intercourse averaging from 70% to 85% and women's orgasm rates averaging 46% to 58% (Gesselman et al., 2024). Related research (Wade et al., 2005) found that among cisgender women, those with more knowledge of the clitoris experienced orgasm more frequently on their own, but possessing this information was *not* related to frequency of orgasm with partners.

The authors point out that this disparity exists in the context of "gender inequality and a social construction of sexuality … that privileges men's sexual pleasure over women's, such that orgasm for women is pleasing, but ultimately incidental" (Wade et al., 2005, p. 118). Cisgender women may not feel empowered or entitled to act on their sexual self-knowledge or to ask for the stimulation that they need for fear of being seen as unfeminine, too demanding, and less desirable to their male partners. The authors continue, "our findings are directly relevant to other means of safeguarding health, such as setting sexual boundaries and using condoms" (Wade et al., 2005, p. 136). The authors clearly demonstrate that gender inequality directly affects not only cisgender women's ability to claim their full sexual pleasure with cismale partners, but their safety from exposure to sexual disease and sexual violence. Sexual dysfunction should never be considered apart from social context.

The situational and relational factors identified make an ongoing and strong case for offering corrective sexual education; addressing sex role expectations; improving sexual communication; and addressing relationship issues concerning sexual initiation, timing, power issues in partners, sharing of familial workload, examining unrealistic expectations, and learning to make sexual interactions more about connection than performance.

Case Study 8.2: Sara, Only Orgasmic on Her Own

Sara, a 33-year-old heterosexual cisgender woman, is in treatment for anxiety and depression, but recently introduced a sexual issue that she wants to address. In her previous sexual relationships, she has never had an orgasm with any partner. However, she is easily able to orgasm on her own during masturbation. She reports typically becoming sexually aroused during partner sex, and sometimes feels that she is close to orgasm. At that point, she becomes self-conscious and "fakes" having an orgasm. Her stated concerns included: embarrassment that she is "taking too long" to orgasm, worries that her partner is becoming bored or tired, worries that she'll be "too much trouble" or "too demanding" as a partner, and fears that her partner may lose interest in her, and that she could lose the relationship. She has never told any previous partner that she didn't have orgasms, having felt trapped if her "lie" were revealed, which would have a negative impact on trust in these relationships.

Therapy to date has included normalizing the challenges for many women in reaching orgasm with partners (not receiving effective stimulation for sufficient duration, not feeling comfortable providing direct feedback to a partner, gender socialization to put others' needs first). Boundary and self-esteem issues were addressed as part of Sara's therapy. Now in a new and promising relationship, Sara has felt empowered to discuss this issue with her new partner *before* they have engaged in sexual contact. She has decided that she deserves to have orgasms when she wants them with a partner, and that she wouldn't want to be with a partner who wasn't equally committed to her sexual pleasure. To his credit, the new partner has offered her reassurance that he will be open to her feedback, and will take as long as she needs. This rewarding outcome is not always guaranteed, but the most important achievement is Sara's changed valuing of herself, and her expectations of future partners.

GENITO-PELVIC PAIN PENETRATION DISORDER

Genito-Pelvic Pain Penetration Disorder (GPPPD) is a new diagnosis for sexual pain disorders in the *DSM-5* and combines the diagnoses of Vaginismus and Dyspareunia in the previous version of the *DSM*. GPPPD subsumes a number of diagnoses, including vulvodynia, vaginismus, and noncoital sexual pain disorder.

Vaginismus and dyspareunia may coexist, or may occur independently of each other, as described in the following. For this reason, these two dysfunctions are discussed separately.

1. Combination of vaginismus and dyspareunia: A medical condition may exist that causes vaginal pain; when penetration is attempted, the association of pain from penetration can result in a secondary pattern of involuntary, reflexive spastic contraction of the vaginal musculature that renders penetration even more painful or impossible, resulting in a combination of both disorders.
2. Vaginismus alone: A client may exhibit the involuntary spastic contraction of vaginal musculature without any organic pathology that renders penetration difficult or impossible.

3. Dyspareunia alone: A client may have a medical condition that causes pain with genital touch and/or penetration, but does not exhibit spastic contraction of the vaginal musculature. Penetrative activity may be painful but not complicated by tightening of the vaginal opening.

VAGINISMUS

Diagnosis and Description

The term *vaginismus* refers to spastic contraction of the circumvaginal musculature (pubococcygeus or PC muscle), such that the penis, or other objects, cannot be admitted to the vagina without great difficulty and great pain. Vaginismus is distinguished from *dyspareunia,* which refers to pain during coitus from any source other than vaginismus. Vaginismus can be situation specific. For example, it may be possible for someone to insert a tampon, but not be able to tolerate a pelvic examination, or the individual may be unable to tolerate intercourse or other penetrative activity, in any combination of these presentations.

However, vaginismus does not preclude someone from experiencing sexual arousal and orgasm. Many people with vaginismus are easily responsive and orgasmic with masturbation and nonpenetrative couple activities. It has been suggested that without the imperative of heterosexual intercourse, that vaginismus would be a nonissue. However, if vaginismus prevents regular PAP testing, this could be a life-threatening condition, as early detection of abnormal cervical cells is highly effective in preventing cervical cancer. A gynocological exam, to the degree possible, is recommended to eliminate the possibility of a coexisting medical condition that requires treatment.

Vaginismus-Related Factors

1. *Negative learning history:* A history of initial painful penetration that results in subsequent involuntary contraction of the PC muscle during subsequent attempts. Many people have unsuccessfully tried to overcome this condition by attempting to engage in intercourse to overcome the symptom. They often mistakenly think that they need to physically stretch the vaginal opening; in fact, the problem is not due to an obstruction in the vaginal opening (assuming this possibility has been ruled out by a gynecological exam). Unfortunately, this repetition of pain associated with penetration only serves to reinforce the association, further solidifying the involuntary contraction of the PC muscle in anticipation of pain. Often people have been forcing penetration attempts on themselves, but partners with penises may have also pressured for intercourse as well. Sometimes a couple attempts penetration in desperation to become pregnant.
2. History of sexual trauma (rape, childhood sexual abuse)
3. Sexual shame and guilt
4. Fear of pregnancy, fear of contracting sexually transmitted infections
5. Ignorance of sexual anatomy and sexual response (i.e., attempted penetration without sufficient arousal and/or lubrication)
6. History of medical conditions that have caused painful penetration in the past (yeast infections, urinary tract infections)
7. Painful childbirth or difficult healing experience from episiotomy or tearing of surrounding tissues—fear of pain may persist even if conditions have resolved.

Treatment Strategies

Relaxation, Dilator Training, Pelvic Floor Physical Therapy

If a careful history and pelvic exam has substantiated the diagnosis of vaginismic response to sexual activity, as opposed to dyspareunia, the client may be appropriately treated using sex therapy techniques. The effective treatment element in resolution of vaginismus is a combination of relaxation training, learning to voluntarily contract and relax the PC muscle, and gradual introduction of progressive-sized dilators performed under the woman's control, at home. The goal of this treatment is to create a new learning association between penetration and no pain, rather than continuing to further engrain the previous association between penetration and pain. This technique has nothing to do with stretching the vaginal opening. Instead, it is based on the client learning to relax the PC muscle enough, often via pelvic floor physical therapy, to accommodate an object, gradually, by tensing and relaxing the PC muscle around the dilator, and never forcing an object into their vagina if at all painful. With each tense and relax contraction, the PC muscle relaxes more to be able to accommodate further insertion of the dilator.

If there is any pain or discomfort, the client is instructed to stop the exercise, relax via deep breathing, and try once more. If there is still pain, the instruction is to stop trying and resume the exercise on another day. In this manner, the client is learning that they can trust themselves not to force a painful activity. The gynecologist, client, or partner forcing a dilator into the vagina and causing pain and discomfort will only make the vaginismus worse, as it confirms the fear that penetration is painful.

The client is encouraged to practice with a graduated progression of different size dilators, initially alone. Dilators are available in soft silicone, as well as more rigid plastic. Many find the soft silicone less threatening to work with in treatment. Utilizing adequate lubrication is always recommended. Once the client has been able to accomplish penetration without pain or involuntary tightening of the PC muscle, a partner may be incorporated into the treatment, initially resting their hand lightly on the client's hand as the client slowly guides the dilator into their vagina. This hand-over-hand procedure can increase trust in the client toward their partner, experiencing penetration under the client's own control, with the partner present. This method can be understood as a form of systematic desensitization.

This progressive dilation program is extremely effective if the client and partner follow it, without rushing progress to larger dilators, finger insertion, and entry of the penis. Ultimately, the couple (if heterosexual) can then try penile penetration. This is best introduced with the client in superior position, so that they can control the pace and depth of penetration.

Systemic Treatment Strategies and Tools

A thorough assessment may uncover relationship issues that need to be addressed before effective intervention can be undertaken for the initial presenting complaint of vaginismus.

As previously mentioned, pelvic issues emerge from a vast etiology of factors. Treatment should be designed to address the complexity of how arousal and desire disorders emerged. Hertlein et al. (2020) note that to be good sex therapists, one needs to be a good couple's therapist; to be a good couple's therapist, one needs to be a good sex therapist. Specific tools include mitigating medical and physical issues, addressing depression and anxiety, treating partners with issues that inspired or are the result of the sexual problem, deconstructing unhelpful messages from family of origin, and having the couple move away from internalizing unproductive and inaccurate myths and messages about sex.

DYSPAREUNIA

Diagnosis and Description

Dyspareunia refers to pain from genital touch that may include painful penetration, although it may not include vaginismus (involuntary contraction of the PC muscle).

Medical Contributing Factors

Medical factors associated with dyspareunia include treated or untreated vaginal infection, history of urinary tract infections associated with spastic urethra or sensitivity at the urethral opening, inflammatory dermatitis, surgical or postdelivery scarring, endometriosis, vulvodynia/vestibulodynia, interstitial cystitis, pelvic floor dysfunction, inadequate vaginal lubrication, estrogen deficiency, or sequalae of medical treatments such as pelvic radiation.

Untreated or persistent yeast or bacterial vaginosis infections can result in intense stinging and burning during and especially after intercourse. Endometriosis can fluctuate during the menstrual cycle, worsening when endometrial tissue enlarges due to higher estrogen during the cycle. Ideally, the client may be able to localize the pain and describe when it is more apparent, hopefully keeping track with a written log.

The use of the vaginal "clock" model can also help, with the 12:00 position corresponding to the front-facing vaginal area, and 6:00 toward the rear, adjacent to the perineal area. Childbirth scarring can affect the perineal area, as well as internal scarring from ligament tearing that has healed with scar tissue. Although not always obvious during a gynecological exam, this can become apparent during sexual arousal, when the internal erectile tissue expands and the uterus is normally pulled upward to elongate the vaginal barrel. Adhesions from scar tissue can pull on adjacent tissue during sexual arousal, as scar tissue is not elastic.

Seemingly idiopathic cases may relate to a history of genital pain, and sometimes a history of abuse or sexual trauma.

Treatment Strategies

Psychoeducation

Education of the client about any medical factors can empower them to report in concrete terms where and when the pain occurs, and may help avoid the symptoms from being dismissed as entirely psychosomatic. It is crucial for the client to have had adequate assessment, diagnosis, and treatment of medical issues associated with dyspareunia.

Medical Intervention

Treatment of dyspareunia may include a variety of medical or physical interventions (Mindyra, 2021, Treated section):

- *Botulinum toxin type A injections:* reduces muscle overactivity through mechanisms such as blocking cholinergic synapses and inhibiting pain-related neurotransmitter release
- *Topical treatments:* may include amitriptyline/baclofen, lidocaine, nifedipine, cromolyn, or fibroblast lysate cream
- *Surgical treatments:* involves excising painful areas
- *Physical therapy:* includes education on vulvar anatomy and muscle function, with techniques like home exercises, biofeedback, and pelvic floor stimulation to reduce pain sensitivity

Cognitive Behavioral Therapy Treatment Strategies and Tools

Treatment of dyspareunia may include (Mindyra, 2021) CBT focused on modification of thought patterns or beliefs that link fears of vaginal penetration or genital touch with pain. Relaxation exercises, mindfulness, and visualization may be incorporated as well.

Systemic Treatment Strategies and Tools

Because relational issues are not necessarily a cause of dyspareunia, the treatment systemically may be related to teaching the partner how to more helpfully respond to the pain the client is experiencing. Sexual pain is a disorder where if the client is pressured for sex, it can create a secondary sexual dysfunction where the person with sexual pain may begin to lose interest or avoid sex.

Eye Movement Desensitization and Reprocessing Therapy Treatment Strategies and Tools

As EMDR therapy follows a standard eight-phase protocol to process distressing, disturbing, or traumatic events and/or symptoms, more detail will be provided toward the end of this chapter. For EMDR therapy specific to pain, targets regarding prior sexual pain, genital shame and/or disgust, erotophobic beliefs and messages, negative thoughts, prior history of trauma or abuse, dissociation, sexual anxiety, and fears and anxiety about communicating sexual needs may help reduce and eliminate some more somatic experiences of pain. In addition to utilizing the standard EMDR therapy protocol, EMDR therapy also has specific pain protocols which can reduce or eliminate pain.

Case Study 8.3 Simona, Using EMDR Therapy to Treat Genito-Pelvic Pain Disorder

By Elena Isola

EYE MOVEMENT DESENSITIZATION AND REPROCESSING THERAPY PHASE 1: HISTORY TAKING

Background History

Simona is a 35-year-old, heterosexual, cisgender woman who was diagnosed with genito-pelvic and penetration pain disorder 2 years earlier. She currently lives alone and holds an administrative job. She has been dating a cismale coworker for a year. They live and work in Italy. Simona sought therapy to resolve sexual difficulties that have been ongoing for many years; she has become aware that her complete rejection of any sexual activity might be causing significant distress. Despite numerous attempts with her current and past partners, Simona has never been able to experience penetrative sexual intercourse. On the rare occasions when she tried, the pain was so unbearable that over time it made her stop trying. She says that if it weren't for her boyfriend, whom she cares about a lot, she would even go without sex.

Additionally, Simona displays a phobic attitude toward touching or looking at her genitals; therefore, experiencing penetration seems even more impossible. She has not been able to receive a gynecological exam. Her current boyfriend has been understanding from the beginning, but recently he has started expressing sexual desire toward her. Both Simona and her boyfriend dream of having children, and therefore, Simona decided to start psychotherapy. She also feared that her boyfriend might cheat on or leave her, finally prompting her to seek help.

Sexological Diagnosis

From the investigation carried out during the first session, enough information emerged to formulate a diagnosis of genito-pelvic pain/penetration disorder (APA, 2013). The motivation that persuaded Simona to pursue this sex therapy was her desire to finally undergo a gynecological examination and to pursue becoming pregnant.

Before starting treatment, Simona was administered the Female Sexual Function Index (FSFI; Rosen et al., 2020) questionnaire. This measure consisted of 19 multiple-choice questions which assessed her satisfaction with her sexual life with her partner and the pain experienced during and after sexual penetration. The questionnaire addressed six main themes: sexual interest, arousal, orgasm, relationship with the partner, lubrication, and symptomatology. Analyzing the six areas, it was observed that the intensity of sexual desire was "low or absent." The intensity of arousal and the lubrication frequency was mainly "low." Additionally, Simona was not able to have an orgasm and had never experienced penetration due to the pain she felt.

Walter, her boyfriend, never pressured or forced vaginal penetration, fearing he would hurt her and traumatize her further. Simona clearly felt muscle contraction throughout her pelvic area when attempting vaginal penetration; she cannot tolerate any type of pain and is terrified at the mere thought of experiencing physical suffering. All attempts at having coitus failed because as soon as he got close, she felt a sharp pain, and he never wanted to force her. Initially, even introducing a finger in the vagina was impossible, but after a few months of EMDR psychotherapy, she managed to tolerate it. However, this progress has not been consistent and varied greatly depending on how her boyfriend approached her. In many cases, she complained about the lack of kisses and foreplay, which were essential for her to relax.

History of the Disorder and Sexuality

Simona began experiencing anxiety symptoms around the age of 11. The triggering event she recalls as particularly stressful was when her father left the house, which was followed by her mother's depressive state. Simona recalls not having received any sexual education. She had her first period at 12 years old and remembers experiencing it poorly, becoming frightened by the sight of the blood. Simona remembers feeling embarrassed by her parents' phone calls to tell their relatives about the event. Her mother had an awkward and concerned approach to sexuality; for example, when there were scenes on television where a man and a woman kissed, her mother would tell her that this is how diseases can be transmitted.

Simona also remembers the shame she felt when she secretly went to her first gynecological visit at 16 years old. In addition to these specific targets, we addressed a series of traumatic events related to Simona's attachment history, including the conflictual relationship between her parents, their separation, and her father's departure. Memories related to her relationship with her mother, who had been anxious, intrusive, and controlling since Simona was a child, were also identified as contributing to her insecurity. Additionally, her mother had strong taboos regarding sexuality.

EYE MOVEMENT DESENSITIZATION AND REPROCESSING THERAPY PHASE 2: PREPARATION

This phase focused on explaining EMDR to enhance Simona's personal motivation. The psychoeducational work aimed at highlighting and explaining the connection between her symptoms and the issues she reported, as well as the link between past and present experiences. The importance of focusing on identifying and strengthening resources was emphasized.

Additionally, it was crucial to explain EMDR and the impact that certain traumatic life experiences might have had on her self-concept, her relationships with others, her sexuality, and her physical responses of rigidity and closure.

Resource Development Installation

Simona participated in three sessions of resource identification and installation, with the purpose of facilitating a stabilization of her current situation and improving her emotional regulation and coping skills (Korn & Leeds, 2002). The first resource installed was the "Safe/Calm Place" (Luber, 2009), to help her modulate and regulate her emotions and anxiety, and to restore a sense of calm and tranquility. Using the resource development installation (RDI) protocol, the perception of being adult and competent, along with the associated feelings and sensations, was installed and reinforced. The resource was identified in a memory of when she was a class representative and successfully convinced her teachers to take the class on a trip abroad. In another session, Simona imagined herself healing, observing her body, returning to previous activities like playing sports, going out freely with friends, and, most importantly, getting closer to her partner, feeling free to do what she wants when she wants. During this phase, we achieved a strong therapeutic alliance.

Psychoeducation

In the psychosexual therapy for vaginismus, the initial phase is dedicated to sexual education, with the purpose of increasing the patient's knowledge of vulva genital anatomy and physiology. Often, people with vulvas, with this condition, have little to no familiarity with their own vulva and are unaware of its structure because their sexual history has been marked by systematic avoidance of both their genitals and any information related to them.

Through this primarily informational sexual education, two simultaneous objectives can be achieved: both bridging the informational gap for the client, as well as enabling them to become more aware of their own sexual body in a calm, relaxed, and nonjudgmental environment. This opens up the possibility for the client to explore their genitals and the sensations associated with them. Through gradual experiences involving observation with a mirror, Simona became able to look at and touch her genitals.

Simona exhibited dissociative aspects, primarily manifesting as a disconnect between her mind and body, where her body was always perceived as a source of problems. The mirror exercise allowed us to focus on the dissociative aspects that were blocking her: control and shame. The first time she tried to observe her genitals with a mirror at home, she came back to the session very agitated, and reported feeling deep shame. I asked her if she was willing to work on these issues, and she agreed, as she no longer wanted to feel blocked. From focusing on the disturbance in the body, Simona was able to trace back to first experiencing the sensations when a volleyball coach sexually abused her at age 11. I provided psychoeducational information about sexual abuse in childhood and about related short- and long-term reactions, explaining the potential development of dissociative symptoms.

EYE MOVEMENT DESENSITIZATION AND REPROCESSING THERAPY PHASES 3 TO 7: PROCESSING TARGETS

The standard EMDR protocol from phase 3 to 7 (assessment of target, desensitization of target, installation of positive cognition, body scan, closure of target and session) was applied to every target memory identified during the history-taking phase, as well as with subsequent targets that emerged. Here is specific information regarding two important targets.

Target Incident: Abuse by the coach, age 11

- *Worst Image:* His hand touching her
- *Negative Cognition (NC) Related to the Incident:* "I am a bad person."
- *Positive Cognition (PC) She Would Rather Believe in the Future:* "I am a good person."
- *Emotions:* Fear, shame
- *SUD (Subjective Units of Disturbance):* Intensity of the distress = 10
- *Location of Distress:* Pelvic area, legs, throat

Target Incident: First Menstrual Cycle, Age 12

- *Worst Image:* Blood on her legs
- *Negative Cognition (NC):* "I am not in control."
- *Positive Cognition (PC):* "I am in control."
- *Emotions:* Agitation, shame
- *SUD (Subjective Units of Disturbance):* 9
- *Location of Distress:* Pelvic area, legs

The positive effects of these initial sessions were evident in the following weeks. For the first time, Simona was able to get closer to her boyfriend without the usual fear and with much less rigidity in her legs. Although the attempt to have intercourse was unsuccessful, she had managed to experience some moments of intimacy. We then reprocessed, in chronological order, the times she had attempted to have intercourse with previous boyfriends and the current one, and it had never worked out, reinforcing her belief that she would never be able to have a normal sexual life.

EYE MOVEMENT DESENSITIZATION AND REPROCESSING THERAPY PHASE 8: REEVALUATION, REINFORCEMENT, AND FUTURE TEMPLATES

Next we installed new resources arising from the prior successful target processing (Korn & Leeds, 2002):

- moments when Simona managed to observe her body in the mirror
- successfully experiencing a gynecological exam, feeling more comfortable
- moments when she was able to tolerate physical contact with her partner without feeling guilty

Lastly, we installed EMDR future templates: (a) the next time she will experience feeling emotionally close to her partner, meeting his gaze, and sustaining physical contact with him; and (b) the next time she will have full penetrative sexual intercourse.

Through processing past events, Simona strengthened her awareness of the connection between her current difficulties and the related past events. She also recognized the regulatory function of the sexual symptoms, which she had used before treatment to cope with her states of anxiety and fear. In the following sessions, Simona began to trust in the possibility of overcoming her difficulties. She felt compassion for her fragile part and felt tenderness toward it. Simona drew her compassionate part, associating it with a positive sensation in her heart. I performed slow bilateral stimulation (BLS) so that she could strengthen this sensation in her body.

SEXOLOGICAL INTERVENTION IMPLEMENTED AND PARTNER INVOLVEMENT

A series of three visits was planned with the team gynecologist to be carried out in a more advanced phase of therapy, as it was first necessary to prepare Simona with an appropriate process of body awareness.

The first visit was to verify the normalcy of the external genitals and confirm the absence of anatomical anomalies (which are very rare but often present in the forms of fears in women with this type of symptom). In the second visit, the woman is encouraged to insert her own finger into her vagina and then allow the doctor to do so as well. In the third meeting, the actual gynecological examination is conducted, including the introduction of the speculum and the Pap smear. Collaboration with the gynecologist is important because the patient usually needs concrete verification from a doctor of the progress made and the real possibility of her vagina "opening" (Isola, 2016).

As expected, the initial phase of therapy primarily revealed Simona's phobic structures and the emotional containment difficulties of her partner. Therefore, individual therapy proceeded where Simona, very gradually, learned to look at and touch her genitals with the help of Kegel exercises. The first gynecological visit, although experienced with much anxiety and apprehension, was very useful because Simona felt reassured about the anatomical normalcy of her genitals. The treatment proceeded quite well: Simona was very serious about performing the assigned tasks, but in each session, her intense feelings of inadequacy emerged, leading her to be very pessimistic and undervalue the progress made. Continuous emotional reinforcement and explanations were essential.

Once Simona learned to insert her own finger into her vagina, it was decided to conduct the second gynecological visit; this was a very important moment for her because the gynecologist positively reinforced her progress. As agreed, the visit was partial (i.e., without the introduction of the speculum, which was postponed to a later meeting). Additionally, since Simona still could not imagine the possibility of having a penis in her vagina, due to the predominance of avoidance defenses, it was found useful to apply Knipe's protocol on avoidance defenses (Knipe, 2017).

As Knipe (2017) indicates, BLS sets enhance associative neural networks and facilitate "slow thinking," allowing the person to abandon the relief of avoidance and assess whether the avoidance strategy is consistent with current life goals. This particular procedure involves using avoidance defense as the target for reprocessing, asking the patient to indicate an image representing the situation being avoided (in this case, the complete insertion of her boyfriend's penis into her vagina), measuring the level of the avoidance impulse (with scores on a scale from 1 to 10; LOUA, level of urge of avoidance), indicating the body part where this impulse is felt, and instructing the patient to follow the therapist's fingers (BLS). As the BLS sets continued, the anxiety and sense of losing control that Simona experienced when imagining penetration completely disappeared; at this point, it was decided to involve the partner in therapy. Walter actively participated in the sessions, diligently performed the assigned tasks at home, carefully noted and reported his emotions, and accepted being encouraged to show greater firmness toward his partner.

After a few attempts, Walter experienced a blockage as he confronted his own anxiety and sense of inadequacy, while Simona no longer assumed full responsibility for what was happening. Guided by her, Walter managed to insert his finger into her vagina without her experiencing pain, instead just some tolerable discomfort. Further sessions followed to consolidate these results and to reflect together on the dynamics of their relationship. In these final sessions, Simona seemed increasingly aware of the contradiction between having a dominant position toward her partner while at the same time demanding greater security and authority from him.

At this point, the third gynecological visit with the introduction of the speculum was carried out without difficulty, and even the Pap smear was completed without obstacles. The suggestion to experiment with penetration was well received, and after a couple of attempts, it was fully successful, as Simona did not experience the much-feared pain. Simona realized she felt more confident and more "womanly." The couple reported that the anxiety surrounding intercourse gradually gave way to a desire to be close that they had never felt before. They appeared relatively comfortable during the final session and reported a further improvement in their situation.

POSTTREATMENT RESULTS

Changes in Sexual Symptoms

The combination of EMDR treatment with pelvic floor rehabilitation, in collaboration with the midwife, resulted in significant benefits for the patient, particularly in terms of symptomatology. Analyzing the six areas of the FSFI questionnaire, administered at the conclusion of therapy, it was observed that the intensity of sexual desire became "moderate," the intensity of arousal and the frequency of lubrication reached "moderate intensity," and Simona was able to experience orgasm without experiencing pain during penetration.

Emotional Regulation

The goal was to enhance Simona's ability to recognize, express, and regulate her emotions concerning sexuality. Progress in emotional regulation was noted, reflecting an improved capacity to manage emotions and engage in intimate relationships with greater confidence and security.

INTEGRATED SEXOLOGICAL TREATMENT *by Elena Isola*

The simple mechanistic treatment of symptoms is not sufficient to resolve sexual problems. The challenge for sexual health clinicians is to integrate all biopsychosocial factors into the treatment protocol, adopting care models developed by a multidisciplinary team capable of holistically addressing the needs of both the patient and the couple.

Patients should be offered a personalized intervention in which they can feel accepted and understood. In these situations, it is essential for professionals to work in an integrated manner, with different treatments used in combination. In addition to the initial phase of sexual education explained earlier, working with a skillful, trauma-informed, and sex-positive gynecologist is very important because it allows the patient to gradually face the fear of gynecological examinations and physically verify the progress made (Simonelli et al., 2019).

After the educational-informative phase, the treatment includes *in vivo* systematic desensitization (Kaplan, 1974) to address the phobia of pain, as well as the use of sensate focus techniques to address anxiety and the fear of penetration. Working on muscle hypertonicity, pain reduction to increase desire and arousal, is also beneficial (Dias-Amaral & Marques-Pinto, 2018; Fugl-Meyer et al., 2013). Other essential interventions include processing traumatic events related to perceived pain and applying Mark Grant's EMDR protocol for pain (Grant, 2012).

Another important treatment modality is pelvic-perineal relaxation and retraining therapy, in collaboration with a midwife (Isola & Maccarrone, 2019). The goal of pelvic floor rehabilitation is to improve awareness and cortical representation of the pelvic floor muscles, enhancing the patient's perception of them. Learning to perceive and control these muscles voluntarily is important during sexual intercourse (Critelli et al., 2016). Positive outcomes include reducing perineal and/or pelvic muscle tension and cognitive distortions related to pain (fewer catastrophic thoughts and greater ability to recognize pain-triggering situations), improving coping strategies (ability to focus on the positive aspects of the sexual experience), and improved sexual functioning (exploring nonpenetrative sexual activities and the ability to communicate needs to a partner; Simonelli et al., 2019).

Penetrative intercourse is not the primary goal but rather the consequence of effective therapy (Dias-Amaral & Marques-Pinto, 2018). The goal of physical treatment on pelvic muscles is to restore muscle and tissue functionality, reduce neural tension, and, in some cases, improve sexual function (Morin et al., 2017; Prendergast, 2017). Pelvic floor physical treatment can be performed with manual techniques (massage, stretching, and trigger point work) or using neuromodulation through TENS, either alone or in combination with vaginal diazepam, or with EMG biofeedback (Rosen et al., 2019).

Working on anxiety reduction is also important. The patient and the couple usually have entered a cycle of avoiding intimacy, discussing the problem, and seeking solutions. It is important to restore confidence in their abilities and active roles. From a cognitive perspective, distorted ideas function to maintain and reinforce the avoidance system. Restoring confidence becomes possible because EMDR therapy has previously worked on the patient's early traumatic experiences and negative cognitions.

OTHER SEXUAL PAIN CONDITIONS

NONCOITAL SEXUAL PAIN

Noncoital sexual pain is a general term referring to discomfort experienced during nonpenetrative intercourse sexual activities (i.e., pain experienced during oral sex, manual stimulation, and/or kissing or other touching).

VULVODYNIA

Vulvodynia is a chronic vulvar pain condition that can include discomforting sensations such as burning or stinging. The pain can occur constantly or irregularly. Causes can be unknown or can be related to hormonal changes, infections, or potentially even nerve damage. For any physical causes, treatment will likely include medical interventions such as medication, physical therapy, or lifestyle changes. Other treatment may involve learning to manage pain, or increasing additional pain-free options for sexual interaction, stimulation, and pleasure.

BLUE VULVA SYNDROME

Blue vulva syndrome (vulvar cyanosis) is characterized by a bluish discoloration of the vulva. Causes can involve increased blood flow to the vulva (engorgement of blood vessels due to arousal or changes in estrogen levels) or venous congestion (blood flow may have difficulty leaving the vulva).

While it can be completely benign, if accompanied by pain, discomfort, or other unusual symptoms, it is important to seek medical evaluation.

SEX HEADACHES

Sex headaches (aka *sexual benign headaches*) comprise an increasing dull background headache that slowly builds and then fades during sexual activity. *Orgasm headaches* involve an intense sharp pain that suddenly occurs as one approaches or experiences orgasm. Orgasm headaches can occur in any gender, but more typically in people with penises, with onset generally between ages 40 and 50. Both sex and orgasm headaches are considered *primary* if benign and harmless, or *secondary* if accompanying a potentially harmful medical condition such as vascular problems. Anyone experiencing them should consult a medical professional to rule out any harmful or dangerous secondary underlying causes. For benign headaches, prophylactic or ongoing migraine medication and management strategies may be recommended. Many sufferers may avoid mentioning these headaches to their doctors out of embarrassment, so it is important for optimal client care to encourage disclosure and medical care.

SUMMARY

People with vulvas and vaginas can experience many pleasures, and many difficulties, regarding sexual interest, arousal, and activity.

Clients seeking sex therapy may report symptoms that indicate any of these diagnoses: desire disorders, arousal disorders, orgasm disorders (preorgasmic, situationally orgasmic), and genito-pelvic pain penetration disorder (e.g., vaginismus, dyspareunia). Sex therapists are trained to treat these disorders. Understanding the broader cultural context in which humans develop their sexual selves is critical to considering a full picture of a particular client's sexual functioning.

Trauma therapists, particularly EMDR therapists, may help sex therapists adjunctly with the processing of any disturbing, traumatic, or difficult material getting in the way of improved sexual functioning.

There is a persistent gendered orgasm gap (individuals with clitorises report fewer orgasms overall than individuals with penises). Correcting myths, engaging in psychoeducation, and prioritizing sexual pleasure for people with clitorises can help reduce this gap.

DISCUSSION QUESTIONS

- Discuss the differences between primary and secondary female orgasmic disorder (FOD) and the type of treatment involved with each.
- What are the challenges in diagnosing and treating female sexual arousal disorder (FSAD), and how can therapists address these challenges in a clinical setting?
- Critically analyze the role client education plays in managing dyspareunia and how therapists can ensure that clients understand and effectively use the information provided.
- Explain how medical, psychological, and relational factors contribute to Genito-Pelvic Pain/Penetration Disorder, and the treatment approaches that can address these factors.

LEARNING ACTIVITIES

CourseConnect

To access self-assessment questions and interactive, competency-based learning activities for this chapter, visit www.springerpub.com/courseconnect. See inside front cover and tear-out card for CourseConnect details.

ADDITIONAL RESOURCES

Additional resources are online and available at www.springerpub.com/courseconnect.

REFERENCES

Althof, S., Meston, C. M., Perelman, M. A., Handy, A. B., Kilimnik, C. D., & Stanton, A. M. (2017). Opinion paper: On the diagnosis/classification of sexual arousal concerns in women. *Journal of Sexual Medicine, 14*(11), 1365–1371. https://doi.org/10.1016/j.jsxm.2017.08.013

American Psychiatric Association. (2013). *Diagnostic and statistical manual of mental disorders* (5th ed.). https://doi.org/10.1176/appi.books.9780890425596

Basson, R. (2002). Women's sexual desire—Disordered or misunderstood? *Journal of Sex Marital Therapy, 28*(Suppl. 1), 17–28. https://doi.org/10.1080/00926230252851168

Bittoni, C., & Kiesner, J. (2022). Sexual desire in women: Paradoxical and non-linear associations with depression and anxiety. *Journal of Sexual Medicine, 19*(Suppl. 3), S5–S6. https://doi.org/10.1016/j.jsxm.2022.05.015

Costa, R. M., Pestana, J., & Costa, D. (2018). Self-transcendence, sexual desire, and sexual frequency. *Journal of Sex & Marital Therapy, 44*(1), 56–60. https://doi.org/10.1080/0092623X.2017.1314397

Critelli, C., Iasevoli, M., & Tripodi, F. (2016). Intervento riabilitativo per il dolore sessuale [Rehabilitation intervention for sexual pain]. *Rivista di Sessuologia Clinica, 1*, 79–81. https://www.torrossa.com/es/resources/an/3187332

Dias-Amaral, A., & Marques-Pinto, A. (2018). Female genito-pelvic pain/penetration disorder: Review of the related factors and overall approach. *Revista Brasileira de Ginecologia e Obstetrícia, 40*(12), 787–793. https://doi.org/10.1055/s-0038-1675805

Dodson, B. (1996). *Sex for one: The joy of self-loving*. Random House.

Ferreira, L. C., Narciso, I., Novo, R. F., & Pereira, C. R. (2016). Partners' similarity in differentiation of self is associated with higher sexual desire: A quantitative dyadic study. *Journal of Sex & Marital Therapy, 42*(7), 635–647. https://doi.org/10.1080/0092623X.2015.1113584

Fugl-Meyer, K. S., Bohm-Starke, N., Peterson, C. D., Fugl-Meyer, A., Parish, S., & Girali, A. (2013). Standard operating procedures for female sexual pain. *The Journal of Sexual Medicine, 10*(1), 83-93. https://doi.org/10.1111/j.1743-6109.2012.02867.x

Gambescia, N., Weeks, G. R., & Hertlein, K. M. (2021). *A clinician's guide to systemic sex therapy* (3rd ed.). Routledge.

Gesselman, A. N., Bennett-Brown, M., Dubé, S., Kaufman, E. M., Campbell, J. T., Garcia, J. R. (2024). The lifelong orgasm gap: Exploring age's impact on orgasm rates. *Sexual Medicine, 12*(3), qfae042. https://doi.org/10.1093/sexmed/qfae042

Ghorayshi, A. (2023, November 9). After antidepressants, a loss of sexuality. *New York Times*. https://www.nytimes.com/2023/11/09/health/antidepressants-ssri-sexual-dysfunction.html

Grant, M. (2012). *Pain control with EMDR: Treatment manual*. Trauma and Pain Management Services.

Heiman, J., LoPiccolo, L., & LoPiccolo, J. (1976). *Becoming orgasmic: A sexual growth program for women*. Prentice-Hall.

Hertlein, K. M., Gambescia, N., & Weeks, G. R. (2019). *Systemic sex therapy* (3rd ed.). Routledge.

IsHak, W. W., Bokarius, A., Jeffrey, J. K., Davis, M. C., & Bakhta, Y. (2010). Disorders of orgasm in women: A literature review of etiology and current treatments. *The Journal of Sexual Medicine, 7*(10), 3254–3268. https://doi.org/10.1111/j.1743-6109.2010.01928.x

Isola, E. (2016). Un viaggio verso l'intimità: Dal matrimonio bianco alla gravidanza, Disturbi sessuali e psicoterapia [A trip towards the intimacy. From the unconsummated marriage to the pregnancy]. *Psicobiettivo*, XXXVI (2), 111–121. https://doi.org/10.3280/PSOB2016-002007

Isola, E., & Maccarrone, B. (2019). *Emdr e Disturbi sessuali [EMDR and sexual disorders]*. Casa Editrice Astrolabio.

Kaplan, H. (1974). *The new sex therapy*. Brunner/Mazel.

Kingsberg, S. A., & Rezaee, R. L. (2013). Hypoactive sexual desire in women. *Menopause, 20*(12), 1284–1300. https://doi.org/10.1097/GME.0000000000000131

Knipe, J. (2017). *EMDR e toolbox: Teoria e trattamento del PTSD complesso e della dissociazione [Theory and treatment of complex PTSD and dissociation]*. Giovanni Fioriti Editore.

Korn, D. L., & Leeds, A. M. (2002). Preliminary evidence of efficacy for EMDR resource development and installation in the stabilization phase of treatment of complex post-traumatic stress disorder. *Journal of Clinical Psychology, 58*(12), 1465–1487. https://doi.org/10.1002/jclp.10099

Laumann, E., Paik, A., & Rosen, R. C. (1999). Sexual dysfunction in the United States: Prevalence and predictors. *Journal of the American Medical Association, 281*(6), 537–544. https://doi.org/10.1001/jama.281.6.537

Lipshultz, L. I., Pastuszak, A. W., Goldstein, A. T., Giraldi, A., & Perelman, M. A. (2016). *Management of sexual dysfunction in men and women: An interdisciplinary approach*. Springer Nature.

LoPiccolo, J., & Lobitz, W. (1972). The role of masturbation in the treatment of orgasmic dysfunction. *Archives of Sexual Behavior, 2*(2), 163–171. https://doi.org/10.1007/BF01541865

Luber, M. (Ed.). (2009). *Eye movement desensitization and reprocessing (EMDR) scripted protocols: Basics and special situations*. Springer Publishing Company (Tr.It. "I protocolli terapeutici dell'EMDR. Condizioni di base e specifiche", Fioriti, Roma).

Masters, W., & Johnson, V. (1966). *Human sexual response*. Little, Brown.

Masters, W., & Johnson, V. (1970). *Human sexual inadequacy*. Little, Brown.

McCabe, M. P. (2016). New concepts in the understanding of female sexual dysfunction. In L. I. Lipshultz, A. W. Pastuszak, A. T. Goldstein, A. Giraldi, & M. A. Perelman (Eds.), *Management of sexual dysfunction in men & women* (pp. 307–314). Springer Nature. https://doi.org/10.1007/978-1-4939-3100-2_26

Meana, M., & Steiner, E. T. (2014). Hidden disorder/hidden desire: Presentations of low sexual desire in men. In Y. M. Binik & K. S. K. Hall (Eds.), *Principles and practice of sex therapy* (5th ed., pp. 42–60). Guilford Press.

Meston, C., & Stanton, A. (2017). Evaluation of female sexual interest/arousal disorder. In W. IsHak (Ed.), *The textbook of clinical sexual medicine* (pp. 155–163). Springer Nature.

Mindyra. (2021). *Female genito-pelvic pain/penetration disorder (GPPPD) in adults*. Mindyra Health Corporation. https://www.mindyra.com/solutions/adults/femalegenito-pelvicpain/penetration

Mintz, L. (2018). *Becoming cliterate: Why orgasm equality matters and how to get it*. HarperOne.

Montejo, A. L., Llorca, G., Izquierdo, J. A., & Rico-Villademoros, F. (2001). Incidence of sexual dysfunction associated with antidepressant agents: A prospective multicenter study of 1022 outpatients. Spanish Working Group for the Study of Psychotropic-Related Sexual Dysfunction. *The Journal of Clinical Psychiatry, 62*(Suppl. 3), 10–21. https://www.psychiatrist.com/jcp/incidence-sexual-dysfunction-associated-antidepressant-2

Morin, M., Carroll, M. S., & Bergeron, S. (2017). Systematic review of the effectiveness of physical therapy modalities in woman with provoked vestibulodynia, *Sexual Medicine Reviews, 5*(3), 295–322. https://doi.org/10.1016/j.sxmr.2017.02.003

Naghibi, S. M., & Hosseini, S. H. (2023). Improved anorgasmia following add-on lamotrigine treatment. *Trends in Pharmaceutical Sciences, 9*(4), 239–242. https://doi.org/10.30476/TIPS.2023.99953.1211

Nagoski, E. (2015). *Come as you are.* Simon & Schuster.

Nguyen, V., Dolendo, I., Uloko, M., Hsieh, T.-C., & Patel, D. (2023). Male delayed orgasm and anorgasmia: A practical guide for sexual medicine providers. *International Journal of Impotence Research, 36*(3), 186–193. https://doi.org/10.1038/s41443-023-00692-7

Perelman, M. A. (2018). Sex coaching for non-sexologist physicians: How to use the sexual tipping point model. *Journal of Sexual Medicine, 15*(12), 1667–1672. https://doi.org/10.1016/j.jsxm.2018.10.010

Prekatsounaki, S., Janssen, E., & Enzlin, P. (2019). In search of desire: The role of intimacy, celebrated otherness, and object-of-desire affirmation in sexual desire in women. *Journal of Sex & Marital Therapy, 45*(5), 414–423. https://doi.org/10.1080/0092623X.2018.1549633

Prendergast S. A. (2017). Pelvic floor physical therapy for vulvodynia: A clinician's guide. *Obstetrics and Gynecology Clinics of North America, 44*(3), 509–522. https://doi.org/10.1016/j.ogc.2017.05.006

Ricky, K. C. A., Tang, V. K. Y., & Walla, P. (2019). The effect of sexual arousal and emotional arousal on working memory. *Cogent Psychology, 6*(1), 1645260. https://doi.org/10.1080/23311908.2019.1645260

Rosen, N. O., Corsini-Munt, S., Dubé, J. P., Boudreau, C., & Muise, A. (2020). Partner responses to low desire: Associations with sexual, relational, and psychological well-being among couples coping with female sexual interest/arousal disorder. *The Journal of Sexual Medicine, 17*(11), 2168–2180. https://doi.org/10.1016/j.jsxm.2020.08.015

Rosen, N. O., Dawson, S. J., Brooks, M., & Kellogg-Spadt, S. (2019). Treatment of vulvodynia: Pharmacological and non-pharmacological approaches, *Drugs, 79*(5), 483–493. https://doi.org/10.1007/s40265-019-01085-1

Simonelli, C., Fabrizi, A., Rossi, R., & Tripodi, F. (2019). *Sessuologia clinica. Diagnosi, trattamento e linee guida internazionali* [Clinical sexology: Diagnosis, treatment, and international guidelines]. Franco Angeli.

Wade, L. D., Kremer, E. C., & Brown, J. (2005). The incidental orgasm: The presence of clitoral knowledge and the absence of orgasm for women. *Women & Health, 42*(1), 117–138. https://doi.org/10.1300/J013v42n01_07

Walen, S. R., & Roth, D. (1987). A cognitive approach. In J. H. Geer & W. T. O'Donohue (Eds.), *Theories of human sexuality* (pp. 335–362). Plenum Press.

CHAPTER 9

Penile and Related Sexual Disorders and Treatment

Wendy Stock, Katherine Hertlein, and Stephanie Baird

LEARNING OBJECTIVES

- Learn about low sexual desire, as well as a variety of treatment strategies related to improving desire levels.
- Learn about erectile disorders, as well as a variety of treatment strategies related to arousal disorders.
- Learn about penile orgasm disorders (premature and delayed ejaculation) as well as a variety of treatment strategies related to orgasm disorders.
- Learn about sexual pain-related concerns and disorders (e.g., sex headaches).

INTRODUCTION

Sexual disorders in people with penises can play a significant role in their well-being and sexual satisfaction, and can contribute to relationship deterioration. With such important implications, it is critical that clinicians have a solid treatment protocol outlined; however, because the etiology can be complex, the most effective treatment for each individual case may be difficult to determine. In this chapter, we identify the physical, psychological, and social elements contributing to men's (which includes cisgender and AMAB [assigned male at birth] transgender diverse/nonconforming) sexual health, along with treatment strategies tailored to each etiology.

MALE HYPOACTIVE SEXUAL DESIRE DISORDER

DIAGNOSIS AND DESCRIPTION

Sexual desire, often colloquially referred to (inaccurately) as *drive*, includes interest in sexual stimuli, wishing for sexual activity, planning for sexual activity, or feeling frustrated when sexual activity does not occur. Many clinicians are using the words *sexual desire* or *sexual interest*, as these words indicate a more temporal state, rather than a permanent or "innate" trait suggested by "drive."

The *Diagnostic and Statistical Manual of Mental Disorders* (5th ed.; *DSM-5*; American Psychiatric Association [APA], 2013) defines Hypoactive Sexual Desire Disorder (HSDD) as persistent or recurrently deficient sexual or erotic thoughts, fantasies, and desire for sexual activity that has persisted for a minimum of 6 months and causes significant distress to the person reporting the difficulty.

The *DSM-5* (APA, 2013) implemented different diagnostic categories for male and female low sexual desire. The male diagnosis has remained the same as in previous *DSM* versions: Male Hypoactive Sexual Desire Disorder (MHSDD).

Clients reporting low desire function quite well sexually by all objective criteria, yet they have no subjective experience of sexual desire. Individuals presenting for treatment of low sexual desire can be characterized as "wanting to want" sex. Low desire can be either global or situational. Some clients have sexual desire but do not want to sexually engage with their partner, yet masturbate regularly. Others do not experience any sexual urges, reporting few or no sexual thoughts or fantasies. Still others may identify as asexual and need permission to embrace this identity.

CONTRIBUTING FACTORS

Biological/Psychopharmacological Factors

Many factors can influence a lower desire and *must* be addressed before implementing specific techniques designed to increase sexual desire. Some factors include hormonal influences (e.g., age related/decrease in testosterone), medication side effects, medical conditions or treatments, and/or substance use.

Individual Factors

A history of untreated trauma or abuse can result in the client having intrusive thoughts or "flashbacks" during sexual activity, eventually resulting in a decrease in interest in sexual activity. Situational HSDD can emerge from adverse life events such as childhood sexual abuse (Hall, 2020). Psychological issues tied to HSDD include anxiety, depression, avoidant attachment styles, and self-concept; i.e. health condition(s) may impair their self-concept (Dosch et al., 2016; Weeks & Gambescia, 2015). In a study of nearly 4,000 cisgender men, primary reduced sexual interest was associated with a higher level of education, more home and relationship disturbances, and an overall healthy body (Corona et al., 2013).

Relational Factors

Relationship conflict and/or poor or absent communication can also impede desire and interest. Clients with penises who are in a relationship over 5 years tend to be more likely to have HSDD, possibly tied to conflict management, since conflict may be managed differently later in relationships versus earlier (Mark & Lasslo, 2018). Other factors include chronic anger and resentment toward one's partner, even when this resentment or anger is at an unconscious level, as well as sexual monotony. Cultural background can play a role (sexual norms often socialize an erotophobic belief that desiring sex is sinful or wrong, resulting in guilt and shame).

TREATMENT AND INTERVENTION TO CREATE/INCREASE SEXUAL DESIRE/INTEREST

For all of the treatment methods that follow, it can be helpful to consider the dual control model of sexual interest, that is, helping the client identify their sexual inhibition system (brakes) and sexual excitation system (accelerators). Once the client can identify brakes getting in the way of potential sexual interest, the treatment strategies that follow may help to reduce or eliminate any specific situational or low-level chronic brakes (e.g., overwork, ongoing stress, prior interfering traumatic material, relational conflict). Additionally, while it may be relatively easy to pinpoint circumstances blocking sexual interest, it may be difficult for some clients to identify potential sexual accelerators. They may need permission to engage in fantasy and erotic exploration to help identify interest-generating context and material (i.e., what they consider a "sexy context"), particularly if they are reporting any shame.

Relational Strategies

Sexual desire is often embedded in a relational context, and it is important to attend to the underlying motivational forces that trigger it. Basson's (2002) nonlinear model of sexual response, discussed in Chapter 3, is a circular rather than the traditional linear model of sexual response. Her model incorporates the need for intimacy; it also acknowledges that desire can be responsive or spontaneous, and may occur either before or after arousal.

Relationship factors impact the cycle and can affect willingness to participate in sex; this is true for cisgender men (and women), transgender clients, and nonbinary clients. Issues of power and control and fear of losing control within a relationship are often psychological factors that contribute to cismen experiencing sexual issues. Conflict in a relationship can also be expressed—either consciously or subconsciously—as sexual dysfunction.

Systemic Treatment Strategies and Tools

Systemic treatments involve assessing and treating any communication issues. This means working with the couple to confront their assumptions about maladaptive communication patterns. Typically, partners with HSDD have had poor experiences with one another when it comes to conflict resolution. These partners avoid having conversations and the problems persist. Partners should be taught to communicate their sexual needs and desires in an appropriately assertive manner, to understand what emotional suppression is and how to avoid it, and to be ready to listen to their partner's needs. Partners may need to be taught how to manage emotions (either individually or conjointly) prior to the communication exercises (Wang et al., 2023).

Cognitive Behavioral Therapy Treatment Strategies and Tools

Cognitive behavioral therapy (CBT) treatment for clients with low sexual desire generally focuses on a "priming" effect of increasing the frequency of sexual thoughts, fantasies, and awareness of sexual stimuli via a desire diary, desire checklist, priming the pump (seeking out erotic material), fantasy time-outs during the day, scheduling sex, and so on. Additionally, most recent writing about sex emphasizes the importance of experiencing and centering pleasure as a way to continue to increase interest in pleasurable activities: "pleasure is the measure" (and pleasure begets more pleasure).

Eye Movement Desensitization and Reprocessing Therapy Treatment

Eye movement desensitization and reprocessing (EMDR) therapy follows an eight-phase protocol to process distressing, disturbing, and/or traumatic events and/or symptoms. For EMDR therapy specific to low desire, identifying and reprocessing targets regarding sexual desire that involve shame, erotophobic and negative cognitions, negative beliefs and messages, prior history of trauma or abuse, and relationship conflict, anxiety, or stress may help reduce blocks to sexual desire.

MALE ERECTILE DISORDER

DIAGNOSIS AND DESCRIPTION

Erectile dysfunction (ED) is the inability to experience an erection, despite the wish to do so. Previously ED was categorized on one scale, as either due to organic or psychogenic conditions. As the field developed, a dual scale was proposed (LoPiccolo & Stock, 1986) that facilitated the understanding that a client may be high on both organic and psychogenic causation of ED, low on both factors, or any combination of high or low on either scale. The implications of this for the therapist is that it is important to assess for causal factors on both axes, organic and psychogenic. It is now recognized that both organic and psychogenic factors can contribute to ED to different degrees for an individual client (LoPiccolo & Stock, 1986).

CONTRIBUTING FACTORS

Biological/Psychopharmacological Factors

It was once thought that ED was predominantly due to psychogenic causes. In 1970, Masters and Johnson stated that 95% of all erectile failure cases were psychogenic in origin and did not involve any physiological pathology. More recent studies, however, have indicated that neurological, vascular (such as cardiovascular disease), and hormonal abnormalities or changes (such as experiencing andropause) are involved in a considerable percentage of cases of ED. Medical conditions (e.g., diabetes) and medications (e.g., selective serotonin reuptake inhibitors [SSRIs] for treating depression, beta-blockers for treating heart conditions) may contribute to erectile issues. There are, however, many cases in which someone has a mild organic impairment, which then makes their erection more vulnerable to being disrupted by psychological, behavioral, and sexual technique factors. If these psychological and behavioral difficulties are eliminated by sex therapy, the client may be able to attain a full erection.

Individual Factors

Individual factors include psychological factors such as the presence of trait depression, maladaptive early cognitive schemas, proneness to sexual inhibition, a lack of proneness to sexual excitation, and one's age. The experience of stress may also impair one's ability to experience an erection. Other individual factors may include stereotypically gendered myths (i.e., "a real man has an erection at will"), any sexual guilt, sexual secrets in the client's family-of-origin, issues with boundaries, and a history of sexual abuse.

Relational Factors

Since anxiety (specifically performance anxiety, that is, the pressure one experiences or perceives to perform sexually) can contribute to ED, relational factors promoting any type of anxiety can be contributors. This includes a demand to perform (often in times of attempted conception with assigned female at birth [AFAB] partners), relational discord, an unconscious (or conscious) desire to withhold pleasure and connection from a partner, impaired communication (especially regarding sexual likes and dislikes), and relationship conflict (Rowland & Kolba, 2018; Yoo et al., 2014). In gay relationships, contributing factors of ED might include impaired sense of maleness/masculinity, internalized homophobia, and being HIV positive (or presence of a transmittable sexually transmitted infection [STI]).

INTERVENTION AND TREATMENTS

Psychodynamic Treatment Strategies and Tools

Prior to the early 1990s, standard sex therapy approaches included deemphasizing the pressure the client put on themselves to produce an erection, and teaching partners to engage in sensual, nondemand touching utilizing the sensate focus exercise. Once the client was able to relax, be present, and connect with their partner, an erection often developed. In many cases, the culturally based demand for people with penises to always be ready for sex, always be able to obtain an erection, and the perceived imperative of penis–vagina intercourse was what created the ED.

Medical Intervention and Treatments

The introduction of Viagra (sildenafil) in 1998 and other similar medications, all phosphodiesterase-5 (PDE5) inhibitors, such as tadalafil (Cialis) and vardenafil, that facilitate erection revolutionized the treatment of ED. Even clients that have medical issues contributing to erectile difficulties often respond to these medications. Tiefer (1988), however, has raised the concern that medicalization of sexuality can obscure the effects of social contributions to people's sexual complaints, including rigid gender roles, unrelenting standards of performance, relationships of unequal power, and histories of sexual victimization. The ability to attain an erection does not address a lack of emotional connection, intimacy, or physical sensuality in a relationship.

Psychoeducation Interventions

Metz and McCarthy (2004) have written an excellent self-help book, *Coping With Erectile Dysfunction,* that offers a psychoeducational approach and guidelines that can be used by the client independently, or in conjunction with sex therapy. The following list highlights the major points covered in their book; these address the social, cultural, and relational factors associated with erectile problems.

1. By age 40, 90% of people with penises will have at least one erectile difficulty. This is a normal occurrence, not a sign of ED.
2. ED can be caused by a wide variety of factors including alcohol, anxiety, depression, vascular or neurological deficits, distraction, anger, side effects of medication, frustration, hormonal deficiency, fatigue, and/or not feeling sexual at that time or with that partner. As clients age, the hormonal, vascular, and neurological systems become less efficient, so psychological, relational, and psychosexual skill factors become more important.
3. ED is a psychobiosocial problem with multiple causes, dimensions, and effects. To comprehensively evaluate medical factors, including side effects of medication, consult a urologist with training in erectile function and dysfunction.
4. Medical interventions, especially the oral medications—sildenafil, tadalafil, and vardenafil—can be a valuable resource to facilitate erectile function; however, they are not a "magic pill. Partners need to integrate the medical intervention into their lovemaking style of intimacy, pleasuring, and eroticism.
5. Do not believe the myth of the "male machine, ready to have intercourse at any time, with any woman, in any situation." The client and their penis are human, not a performance machine; this myth is dehumanizing for all involved.
6. View the erectile difficulty as a situational problem; do not overreact and label oneself "impotent" or put oneself down as a "failure."
7. A pervasive myth is if someone loses their initial erection, it means they are sexually turned off. It is a natural physiological process for erections to wax and wane during prolonged pleasuring.
8. In a 45-minute pleasuring session, erections will wax and wane two or more times. Subsequent erections, intercourse, and orgasm can be quite satisfying.
9. A penis is not needed to satisfy a partner. Orgasms can occur manually, orally, with sex toys, or with rubbing stimulation. If one has difficulty getting or maintaining an erection, do not stop the sexual encounter. Many find it arousing to have their partner's fingers, tongue, or penis (erect or flaccid) used for stimulation.
10. Actively involve oneself in giving and receiving pleasurable and erotic touching. Erection is a natural result of pleasure, feeling turned-on, and getting into an erotic flow.
11. One cannot will or force an erection. Do not be a "passive spectator" who is distracted by the state of the penis. Sex is not a spectator sport; it requires active involvement for all partners.
12. Allow the partner to initiate intercourse and guide the penis into their vagina (or other orifice). This reduces performance pressure and, since they are the expert on their orifice, is the most practical procedure.
13. Feel comfortable saying, "I want sex to be pleasurable and playful. When I feel pressure to perform, I get uptight and sex is not good. We can make sexuality enjoyable by taking it at a comfortable pace, enjoy playing and pleasuring, and being an intimate team."
14. Erectile problems do not affect the ability to ejaculate (people can ejaculate with a flaccid penis). Ejaculation to the cue of an erect penis can be relearned.
15. One way to regain confidence is through masturbation. During masturbation, one can practice gaining and losing erections, relearn ejaculation with an erection, and focus on fantasies and stimulation, which can transfer to partner sex.
16. Do not try to use a waking erection for quick intercourse. This erection can be associated with rapid eye movement (REM) sleep and can result from dreaming and being physically close to the partner. People try vainly to have intercourse with the morning erection before losing it. Remember: arousal and erection can be regained. Morning can be a good time to be sexual.
17. When sleeping, erections occur every 90 minutes (an estimated three to five erections per night). Sexual response is a natural physiological function.

18. Make clear, direct, assertive requests (not demands) for preferred erotic stimulation. Verbally and nonverbally guide partners in how to provide pleasure and arousal.
19. Trying to stimulate one's penis when it is flaccid is counterproductive, as the person can become distracted and obsessed with the state of their penis. Engage in sensuous, playful, nondemand touching. The base of sexual response is relaxation and sensuality. Enjoy giving and receiving stimulation rather than trying to "will an erection."
20. Anticipatory anxiety, performance anxiety, distraction, and/or putting yourself down can reduce or block erections. Give oneself (and one's partner) permission to enjoy the pleasure of sexuality. Attitudes and self-thoughts affect arousal. The key is "sex and pleasure" not "sex and performance."
21. A sexual experience is best measured by pleasure and satisfaction, not whether one had an erection, how hard it was, or whether the partner was orgasmic. Some sexual experiences will be great for all, some better for one than the other, some mediocre, and others not enjoyable. Do not put sexual self-esteem on the line at each experience. The "good enough" model of sexual pleasure is much healthier than the perfect intercourse performance criterion.

Systemic Treatment Strategies and Tools

The complexity of ED alongside the social and cultural factors and myths around cisgender men's sexuality compels that a therapist gives "go slow" messages to the client. The therapist should evaluate any barriers to treatment (including individual fears, myths, deeply held negative beliefs about sex, and recovery from trauma) prior to beginning the work. Therapists should work on reducing anxiety and helping the couple to focus on pleasure and sensuality, rather than orgasm, as the goal for a sexual experience. As the couple moves toward greater levels of intimacy, the therapist can pair sexual activities with desensitization in a sensate-focused manner.

Cognitive Behavioral Therapy Treatment Strategies and Tools

For ED related to anxiety or stress, learning and practicing relaxation techniques can go a long way toward restoring pleasure and confidence. Taking the time to learn and experience deep relaxation in the pelvic and genital region, as well as addressing the issue causing the problem, can be life-changing. In many cases, ED is the result of performance anxiety. The more anxious one becomes as sexual situations approach, the more likely ED will emerge. Another element of CBT is when the erectile issues are supporting or reflecting a problematic negative cognition. It is well-demonstrated that negative cognitions (e.g., "I am damaged," "I am not good enough"), as well as automatic negative thoughts, contribute to the development and maintenance of ED (Carvalho & Nobre, 2011). Effective CBT strategies would address the negative cognitions to reduce the performance anxiety and enable more satisfactions and functioning.

New England Sex Therapy developed a handout on "relaxing your pelvic muscle" for easy erections, adapted from Metz and McCarthy's 2004 book Coping with Erectile Dysfunction (Timberlake, J.C.). Essentially, folks with penises can locate the contraction of this muscle by trying to stop the flow of urine briefly, or by "twitching" the penis. Once this muscle group is located, initially spend about 3 seconds tensing this area, then release that tension, spending another 3 seconds in the relaxed state. Continue lengthening the time of relaxation between contractions, as well as developing a continuum of awareness from 0 (relaxed) to 10 (tight).

Eye Movement Desensitization and Reprocessing Therapy Treatment

For EMDR therapy specific to ED, identifying and reprocessing targets regarding sexual desire that involve shame, shame about perceived "sexual failure," erotophobic and negative cognitions, negative beliefs and messages, prior history of trauma or abuse, history of feeling betrayed, and relationship conflict, anxiety, or stress may help reduce blocks to sexual desire and subsequent erections.

Case Study 9.1: Treatment of Paul's Erectile Dysfunction With Eye Movement Desensitization and Reprocessing Therapy

By Nicola Pinder, MSc (EMDR Therapy), Psychosexual Therapist, Supervisor and EMDR Consultant

Details of this case have been altered to protect the client's confidentiality.

EYE MOVEMENT DESENSITIZATION AND REPROCESSING THERAPY PHASE 1: HISTORY AND TREATMENT PLANNING

Paul is a cisgendered White British heterosexual man married to his wife, Sue, for 16 years. They have been together for 19 years, and are in a monogamous relationship. He was 43 years old when he presented for help regarding the inability to get erections in partnered sex. His erections were good on his own for masturbation, and he would usually wake with an erection in the morning. There had been a sudden onset of erection difficulties about 6 months ago, and Paul was now desperate to get this situation resolved.

Paul had no health issues, enjoyed going to the gym, and was usually quite a positive person. Paul described his relationship with Sue as very close and loving. They worked together in a clothing business they owned and shared the household tasks well. They had two sons, aged 13 and 9.

Paul's history indicated that his childhood was good; he did well at school, was popular, and got on well with his older sister and brother, which they still did as adults. He did not use any recreational drugs growing up or now, drank alcohol infrequently, and had a good network of friends. His parents divorced when he was 8 years old. He and his siblings stayed in the family home with their mother while their father moved out. Only as adults did they learn that their father had an affair, which led to the breakdown of the relationship and subsequent divorce.

As an EMDR-trained psychosexual therapist, alongside taking a comprehensive history from a new client, we also assess a person's ability to regulate their emotions. This is important as many psychosexual presentations are rooted in anxiety and self-criticism; therefore, helping people learn or develop their ability to calm their body and mind can be very helpful. In Paul's case, his penis was very much his emotional barometer and was an external marker of his anxiety about sexual contact with his wife.

EYE MOVEMENT DESENSITIZATION AND REPROCESSING THERAPY PHASE 2: PREPARATION

We discussed a positive visualization that Paul could access in his mind's eye, a calm place where he felt peaceful and relaxed. For him, it was a beautiful beach with white sand, clear water, and just the right temperature. It was quiet, with the gentle sound of the waves coming in and out. He was advised to "visit" this calm place daily and notice its soothing effect on his nervous system. The addition of slow alternating bilateral stimulation (BLS; his hands tapping on his knees, from one side to the other) was added to deepen his sense of calm and introduce this key EMDR BLS feature.

Paul could focus when he was at work and could also be present with his family, yet the overwhelming panic when he began to think about becoming intimate with his wife caused him great concern. Sue, Paul's wife, supported him during this time; she knew he was attending therapy and was keen to help however she could. I recommended that they take the pressure off themselves and stop trying to have penis–vagina intercourse or sexual activity for the time being. Instead, they should focus on their closeness and connection via nonsexual hugging and touching.

I explained to Paul that we would utilize EMDR therapy to reduce his level of anxiety that had become associated with the thought of sexual intimacy with his wife. EMDR therapy is an evidence-based approach for treating the symptoms of posttraumatic stress disorder (PTSD); more recently, research has demonstrated its effectiveness in treating conditions other than PTSD, such as depression, pain conditions, addictions, and more. See Scelles and Bulnes's (2021) systematic review for more information on this.

When we think about making sense of someone's presentation from an EMDR perspective, we seek to explore when the adaptive thoughts, feelings, or behaviors began and what they might be linked to. In Paul's case, there was a sudden onset 6 months earlier. Through discussion, Paul said he and Sue had decided to have intimate time together as their oldest son was out and the younger one was asleep. As Sue went to the bathroom before they got intimate, Paul noticed an expression on Sue's face that filled him with dread, and from that point, he had been unable to get an erection. He did not understand this response, and yet it seemed so powerful. He was sure he would lose his wife if he could not regain his erections, which was contrary to the love and support Sue offered.

I discussed with Paul the idea that we should explore what that facial expression meant to him so we could understand the reaction he was experiencing. I asked Paul to see that facial expression in his mind's eye, notice his emotional response, and notice if he had any sensations in his body that also went with it. Paul reported fear, distress, and a "black hole in the pit of (his) stomach." I asked him to bridge or float back in time in his mind and see where he landed, the very first place, without analysis or conscious thought, associated with his reported emotions and sensations. Paul spoke of when his father left the family home when Paul was young. His mother and father were standing on the driveway; Paul was up in his room watching through the window. His mother stood on the driveway as his father drove off; she turned to come back to the house and saw Paul in the window; it was his mother's face at that moment that he had seen on his wife's face 6 months earlier.

We discussed adaptive information processing (AIP), the theory underpinning EMDR therapy, and how, in overwhelming moments, fragments of information get stuck and cannot fully be made sense of and processed, but remain in our nervous system. They potentially become triggered in the present when something feels familiar to the unprocessed old memory. This became our target memory to process with EMDR therapy.

We needed some key information, gathered in EMDR therapy Phase 3 (Assessment), to activate the memory network, move the memory from its stuck place to a more adaptive resolution, and resolve the distress associated with it.

Target Image: (*"What image holds the most energy for you in that memory?"*) "Mom looking up at me with that face."

Negative Cognition: (*"What's the negative belief about yourself right now related to that image, 'I'm ...'?"*) "I'm not a good enough husband."

Positive Cognition: (*"What would you want to believe about yourself?"*) "I am a good enough husband."

Validity of Cognition: (VOC; *"How true does that positive belief seem to you now on a scale of 1 to 7, 1 being false and 7, true?"*) "A 3 out of 7."

Emotions: ("What emotions are part of this for you?") "Fear, upset, confusion."

Subjective Units of Distress: (SUD; *"How upsetting is this on a scale of 0 to 10 where 0 is neutral, no distress, and 10 is the worst distress you can imagine?"*) "It's a 9."

Body: (*"What do you notice in your body?"*) "I feel an emptiness in my stomach, and my heart is beating fast."

EYE MOVEMENT DESENSITIZATION AND REPROCESSING THERAPY PHASES 4 TO 7: DESENSITIZATION, INSTALLATION, BODY SCAN, CLOSURE

With this information, we began processing the memory. Information had been given to Paul about what to expect during the processing sessions, that he was in control and could stop if it felt like too much at any point by giving me a signal we had discussed. Many insights came to Paul during the processing, the key ones being sadness at the split between his parents, which he did not want for himself; the realization "I am not my father," "I am a good and loving husband," "Sue loves me, and we're a great team." The memory was processed until the SUD was a zero. Paul's positive belief was checked for accuracy (in case something else felt more appropriate) and was installed and strengthened with further positive insights coming to mind until it was a 7 out of 7. He scanned his body for any residual unpleasant sensations; none were reported, and he reported feeling calm and whole.

EYE MOVEMENT DESENSITIZATION AND REPROCESSING THERAPY PHASE 8: REEVALUATION

The process was concluded with a future template, an imagined rehearsal of everything working as he would like in a visualised run-through of he and Sue being intimate. No disturbance was noted and Paul shared that he felt like himself again.

Processing this one key memory resolved the issue Paul was having experiencing an erection in partnered sex. This provides an example of the benefits of using EMDR therapy and conceptualizing the case from an AIP perspective, to treat issues related to sexual functioning. This approach differs from psychosexual "treatment as usual," as links between maladaptively stored memories are processed to reduce the distress held and, therefore, resolve associated symptomology.

ORGASM DISORDERS

PREMATURE EJACULATION

Diagnosis and Description

The cause of premature, or early, ejaculation (PE) is not well understood. It should be noted that what defines this dysfunction is culturally relative. Many clients hold themselves to unrealistic standards for how long they believe they should last before ejaculation during intercourse. It is important to assess how the client is defining this problem when this is the presenting complaint. For some, anxiety may contribute to worsening this tendency, and for others, having gone a long time without orgasmic release may also contribute. Many clients with this problem, however, have tried reducing their anxiety by masturbating before a sexual encounter, with unreliable success.

Contributing Factors

Biological/Psychopharmacological Factors

Biological factors of PE include abnormalities in the nervous system and condition which cause issues in the vascular system. Alcohol use may reduce ejaculatory control. Hormonal, thyroid, prostate, or urethra issues, or neurotransmitter imbalances (e.g., low serotonin) may also impact control (Mayo Clinic Staff, 2022). In addition, clients who are physically active at least six times per week are less likely to have PE (Herkommer et al., 2024).

Individual Factors

Emotional issues such as depression, anxiety, guilt, shame, low self-esteem, and stress can contribute to PE. From a learning perspective, some clients may not have much experience in dating or interpersonal relationships, and are not yet able to control their ejaculatory response.

Relational Factors

Relational factors that contribute to PE include the interactional and relational conflicts that exist within the relationship. Power struggles that manifest in sexual demand struggles, poor communication, fear of commitment, fear of intimacy, and unrealistic expectations of the relationship and experience regarding sexual performance have been cited as potential causes of PE. Further, the family of origin may have conflicts that shape the way a client handles conflict in their own adult relationships. The cultural or environmental context can also contribute to PE, due to practices around circumcision and effects relating to penile sensitivity, religious values, and moral codes around sex.

Intervention and Treatments

Psychoeducation Interventions

It is helpful to normalize this condition as existing on a normal continuum of latency to orgasmic threshold. Latency to ejaculation appears to be distributed on a normal curve in the human population, similar to many other human traits. The basic treatment resets the brain to accommodate to a longer period of intensity of stimulation without triggering the orgasmic reflex. Metz and McCarthy (2003) have written an excellent self-help book, *Coping With Premature Ejaculation*, which offers a psychoeducational approach and guidelines that can be used by the client independently, or in conjunction with sex therapy.

The major points covered in their book that address the social, cultural, and relational factors associated with erectile problems include the following:

1. Premature (rapid) ejaculation is the most common penile sexual problem. The majority of people with penises begin as rapid ejaculators in adolescence, and 30% of adults with penises complain of PE. Lack of ejaculatory control is not a bad problem to have, because sex therapists have been very successful in resolving it. With treatment, 80% to 90% of clients learn better control in therapy, provided they are willing to devote the necessary time and energy. Ejaculatory control is a skill or habit that can be learned in 8 to 20 weeks by following the exercises described in the text that follows.
2. "Do it yourself" techniques to reduce arousal (bite one's lip, focus on nonsexual thoughts like how much money is owed to one's mother-in-law, using two condoms or a penile numbing cream) do not teach ejaculatory control. By reducing arousal, these techniques can cause ED.
3. Learning ejaculatory control involves learning two skills:
    a. The ability to attend more fully to one's own sensations of arousal and tension.
    b. The ability to make changes in behavior that will prevent or delay ejaculation.
    The result of treatment is having more time to enjoy being aroused and the sexual interaction before reaching the PEI (point of ejaculatory inevitability). One learns to increase the amount of time spent in the zone of arousal and lengthen ejaculatory latency.
4. Ejaculatory control can be learned both through self-stimulation as well as through partner stimulation. Practicing new sexual skills with self-stimulation develops awareness, comfort, and confidence, and is the best place to start to learn ejaculatory control. Once learned on one's own, it is much easier to transfer those skills into partner sex. Ejaculatory control during partner sex, especially intercourse, is more complex and challenging.
5. The most effective technique is the ***stop–start technique***. This strategy in learning ejaculatory control may seem counterintuitive. Rather than attempting to decrease stimulation or sexual arousal, the approach is to increase comfort and awareness of arousal level, and then increase the ability to experience increasing intensity of stimulation without climaxing.
    a. Stop–start technique with self-stimulation:
        i. Plan on a 15-minute practice period.
        ii. Stimulate oneself until highly aroused, but not on the verge of having an orgasm.

   iii. Stop stimulation when highly aroused, and when one knows that if one continues, one will reach the "point of no return," otherwise known as the PEI.
   iv. Pause until one can continue stimulation without immediately reaching the PEI. The pause is likely to be from 15 to 60 sec.
   v. Resume stimulation and stop again slightly before the PEI.
   vi. Pause.
   vii. Resume.
   viii. Repeat this sequence with as many pauses as you need to get to the end of the 15-minute practice period.
   ix. One can finish this exercise by having an orgasm.
b. With self-stimulation, it is recommended to start using one's hand without any lubrication. Once the exercise can be completed with only 3 to 4 pauses within 15 minutes, then add a lubricant. Once the exercise, with lubricant, can be completed with only 3 to 4 pauses in 15 minutes, then add more arousing sexual fantasy. The idea is to challenge oneself with increasing levels of stimulation, essentially retraining the brain to enjoy stimulation without immediately triggering the orgasmic reflex.
c. The stop–start technique with a partner:
   i. Again, the idea is to start with the least challenging, and to move to the most challenging form of partner stimulation, as ejaculatory control increases.
   ii. The stop–start technique is used first with manual stimulation, then oral stimulation, and then during intercourse.
   iii. Learning ejaculatory control is a gradual process requiring practice and feedback, and a generous, patient, and cooperative partner.
   iv. The client signals the partner to stop stimulation as they approach the point of inevitability. Stimulation stops for 15 to 60 seconds, until the client no longer feels the need to ejaculate. Then resume stimulation.
   v. Initially, the client stops movement or withdraws. As awareness and confidence increase, the strategy is to use slower, longer, or circular thrusting.
   vi. Typically, ejaculatory control exercises during heterosexual intercourse begin with the "woman on top" position using minimal movement (the quiet vagina exercise), guiding intromission and controlling thrusting.
   vii. Most couples prefer this rather than the traditional "squeeze" technique, which can feel awkward and mechanical, and has no advantage in terms of efficacy.

6. Realistic expectations and goals are crucial. The typical lovemaking experience extends from 15 to 45 minutes, of which only 2 to 7 minutes involves penetrative intercourse. Contrary to stereotypical male bragging and media myths, intercourse seldom lasts longer than 10 minutes, with 5.4 minutes being the average according to one study (Waldinger et al., 2005).

7. Only one in four people with vulvas has the same response pattern as people with penises (i.e., a single orgasm during intercourse without additional stimulation). One in three people with vulvas is never orgasmic during intercourse. Improved control increases pleasure and eroticism for the person with the penis, as well as their partners. The goal of ejaculatory control is not to guarantee that other partners have an orgasm during intercourse.

8. With continued practice, other intercourse positions are added. Utilize longer, slower thrusting or circular thrusting. Alternate which partner controls the thrusting. Ejaculatory control is most difficult in the heterosexual "man on top" position with short, rapid thrusting. With practice, new methods can be learned that allow enjoyment of higher levels of arousal without immediately climaxing. For example, thrusting can change from faster to slower, or one can stop moving altogether for a few seconds or longer. (It is considerate to let partners know what one is doing.) Perhaps one can move their hips slightly to change the angle of thrusting, or do circular movements, rather than thrusting, for a few minutes.

Monitor one's breathing and take some slow, deep breaths. If holding one's partner's hips or looking at their face is orgasm-producing, try avoiding specific orgasm triggers until one wants to climax. By making these adjustments, one can stay in the shaded area for a longer time, while enjoying sensations, until ready to climax.

9. Try to maintain ejaculatory control for 10 to 15 minutes with nonintercourse stimulation (self-stimulation and partner manual or oral stimulation). Try to maintain ejaculatory control with 4 to 7 minutes of intercourse stimulation.
10. Upon ejaculation, whether rapidly or voluntarily, enjoy the feelings and sensations; do not become upset or angry. "Beating up" on oneself does not facilitate ejaculatory control. Expect there will be occasional miscalculations as the ability to tune in to arousal level and pausing is refined. This treatment involves a learning curve, so even going over the edge sooner than wished constitutes a learning experience.
11. The feelings and sensations of orgasm begin at the point of ejaculatory inevitability and last 3 to 10 seconds.
12. The partner's emotional and sexual feelings are very important. Their role is as an intimate, involved partner. They can be pleasured to arousal and orgasm with manual, oral, rubbing, or vibrator stimulation. Most partners prefer this after the ejaculatory control exercise, but some prefer it before. Sex need not end when someone ejaculates (or orgasms).
13. Remember, do not try to reduce stimulation or feeling "turned on." This could lead to an arousal problem (i.e., ED). Focus on comfort, awareness, pleasure, and arousal, without moving rapidly to ejaculation.
14. Sexuality is about giving and receiving pleasure, not a perfect performance. Partner sex is inherently variable. The "good enough" pleasure model is that 85% of the time ejaculatory control is enjoyed during intercourse. Enjoy and share the entire sexual experience: intimacy, pleasure, eroticism, arousal, intercourse, and outercourse.

Medical Intervention and Treatments

Some clients choose to utilize medication, either at a low dose continuously or a moderate dose 2 hours before intercourse, to promote ejaculatory control. Supplements and medications such as sertraline may be helpful for some clients. However, success may become dependent on remaining on medication, while the stop–start technique—once mastered—is a lifelong skill.

The preferred strategy is to use medication as an additional resource. The client should integrate the medical intervention into their couple style of intimacy, pleasuring, and eroticism. This protocol would involve practicing ejaculatory control exercises while taking medication and then gradually phase out the medication.

Increasing physical health (through regular exercise and other healthy lifestyle choices) and decreasing or eliminating performance anxiety may also improve ejaculatory control.

Systemic Treatment Strategies and Tools

When there are comorbid sexual dysfunctions, ED and HSDD should be treated first (Gambescia et al., 2020). Therapists need to identify the presence, if at all, of contradictions in the relationship. Betchen and Davidson (2018) developed a framework called *master conflict theory*. Couples may experience unconscious conflicts that play out in the bedroom as they each try to balance out the "conflict" scorecard. The goal of the therapy is to uncover and address the conflict.

Cognitive Behavioral Therapy Treatment Strategies and Tools

The treatment of PE requires that men obtain an awareness of sensations again, and then regulate the degree of arousal they experience. CBT techniques should center on starting with at-home exercises for the client to practice. Specific behavioral interventions include sensate focus, stop and start, stop and slow technique, and the squeeze technique developed by Masters and Johnson (1970). In this approach, one partner squeezes the other partner's penis as a way to delay orgasm.

Eye Movement Desensitization and Reprocessing Therapy Treatment

For EMDR therapy specific to PE, similar to ED, identifying and reprocessing targets regarding sexual desire that involve shame, shame about perceived "sexual failure," erotophobic and negative cognitions, negative beliefs and messages, prior history of trauma or abuse, history of feeling betrayed, and relationship conflict, anxiety, or stress may help reduce any distress regarding PE incidents.

DELAYED/INHIBITED EJACULATION

Diagnosis and Description

Inhibited/Delayed ejaculation (DE) has received very little attention in the therapeutic literature. As initially reported by Masters and Johnson (1970), this remains a relatively rare dysfunction, and the etiology remains unclear. This dysfunction may be global or situational, with most of these clients being able to ejaculate during masturbation, sometimes with partner stimulation, but most commonly not during penetrative sexual activity.

Contributing Factors

Biological/Psychopharmacological Factors

Inhibited ejaculation can result from physiological conditions such as multiple sclerosis. Similarly, several medications, including antihypertensives, sedatives, antianxiety, and antipsychotic agents, may have the side effect of preventing ejaculation.

Individual Factors

Clinical case studies suggest a variety of psychological factors, but there is virtually no supporting empirical research. Michael Perelman notes a contributing factor to DE as well as other sexual dysfunctions is that the individual with DE is not stimulated enough and has not reached the "tipping point" (Perelman & Watter, 2016). There may be an issue where clients masturbate in a specific way to achieve an orgasm, and because of the specificity in their masturbation patterns, it is difficult for them to achieve ejaculation with a partner in situations that do not fit the exact script of their masturbation practices.

Relational Factors

Relationship problems contributing to DE include fears of intimacy and communication, desire discrepancies, poor communication, and health issues (Perelman & Watter, 2016). Clients may also have fears about pregnancy, hostility toward partners, prior traumatic history, or even an unacknowledged sexual orientation. Many couples present to therapy with DE at a time of failed conception. It is also common for the partner of the person with DE to blame themselves for not being attractive enough. Intergenerational factors may include coming from households where there is aggression (and withholding sex and/or or ejaculation as a pattern to manage conflict) and/or the myth that people with penises should go "all night" (Hertlein et al., 2020).

Intervention and Treatments

Psychoeducation Interventions

Providing psychoeducation similar to the earlier sections can help break myths clients may hold about ejaculation timing. For instance, a client may report that it takes them 8 minutes of intercourse to ejaculate, and may think this is too long, or be told by a partner it is too long, when in actuality it is well within the normal range. Also providing clarifying information about pregnancy prevention, STI prevention, or other information specific to a client's fears may help alleviate anxiety, allowing for a more sensual and relaxed experience of sexual activity.

Medical/Physical Interventions

The client's physician can assess for and treat any potentially interfering medical concerns that may reduce arousal or delay ejaculation. The client, along with their physician, can evaluate the presence of interfering medications and may consider reducing or eliminating an interfering medication, or switching to other less interfering medications.

Psychodynamic Treatment Strategies and Tools

This author (W. Stock) has treated several cases of inhibited ejaculation during sexual interaction with a partner that occurred following a devastating betrayal of trust by a partner. In these cases, addressing the emotional trauma and loss of trust in therapy resulted in remission of inhibited ejaculation. Reducing performance anxiety and increasing physical stimulation remain the major treatment elements for inhibited ejaculation (LoPiccolo, 1977).

Systemic Treatment Strategies and Tools

Relationship treatment includes sexual skill building and decreasing the pressure on performance. Couples are taught to be more flexible and spontaneous as well as being more supportive of one another. Hertlein et al. (2020) suggest clients borrow competencies in other parts of their relationships and bring those skills into new parts of their relationship—like sex—where a great deal of weight is placed on the relationship. In addition, the couple needs to move toward building more sensuality in order to improve intimacy and take the pressure off the sexual portion of the relationship. Therapists can also prescribe sensate focus to help partners focus on their needs, desires, and improve communication on what they want sexually.

Cognitive Behavioral Therapy Treatment Strategies and Tools

CBT strategies work to decouple internalized messages generated from not being able to ejaculate in a timely manner. Examples of negative cognition and emotional states that may be common in DE include lack of confidence, impaired body image, anxiety, and trauma (Perelman, 2016). Relationship factors and stressors can also be a contributing factor. CBT strategies can include reduction of anxiety through relaxation pairing with more adaptive cognitions, evaluating the evidence behind negative judgments about oneself, and skills in effective relational communication.

Eye Movement Desensitization and Reprocessing Therapy Treatment

For EMDR therapy specific to DE, similar to ED, identifying and reprocessing targets regarding sexual desire that involve shame, shame about perceived "sexual failure," erotophobic and negative cognitions, negative beliefs and messages, prior history of trauma or abuse, history of feeling betrayed, relationship conflict, anxiety, and/or stress may help reduce any distress regarding PE incidents.

Case Study 9.2: Mitchell, Experiencing Delayed Ejaculation

Mitchell, a cisgender Black pansexual man in his mid-thirties, sought therapy to process the fallout from a high conflict divorce from his cisgender White husband of similar age. Both worked in business settings and enjoyed professional success. They had one child via surrogacy and had been engaged in a very contentious custody battle for some time over this child. During the first 2 years of the separation Mitchell had no time or energy to date.

As therapy progressed over 6 months (focused on processing the divorce and custody conflict), he met and began dating a new partner, a ciswoman, but soon discovered he was now experiencing DE. As this was a surprise to himself, he brought it up during the next therapy session. The therapist, in the intake session, had mentioned that any and all concerns can be addressed during the course of therapy, including intimacy and sexuality concerns. He had filed this piece of information away, laughing it off at the time that he did not "anticipate dating anytime soon."

Once the DE was understood in greater detail, he was provided with validating and normalizing psychoeducation, as well as mindfulness suggestions. Despite overall improvement, he continued to experience occasional DE instances. Upon further exploration, the therapist learned that his ex-husband used to sometimes complain if Mitchell was "taking too long" to orgasm. His new partner was quite supportive of Mitchell and stated that she enjoyed the longer intercourse overall, although she occasionally reached a point of feeling a little sore.

The negative messages from the ex-husband became EMDR therapy targets, along with accompanying negative self-image and shame, and were all processed to completion. Additionally, Mitchell had a fear of getting his new partner pregnant. Pregnancy prevention was discussed and instituted (birth control pills and condoms). EMDR future templates were also used to help Mitchell fully strengthen positive cognitions of "My partner and I get to enjoy our sexuality for any length of time" and "I deserve support and respect." Mitchell was then able to enjoy sexual activity with his new partner with varying lengths of sexual activity and intercourse.

PENILE, TESTICULAR AND OTHER SEXUAL PAIN ISSUES

PENILE PAIN

Penile pain can come from untreated STIs, too tight foreskin (if uncircumcised), Peyronie disease (scar tissue causing a painful bend in the penis), abnormal curvature of the penis, cysts or lesions, allergies to some contraception or vaginal fluids, hypersensitivity postcoitus, and/or skin disorders such as lichen sclerosus (which can also occur to vulvas). Some folks may also experience priapism, where a nonsexual, sustained, and painful erection can occur.

TESTICULAR PAIN

Pain can also occur in the testicles. While "blue balls" is usually something giggled about in middle school, epididymal hypertension (EH; pain in the testicles) can occur with a sustained erection not accompanied by an orgasm. If someone experiences this, their partner is under no obligation at all to help them relieve their EH. If one partner no longer wants to continue sexual activity, provide the person with testicular pain privacy to orgasm if they wish. If a bit of blueish or purplish color develops in the testicles, then the EH might be heading toward testicular torsion, which is serious and likely necessitates an immediate visit to the emergency department for possible emergency surgery. Also, if a client experiences ongoing testicular pain, when not sexually aroused, they should visit a doctor as soon as possible to rule out potential causes like cancer, kidney stones, prostatitis, and so on. Tight pants can contribute to testicular pain and potential issues.

SEX HEADACHES

Sex headaches (aka *sexual benign headaches*) comprise an increasingly dull background headache that slowly builds and then fades during sexual activity. *Orgasm headaches* involve an intense sharp pain that suddenly occurs as one approaches or experiences orgasm. Orgasm headaches can occur in any gender, but more typically in people with penises, with onset generally between ages 40 and 50.

Both sex and orgasm headaches are considered *primary* if benign and harmless, or *secondary* if accompanying a potentially harmful medical condition such as vascular problems. Anyone experiencing them should consult a medical professional to rule out any harmful or dangerous secondary underlying causes. For benign headaches, prophylactic or ongoing migraine medication and management strategies may be recommended. Many sufferers may avoid mentioning these headaches to their doctors out of embarrassment, so it is important for optimal client care to encourage disclosure and medical care.

TREATMENT

Refer clients to their physicians or urologists to assess and treat penile or testes pain or other sex-related pain issues. Medical intervention and treatment may easily and successfully resolve the pain. For any lingering emotional or psychological distress regarding the pain, as well as chronic (managed) pain, EMDR therapy can target this residual distress. Pelvic floor physical therapy can also help reduce any tension built up over time that may be contributing to any genital or other pain. The EMDR therapy pain protocol may also help to reduce any chronic pain.

SUMMARY

People with penises and testes can experience many pleasures, and many difficulties, with sexual activity.

Clients seeking sex therapy may report symptoms that indicate any of these diagnoses: desire disorders (low interest), arousal disorders (ED), orgasm disorders (PE, DE), and penile, testes, or other sex-related pain. Sex therapists are trained to treat these disorders. Accounting for any potential physical, medical, or physiological factors, and understanding the broader relational, systemic, and cultural context in which clients experience their sexual selves, is critical to considering a full picture of a particular client's sexual functioning.

Lastly, trauma-informed therapists, such as EMDR therapists, may adjunctly help sex therapists with the processing of any disturbing, traumatic, or difficult material getting in the way of improved sexual functioning.

DISCUSSION QUESTIONS

- What psychological or relational elements might contribute to ED or DE?
- What are some individual and societal factors that may contribute to lower sexual desire for people with penises?
- Critically analyze the different CBT and psychodynamic intervention strategies and what instances they may not be effective on individuals exhibiting any one of the mentioned penile disorders.

LEARNING ACTIVITIES

CourseConnect

To access self-assessment questions and interactive, competency-based learning activities for this chapter, visit www.springerpub.com/courseconnect. See inside front cover and tear-out card for CourseConnect details.

ADDITIONAL RESOURCES

Additional resources are online and available at www.springerpub.com/courseconnect.

REFERENCES

American Psychiatric Association. (2013). *Diagnostic and statistical manual of mental disorders* (5th ed.). https://doi.org/10.1176/appi.books.9780890425596

Basson, R. (2002). Women's sexual desire—Disordered or misunderstood? *Journal of Sex Marital Therapy, 28*(Suppl. 1), 17–28. https://doi.org/10.1080/00926230252851168

Betchen, S. J., & Davidson, H. L. (2018). *Master conflict therapy: A new model for practicing couples and sex therapy*. Routledge.

Carvalho, J., & Nobre, P. (2011). Biopsychosocial determinants of men's sexual desire: Testing an integrative model. *The Journal of Sexual Medicine, 8*(3), 754–763. https://doi.org/10.1111/j.1743-6109.2010.02156.x

Corona, G., Rastrelli, G., Ricca, V., Jannini, E. A., Vignozzi, L., Monami, M., Sforza, A., Forti, G., Mannucci, E., & Maggi, M. (2013). Risk factors associated with primary and secondary reduced libido in male patients with sexual dysfunction. *The Journal of Sexual Medicine, 10*(4), 1074–1089. https://doi.org/10.1111/jsm.12043

Dosch, A., Rochat, L., Ghisletta, P., Favez, N., & Van der Linden, M. (2016). Psychological factors involved in sexual desire, sexual activity, and sexual satisfaction: A multi-factorial perspective. *Archives of Sexual Behavior, 45*(8), 2029–2045. https://doi.org/10.1007/s10508-014-0467-z

Hall, K. (2020). Male hypoactive sexual desire disorder. In K. M. Hertlein, G. R. Weeks, & N. Gambescia's (Eds.), *Systemic sex therapy* (3rd ed., pp. 41–59). Routledge.

Herkommer, K., Meissner, V. H., Dinkel, A., Jahnen, M., Schiele, S., Kron, M., Ankerst, D. P., & Gschwend, J. E. (2024). Prevalence, lifestyle, and risk factors of erectile dysfunction, premature ejaculation, and low libido in middle-aged men: First results of the Bavarian Men's Health-Study. *Andrology, 12*(4), 801–808. https://doi.org/10.1111/andr.13524

Hertlein, K. G. Weeks, & Gambescia, N. (2020). *Systemic sex therapy* (2nd ed.). Routledge/Taylor & Francis Group.

LoPiccolo, J. (1977). Direct treatment of sexual dysfunction in the couple. In J. Money & H. Musaph (Eds.), *Handbook of sexology* (pp. 1227–1244). Excerpta Medica.

LoPiccolo, J., & Stock, W. E. (1986). Treatment of sexual dysfunction. *Journal of Consulting and Clinical Psychology, 54*(2), 158–167. https://doi.org/10.1037/0022-006X.54.2.158

Mark, K. P., & Lasslo, J. A. (2018). Maintaining sexual desire in long-term relationships: A systematic review and conceptual model. *The Journal of Sex Research, 55*(4-5), 563–581. https://doi.org/10.1080/00224499.2018.1437592

Masters, W., & Johnson, V. (1970). *Human sexual inadequacy*. Little, Brown.

Mayo Clinic Staff. (2022, July 14). *Premature ejaculation*. https://www.mayoclinic.org/diseases-conditions/premature-ejaculation/symptoms-causes/syc-20354900

Metz, M., & McCarthy, B. (2003). *Coping with premature ejaculation: Overcome PE, please your partner, and have great sex*. New Harbinger Publications.

Metz, M., & McCarthy, B. (2004). *Coping with erectile dysfunction: How to regain confidence and enjoy great sex*. New Harbinger Publications.

Perelman, M. A. (2016). Psychosexual therapy for delayed ejaculation based on the sexual tipping point model. *Translational Andrology and Urology, 5*(4), 563–575. https://doi.org/10.21037/tau.2016.07.05

Perelman, M. A., & Watter, D. N. (2016). Delayed ejaculation. In S. Levine (Ed.), *Handbook of clinical sexuality for mental health professionals* (3rd ed., pp. 150–163). Routledge, VitalBook file.

Rowland, D. L., & Kolba, T. N. (2018). The burden of sexual problems: Perceived effects on men's and women's sexual partners. *Journal of Sex Research, 55*(2), 226–235. https://doi.org/10.1080/00224499.2017.1332153

Scelles, C., & Bulnes, L. C. (2021). EMDR as treatment option for conditions other than PTSD: A systematic review. *Frontiers in Psychology Journal, 12*, 644369. https://doi.org/10.3389/fpsyg.2021.644369

Tiefer, L. (1988). A feminist perspective on sexology and sexuality. In M. Gergen (Ed.), *Feminist thought and the structure of knowledge* (pp. 16–26). NYU Press.

Timberlake, J. C. (n.d.). *Relaxing your pelvic muscle* [Handout]. New England Sex Therapy Associates.

Waldinger, M. D., Quinn, P., Dilleen, M., Mundayat, R., Schweitzer, D. H., & Boolell, M. (2005). A multinational population survey of intravaginal ejaculation latency time. *The Journal of Sexual Medicine, 2*(4), 492–497. https://doi.org/10.1111/j.1743-6109.2005.00070.x

Wang, G. A., Corsini-Munt, S., Dubé, J. P., McClung, E., & Rosen, N. O. (2023). Regulate and communicate: Associations between emotion regulation and sexual communication among men with hypoactive sexual desire disorder and their partners. *Journal of Sex Research, 60*(3), 325–335. https://doi.org/10.1080/00224499.2022.2092588

Weeks, G., & Gambescia, N. (2015). Definition, etiology, and treatment of absent/low desire in women. In K. Hertlein, G. Weeks, & N. Gambescia (Eds.). *Systemic sex therapy* (2nd ed., pp. 125–151). Routledge/Taylor & Francis Group.

Yoo, H., Bartle-Haring, S., Day, R. D., & Gangamma, R. (2014). Couple communication, emotional and sexual intimacy, and relationship satisfaction. *Journal of Sex & Marital Therapy, 40*(4), 275–293. https://doi.org/10.1080/0092623X.2012.751072

SUPPLEMENTAL MATERIALS FOR CLINICIANS AND CLIENTS

For PDF versions of this material, access the "Downloads" feature on Course Connect (www.springerpub.com/courseconnect).

Stop–Start Technique

The most effective technique to increase ejaculatory timing and control is the stop–start technique. This strategy in learning ejaculatory control may seem counterintuitive. Rather than attempting to decrease stimulation or sexual arousal, the approach is to increase comfort and awareness of arousal level, and increase the ability to experience increasing intensity of stimulation without climaxing.

I. Stop–start technique with self-stimulation:
   1. Plan on a 15-minute practice period.
   2. Stimulate oneself until highly aroused, but not on the verge of having an orgasm.
   3. Stop stimulation when highly aroused, and when one knows that if one continues, one will reach the "point of no return," otherwise known as the PEI (point of ejaculatory inevitability).
   4. Pause until one can continue stimulation without immediately reaching the POIE. The pause is likely to be from 15 to 60 sec.
   5. Resume stimulation and stop again slightly before the POIE.
   6. Pause.
   7. Resume.
   8. Repeat this sequence with as many pauses as you need to get to the end of the 15-minute practice period.
   9. One can finish this exercise by having an orgasm.

II. With self-stimulation, it is recommended to start using one's hand without any lubrication. Once the exercise can be completed with only 3 to 4 pauses within 15 minutes, then add a lubricant. Once the exercise, with lubricant, can be completed with only 3 to 4 pauses in 15 minutes, then add more arousing sexual fantasy. The idea is to challenge oneself with increasing levels of stimulation, essentially retraining the brain to enjoy stimulation without immediately triggering the orgasmic reflex.

III. The stop–start technique with a partner:
   1. Again, the idea is to start with the least challenging, and to move to the most challenging form of partner stimulation, as ejaculatory control increases.
   2. The stop–start technique is used first with manual stimulation, then oral stimulation, and then during intercourse.
   3. Learning ejaculatory control is a gradual process requiring practice and feedback, as well as a generous, patient, and cooperative partner.
   4. The client signals the partner to stop stimulation as they approach the point of inevitability. Stimulation stops for 15 to 60 seconds, until the client no longer feels the need to ejaculate. Then resume stimulation.
   5. Initially, the client stops movement or withdraws. As awareness and confidence increase, the strategy is to use slower, longer, or circular thrusting.
   6. Typically, ejaculatory control exercises during heterosexual intercourse begin with the "woman on top" position using minimal movement (the quiet vagina exercise), guiding intromission and controlling thrusting.
   7. Most couples prefer this rather than the traditional "squeeze" technique, which can feel awkward and mechanical, and has no advantage in terms of efficacy.

Realistic expectations and goals are crucial. The typical lovemaking experience extends from 15 to 45 minutes, of which only 2 to 7 minutes involve penetrative intercourse. Contrary to stereotypical male bragging and media myths, intercourse seldom lasts longer than 10 minutes, with 5.4 minutes being the average according to one study (Waldinger et al., 2005).

CHAPTER 10

Sexual Violence, Trauma, and Victimization

Stephanie Baird and Wendy Stock

LEARNING OBJECTIVES

- Learn basic information about sexual violence, including definitions and statistics, as well as diagnoses and nervous system information related to traumatic experiences.
- Understand that trauma treatment is important to complete before addressing sexual concerns.
- Explore information regarding the sexual marketplace (i.e., sex workers), as well as the potential impact of pornography on sexual health. Case studies are included.
- Learn about the traumatic impact of sex trafficking, illustrated with a true case study.
- Learn about "out of control" sexual behaviors. One EMDR therapy case study is shared.
- Learn basic information about identifying and working with offenders.
- Learn about the potential of vicarious traumatization when working with traumatic clinical content.

INTRODUCTION

SEXUAL VIOLENCE DEFINITIONS

Trauma in the form of *sexual violence* (SV) continues to be pervasive. The Centers for Disease Control and Prevention (CDC) defines SV as "sexual activity when consent is not obtained or freely given. … Anyone can experience or perpetrate [SV]" (2024, What Is Sexual Violence), but most victims are (cis)female. The person responsible for the violence is (often) (cis)male and usually someone known to the victim. SV includes sexual assaults such as nonconsensual penetrative intercourse, molestation, and unwanted touching of body parts, as well as verbal and/or written sexual harassment (including receiving or experiencing unwanted sexually explicit digital content in the form of texts, emails, social media posts, or images).

SEXUAL VIOLENCE STATISTICS

Most therapists are too familiar with the longstanding general statistics that one in three females, one in six males, and one-half of all transgender individuals experience SV at some point in their life (often before the age of 18). The World Health Organization (WHO) more recently reported that 20% of ciswomen and 5% to 10% of cismen have been sexually abused as children, slightly lower than the statistics from 20 years ago, but still unsettlingly high.

FEMALE GENITAL MUTILATION

Many of us have heard of female genital mutilation (FGM) practices, most commonly occurring in Africa, the Middle East, and Asia, and even in very religiously conservative sects in the United States and other "developed" countries. These practices involve partially or fully removing external vulva-related genitalia (including the clitoral glans) for nonmedical reasons, resulting in reduced sensations of sexual arousal pleasure (Types 1 and 2). Type 3 involves infibulation—the narrowing of the vaginal opening through cutting, repositioning, and stitching of the labia majora, labia minora, and/or clitoral glans, prepuce, and hood.

Groups, societies, religions, and individuals that perform these surgeries justify them by citing these possible reasons: tradition, cultural norms, rite of passage for girls, preparing girls for marriage, enhancing beauty, and hygiene. The WHO (2025) estimates that over 230 million people alive today have been subjected to some form of FGM with around four million youth with vulva currently at risk. All types of FGM are recognized internationally as human rights violations; they are seen as having no health benefits and, in fact, frequently result in short-term and long-lasting negative outcomes such as severe bleeding, urinary problems, vaginal problems, menstrual problems, cysts, infections, painful intercourse, scar tissue, ongoing mental health problems (including posttraumatic stress disorder [PTSD]), complications in childbirth, and even death (2024).

Thankfully, much activism has brought attention to and reduced these torturous and debilitating cliterectomy practices. On February 6, 2023,

> The Criminal Division's Human Rights and Special Prosecutions Section (HRSP) joined federal partners, including the U.S. Immigration and Customs Enforcement's (ICE) Human Rights Violators and War Crimes Center (HRVWCC), the FBI's International Human Rights Unit, non-governmental organizations, and others in recognizing the International Day of Zero Tolerance for Female Genital Mutilation (FGM). (Office of Public Affairs, 2023, para. 1)

You may certainly encounter a client who has experienced such an atrocity. Expect to provide comprehensive trauma treatment, as well as extensive psychoeducation about sexual rights, including their right to sexual pleasure. Part of the healing process may involve the client reclaiming their sexuality and finding new pathways to experience erotic pleasure.

ADVERSE CHILD EXPERIENCES STUDY

The adverse childhood experiences (ACE) study looks at the impact of particular childhood difficulties on the future adult's physical and mental health. The ACE questionnaire is a simple list of 10 items a child may experience before turning 18. These 10 items include five related to direct adverse experiences on the child such as physical, verbal, or sexual abuse; physical neglect (not enough to eat, dirty clothes, etc.); and emotional neglect (i.e., "No one in your family thought you were special"). Five items relate to other family members: a parent who abused alcohol or street drugs, a person who was a victim of domestic violence, a family member in jail or diagnosed with a mental illness, and losing a parent through divorce, death, or abandonment. Each type of adverse experience counts as one point.

There has been recent criticism that the ACE study does not accurately capture and account for social and structural inequities, the length of time a person may have been exposed to the events, or the presence of intergenerational trauma (impact of trauma passed from one generation to the next).

The CDC and Kaiser Permanente teamed up to conduct the largest study to date of 17,000 individuals, finding that "[a]lmost two-thirds of study participants reported at least one ACE, and more than one in five reported three or more ACEs (CDC, n.d., Major Findings). These results confirm what therapists have known for a long time: ACEs are much more common than previously thought. Simply consider the rates of sexual trauma mentioned earlier. In fact, most of our psychotherapy caseloads are overwhelmingly composed of sexual trauma survivors. Yet, sexuality is still frequently relegated to specializations such as sex therapy. It is estimated that sexual problems affect 40% to 45% of ciswomen and 20% to 30% of cismen (Lewis et al., 2010), with a noticeable correlation between trauma and adult sexual issues (Yehuda et al., 2015); these include concerns such as low or lower sexual interest, arousal, orgasms, and sexual satisfaction (Neumann et al., 1996).

THE CASE TO INCLUDE SEXUAL HEALTH WITHIN TRAUMA TREATMENT

Most psychotherapists (including trauma specialists such as eye movement desensitization and reprocessing [EMDR] therapists) often complete therapy with sexual trauma survivors without ever broaching the concepts of client sexual health (Baird, 2023). This possibly premature discharge is due to many reasons, including a lack of sexual health classes in graduate school, our general erotophobic culture, and worries about therapist/client boundaries.

Many mental health clients want permission to explore and discuss their sexual health and how their prior history of disturbing events may have negatively impacted their sexual health. According to Gallagher (2014), overall research shows that many clients want to bring up and discuss sexual concerns, yet most prefer their providers inquire first. Gallagher noted that most clients rarely ever bring up their concerns at all, likely due to concerns about whether they are "normal."

Unfortunately, this general silence should not be surprising given the sorry state of sex education in the United States. Only about 20 states mandate some amount of public school sex education, usually equaling a handful of hours. Even my (S. Baird) progressive home state of Massachusetts does not require any official sex education in public schools. Psychology related graduate programs typically only offer one or two graduate classes in human sexuality, often as an elective (which is probably why you are reading this book right now).

Additionally, van der Hart et al. (2006) often describe healing from trauma as a three-phase comprehensive approach. Phase one involves stabilization (resourcing, skill-building, support-system building, grounding, etc.). Phase two includes the nitty-gritty of treatment (including EMDR therapy and trauma-informed cognitive behavioral therapy (CBT) therapy). Phase three of overall trauma treatment includes supporting our clients to experience positive and healthy intimacy, sexual health, and self-actualization. Any of these phases can take several weeks to several years, depending on the severity of the traumatic history and symptoms. Psychoeducation can be a big part of all three phases and may be metabolized much easier in Phase three.

SEX THERAPY WITH SEXUAL TRAUMA SURVIVORS

INTRODUCTION

Rather than addressing this area at the end of a section on treatment of sexual dysfunctions, as if it were an unusual and separate issue, it is crucial to emphasize here that implementing treatment of sexual problems is unlikely to work in cases where there is unprocessed sexual trauma. Given the relatively high frequency in the general population of childhood sexual abuse and sexual assault, we know that these experiences put people at higher risk of having mental health sequelae. This population is overrepresented in the clinical population, which also applies to those seeking sex therapy. Common presentations includes sexual interaction triggering memories of abuse, states of dissociation ranging from feeling present but disconnected, and/or mild depersonalization (sensation of watching oneself as if from outside one's body). A brief loss of awareness during a sexual encounter can be common.

Some survivors of childhood sexual abuse report the ability to feel initial sexual arousal, but as they approach high arousal and potential orgasm, sexual arousal dissipates suddenly. Some of these individuals experience a fear of loss of control of their bodies. An excellent example of this response is depicted by the main character Molly in the Hulu/Disney+ series "Dying for Sex" (Meriwether & Rosenstock, 2025).

For most survivors of sexual assault and abuse, the trauma must be addressed therapeutically before anything is done in sex therapy. Even with a supportive partner, the individual with unprocessed trauma will likely not be able to respond well to sex therapy interventions. Sex therapists may refer these clients for trauma-focused therapy; therefore, it is helpful to be familiar with the information throughout this chapter (and book) in the joint goal of improving client sexual health.

SYMPTOMS AND DIAGNOSES RELEVANT TO SEXUAL VIOLENCE

Many *survivors* of sexual abuse, assault, and/or violence may experience a multitude of traumatic responses to the perceived frightening or violent event, ranging from mild to severe symptomatology.

Posttraumatic Stress Disorder

PTSD is the most common diagnosis for survivors of violence (and historically refers to symptoms in response to a single or acute incident). An abuse survivor (individuals often prefer the term *survivor*, versus *victim*) reporting at least a month of experiencing most of the following potential symptoms can likely be diagnosed with PTSD:

- *avoidance:* avoidance of details and information related to the event and/or assailant
- *reexperiencing of the event:* interfering thoughts related to the event and/or assailant, nightmares, and/or flashbacks (feeling like the event is happening all over again, in the current moment)
- *hyperarousal:* hypervigilance, exaggerated startle response, increased anxiety and/or irritability, difficulty with sleep
- *negative changes in mood and cognition:* feeling guilt-ridden, hopeless, trouble remembering some elements of the event

Complex Posttraumatic Stress Disorder

Complex PTSD (C-PTSD) is a more recent development, arising from the recognition over decades of research and clinical work, initially posited by trauma researcher Judith Herman, that some individuals who have experienced ongoing abuse and/or traumatic events manifest additional symptoms beyond the previously defined PTSD diagnosis. These additional symptoms include emotional dysregulation, interpersonal relationship dysregulation, and negative self-concepts (WHO, 2019/2021).

All these possible symptom constellations and client reports are important to heed, as any of them can impact healthy and positive sexual functioning.

POLYVAGAL THEORY AND NERVOUS SYSTEM STATES ***by Sarah Burnham, LICSW with thanks to Ellaine Miller-Karas and the trauma resiliency model***

Polyvagal theory [PVT], developed by Steven Porges in 1994 (Porges, 2011), is a framework for understanding how human nervous systems respond to cues of danger and cues of safety, as well as how this impacts behavior. The vagus nerve, the longest cranial nerve, runs from the brain to the large intestine and is involved in involuntary responses in the face, lungs, heart, diaphragm and stomach; for example, it plays a role in breathing, heart rate, digestion, and facial expressions. The *sympathetic response* activates energy, like an accelerator. The *parasympathetic response* decreases energy, like a break.

PVT posits that humans have three possible nervous system states. The scientific names for the three states are *ventral vagal, sympathetic,* and *dorsal vagal.* The last two are commonly referred to as fight/flight and freeze/numb.

Ventral vagal is the state we are in when we have sufficient cues of safety, that is, when we feel safe enough. The sympathetic accelerator and parasympathetic brake are in balance, adjusting our energy throughout the day so we have more energy when we need it—for example, to complete a task or when laughing with friends—and less energy when we need to downshift (i.e., rest and digest). We feel present and able to connect with ourself and to others. This internal "checking in" with the external environment is called *neuroception* and plays an important role in self-regulation. However, the ventral vagal state is not synonymous with a "happy place." We may feel any variety of emotion, but it is a manageable amount of emotion. In this *resilient zone* we experience emotions in waves; they crest and ebb. We are able to think about our response *before* acting. In this state, our frontal lobe, aka thinking brain, is fully on line.

In sympathetic response arousal, our bodies prepare to run from or fight a threat. In fight/flight we feel jittery, hypervigilant, and heated. We often react without thinking and feel irritable or angry. Our sleep is poor. When we are stuck in fight/flight, these "feelings" do not seem to pass the way emotions normally do when we are in our resilient zone, as they are a reflection of a sustained nervous system state. If we stay in that state, we will continue feeling them.

Dorsal vagal is the system that gets activated when a threat is perceived by our nervous system as being too big to fight or flee. In this system, we often feel numb, checked out, or zoned-out. We feel tired, sluggish, and cold. When people stay in freeze too long, they often feel depressed.

In both sympathetic and dorsal vagal states, the more bumped out of our resilient zone we are, the more our thinking brain goes off line.

With PTSD and C-PTSD, we spend more time bumped out of our resilient zone, feeling angry and anxious, or shut down and depressed. Sometimes people describe feeling as if they are bouncing between fight/flight and freeze. Like a smoke detector which is too sensitive, our nervous system can become hypersensitive to signals of threat. Depending on the messages we grew up with, we can be afraid of feeling certain emotions, and those emotions can be perceived as threatening. This happens most often with sadness, anger, and shame. Additionally, *memory capsules* open when we are reminded of past experiences, including traumas. When they open, we feel what we were feeling the last time that memory capsule was open.

Trauma treatment involves widening our resilient zone, learning how to return to it faster when we do get bumped out, and approaching, rather than avoiding, trauma memories. Over time, they will become less charged and easier to sit with, as is the case with all our emotions. Trauma-specific therapies such as EMDR therapy also help reprocess the information in the memory capsules, eliminating any disturbance associated with it.

TRAUMA PROCESSING *FIRST* WITH SEXUAL TRAUMA SURVIVORS: TWO APPROACHES

The following is a very brief description of two well-known approaches to the treatment of trauma. A longer discussion of these approaches, and others not included here, would exceed the scope of this chapter. It is helpful to provide clients information about these approaches. Several handouts available via open access online are referred to in this next section.

Trauma-informed therapy overall involves these five principles: (a) *safety* (physically and emotionally safe environment), (b) *trustworthiness* (clinician transparency and consistency), (c) *empowerment* (client autonomy and choice), (d) *collaboration* (developing goals and strategies together), and (e) *intersectionality* (acknowledging societal, historical, racial, gender issues, and other intersections of identity).

Trauma-Focused Cognitive Behavioral Therapy

Trauma-focused cognitive behavioral therapy (TF-CBT) shares a great deal of common features with other empirically validated cognitive processing approaches to trauma, including those developed by Herman (1992), Christine Courtois's work on treatment of complex trauma (2004), and Edna Foa et al.'s (2008) model of prolonged exposure therapy.

The cognitive processing approach is based on the idea that when trauma is not fully processed, the trauma remains in active memory, more easily triggered by trauma-associated cues, and remains a drain on mental energy for the client (Ehlers & Clark, 2000). The memories follow an intrusion-avoidance pattern, but the exposure is never long enough to process or desensitize the traumatic memory.

TF-CBT involves a trust-based relationship with the therapist and trains the client in emotional regulation techniques, thus creating a stable base to support the active processing of the traumatic memory. Writing and other expressive techniques provide the brain with an opportunity to integrate the narrative and affective components of the traumatic memory.

What Is TF-CBT? (Psychology Tools, n.d.-b) is an information sheet describing the key principles of TF-CBT and is available at www.psychologytools.com/resource/what-is-tf-cbt. It outlines the differences between trauma and PTSD, describing some of the key components of CBT for PTSD.

CBT is a collaborative form of therapy: The client and therapist first form a trusting working relationship.

Components of Trauma-Focused Cognitive Behavioral Therapy

Grounding and Stabilization—Relaxation and/or other techniques

Work With Memories—Talking, writing, drawing, and so forth

Work With Beliefs—Making sense of what the client thought at the time of the trauma and questioning what is a fair and rational way to think about themselves and their current situation (Grey et al., 2002)

Reclaiming Your Life (sometimes referred to as the "Resilience Phase" of trauma therapy)—PTSD often has the effect of stealing people's lives; it is common after trauma to start avoiding things that cause emotional discomfort. However, this can have the effect of shrinking their world. Effective therapy is directed at taking back the things that the client used to enjoy, and building a new life that they can value.

Eye Movement Desensitization and Reprocessing Therapy

EMDR therapy originated in the late 1980s by Francine Shapiro's discovery that moving her eyes back and forth helped reduce emotional disturbance. This discovery drove decades of validating research, particularly regarding the treatment of PTSD, that continue today (Shapiro, 2001; Solomon & Shapiro, 2008).

EMDR therapy is commonly used to treat PTSD. Both the American Psychological Association (since 1995) and the National Institute for Health and Care Excellence (NICE; UK) recommend it as an effective treatment. In addition, both the WHO and the Department of Veterans Affairs also officially endorse EMDR therapy as an effective treatment of PTSD and trauma.

When Francine Shapiro began developing EMDR therapy in the late 1980s, she initially posited a theoretical model called "accelerated information processing" to explain the framework and efficacy of EMDR therapy. Over time, the name evolved to adaptive information processing (AIP) while retaining many of the original hypotheses and principles (Shapiro, 2018).

The AIP theory is that many psychological difficulties are the result of distressing life experiences that have not been stored properly in memory and are unprocessed or blocked. These traumatic memories may need help to become processed, and EMDR therapy is one method. The main tenets of the AIP model focus on healing using the client's resources and innate ability to process maladaptive information to complete integration. Ideally, a human brain can usually process information satisfactorily, filing that data away appropriately and neatly, like in a file cabinet, in a part of the brain called the hippocampus. The hippocampus is like a librarian that catalogues (processes) events and stores them in the right place.

However, some traumatic events (such as accidents, abuse, disasters, or violence) are so overwhelming that the hippocampus does not do its job properly and the "information processing system is impaired." When this happens, trauma memories are stored in their "raw, unprocessed, and maladaptive form" (Hase et al., 2017, The AIP Model).

This means that this disturbing event will have difficulty connecting to other memory networks that hold adaptive information. Therefore, "when a memory is encoded in such excitatory, state-specific form, the original perceptions can be triggered by a variety of internal and external stimuli" (Hase et al., 2017, The AIP Model). These dysfunctionally stored memories then form the basis for future maladaptive responses and possible psychopathology. Activating these memories, even years later, can lead to a variety of symptoms from PTSD to anxiety to "barely noticeable intrusions" (Hase et al., 2017, The AIP Model).

These trauma memories are often easily triggered, leading them to replay and cause distress over and again. This often shows up in the form of flashbacks and interfering thoughts (particularly during intimate sexual encounters).

Additionally, EMDR therapy is increasingly being used to treat other conditions in which disturbing memories occur, such as anxiety, phobias, and depression. *What Is EMDR?* (Psychology Tools, n.d.-a) is a one-page information sheet describing the key principles of EMDR available at www.psychologytools.com/resource/what-is-emdr. It is helpful to use this as a handout for clients who may want information before choosing between EMDR and TF-CBT.

The Eight Phases of Eye Movement Desensitization and Reprocessing Therapy

From the early supportive research, EMDR therapy evolved into a distinct eight-phase therapeutic approach that uses *bilateral stimulation* (BLS)/*dual attention stimulus* (DAS; i.e., eye movements) to aid the integration (processing) of distressing and/or traumatic information. Briefly, the eight phases are

1. *History Taking and Treatment Planning*: This involves obtaining information from the client about their presenting concern and collaborating to develop treatment goals and steps.
2. *Preparation*: This involves establishing trust and rapport, thereby teaching the client grounding, visualization, relaxation, and other emotional stabilization techniques, and laying the groundwork to work on difficult/traumatic material.
3. *Assessment*: This involves identifying a distressing target/memory to work on in EMDR therapy, as well as the related image and negative and positive cognitions that accompany it, plus how disturbing it currently feels (the subjective unit of distress).
4. *Desensitization*: This involves the actual processing of the memory/target utilizing BLS/DAS to reduce the distress associated with it.
5. *Installation:* Once the target is no longer distressing, positive beliefs and cognitions developed with the client are then installed with BLS.
6. *Body Scan:* The body is scanned for any remaining disturbance associated with the target; if present, it is processed with additional BLS.
7. *Closure:* The session is closed and the client is brought back to equilibrium via relaxation/grounding techniques.
8. *Reevaluation:* When the client returns for the next session, their progress is reviewed, including the strength of their new positive cognition/belief, as well as anything that may have arisen since the previous processing session.

Integrating Sexual Health into the Adaptive Information Processing Model

The AIP model helps us understand how a client's sexual health can be negatively impacted at any point in time, leading to sexual unease, discomfort, or dysfunction. From a yet-to-be-born child experiencing domestic violence vicariously through their parent's stress hormones, to a child witnessing a parent's sexual coercion, to a preteen noticing the lack of physical affection from or between parents, these are all events and atmospheres that can negatively impact a client's sexual health. Add in a shaming and sexually punitive society, and it's a miracle that any child can make their way to adulthood with an empowered pleasurable sex life.

EMDR therapy has been a remarkable force of good in righting numerous wrongs, via alleviating suffering and unlocking adaptive cognitions and futures for clients, particularly related to sexual traumas. However, we all can do better to look for the thousand tiny cuts our clients have likely sustained from negative messaging around sexuality, and find targets related to early misinformation, lack of information, shaming of emerging sexuality, and the million other ways our puritanical and erotophobic culture shames individuals for being sexual beings.

Here is just a small list of potential EMDR targets related to negative sexual socialization or lack of appropriate sexuality education, which can negatively impact someone's sexual health:

1. An adult cismale client reveals he was caught masturbating as a youth and remains mortified.
2. An adult cisfemale client recalls an abusive first boyfriend who criticized her "slutty" outfits in public.
3. An adult discloses first learning about sex through pornographic magazines discovered in the woods, resulting in continued confusion.
4. A nonbinary who went to religious primary school mentions how there was no sex education at all. When they began menarche, they were treated with scorn.
5. A gender nonconforming assigned female at birth adult described how their parents simultaneously shamed their growing interest in dating AND emphasized and enforced feminized notions of beauty (makeup, dresses, body shape, etc.), creating confusion and shame.

TREATMENT OF SEXUAL PROBLEMS IN SEXUAL TRAUMA SURVIVORS: AFTER TRAUMA PROCESSING

Once the treatment of trauma processing has occurred, clients are in a better position to work directly on the effects of trauma on their sexuality. Wendy Maltz, MSW, has written and created excellent self-help resources for survivors of sexual trauma. These can be used in conjunction with a trauma therapist, individually, and/or with their partners in sex therapy. Her materials are available on her website, healthysex.com, and include the books *Incest and Sexuality* (Maltz & Holman, 1987) and *The Sexual Healing Journey* (Maltz, 2012), and the videos *Partners in Healing* (Maltz, n.d.-a) and *Relearning Touch* (Maltz, n.d.-b). Full versions of both videos are available on her website. As described on Maltz's website, *The Sexual Healing Journey* helps survivors to identify the sexual effects of their abuse; create a positive meaning for sex; develop a healthy sexual self-concept; gain control over upsetting reactions to touch and sex; improve partner intimacy; incorporate nondemand, sensual touch with sex; and address sexual functioning concerns.

Maltz's approach also addresses helping survivors heal from having unwanted sexual fantasies. This can include the survivor taking themselves through a repatterning of the process of sexual socialization (e.g., engaging in nondemanding and consensual touch with a partner) and developing fantasies that do not involve unwanted sex. Maltz emphasizes the importance of sexual communication and boundary setting in her work with survivors.

TRAUMA REENACTMENT VERSUS TRAUMA PLAY

Some professionals assume kink/BDSM (bondage, discipline/domination, submission/sadism, masochism) behavior is pathological and/or trauma reenactment. BDSM activities were removed as disorders from the *Diagnostic and Statistical Manual of Mental Disorders* (5th ed.; *DSM-5*, American Psychiatric Association [APA], 2013) in 2013.

"*Trauma reenactment* [emphasis added] is when people recycle the events and relationships from childhood, repeating old wounds by placing themselves at emotional risk or in physical danger in a compulsory mimicry of the past" (Kort, n.d., para. 4). An example is someone who was emotionally and verbally abused by a parent, then suffered successive abusive relationships as an adult.

Trauma play involves learning "how to 'play' with their childhood traumas without putting themselves in danger or stunting emotional growth" (Kort, n.d., para. 4). For example, someone who had their knuckles hit by a ruler-wielding teacher may now, as an adult, notice, experience, and purposely enhance sexual arousal in a sexual role-play where their partner pretends to be their teacher.

Clients who engage in kink/BDSM do not have higher rates of trauma than the general population, and very often insightfully understand and communicate their trauma-free interest in kink/BDSM. For BDSM, the practitioners purposely play with the particular act to enhance a sexual experience.

Jack Morin's book *The Erotic Mind* (1996) explores and examines how childhood experiences and relationships shape adult preferences and fantasies (for all individuals, whether vanilla/mainstream or kinky). He encourages people to explore favorite and peak sexual experiences and fantasies to help discern *core erotic templates* (CETs). CETs are our arousal imprints, and "the purpose is to use old wounds and conflicts as aphrodisiacs" (Morin, 1996, p. 142). His approach is sex-affirming and erotic-positive, seeing our CETs not as problems, but solutions. It is helpful to keep all of this in mind when clients disclose interests and activities that diverge from mainstream heteronormative, vanilla, and erotophobic culture.

If clients arrive for therapy unsure of whether their sexual behavior (including kink/BDSM) is "unhealthy" (potentially *reenactment*) or "healthy" (*play*), processing any prior, lingering traumatic material first will help provide a clear path to understanding their relationship to current or future sexual activities (including vanilla and/or kink/BDSM activities).

SEXUAL MARKETPLACE

SEXUALLY EXPLICIT MATERIAL (PORNOGRAPHY, EROTICA, ETC.)

Definitions, Statistics, Internet, Usage

Sexually explicit material (SEM; which includes erotica as well as pornography) has a complicated existence and is best understood in book-length examinations. Poll anyone on the street and you will get a wide array of definitions, opinions, and emotional responses.

Pornography is generally defined as showing sexually explicit content (photographs, film/videos, writings in magazines and books, etc.) with the purpose of stimulating sexual excitement. Some pornography can also include a *supernormal stimulus* nature of more violent or extreme content specifically designed to quickly shock recipients into having an intense physiological and/or emotional response, in some cases numbing said viewers over time more and more to the extreme depictions of degradation.

Sociologists, psychologists, evangelists, feminists, parents, lawyers, and justices have weighed in on what constitutes pornography versus something more "socially acceptable" that might land in the "erotic" category (e.g., the well-known *Fifty Shades of Grey* book series, as well as the *Bridgerton* Netflix series).

Gloria Steinem argued in 1977 that if a ciswoman and a cisman engaging in sex were shown as having equal power, equal pleasure, and equal choice, and the imagery is egalitarian, non-coercive, and nondegrading, this should not be termed pornography, but *erotica*.

At this point, most people acknowledge that porn exists and will likely continue to exist in some form. Since humans could first make marks on walls and observe ourselves and each other, we have attempted to depict our sexuality, going back to images and sculptures of genitals in the Paleolithic and Mesolithic periods (upwards of 30,000 years ago) such as the Venus of Willendorf.

Additionally, many folks assume that most internet activity involves searching for porn. In reality, porn represents only 4% of the top million sites, and about 13% to 25% of web searches. One in three viewers of porn identifies as a woman. The online adult entertainment market is currently estimated at a revenue of 76.17 billion in 2024 and 81.86 billion in 2025, growing at a rate of around 7.6% (Research and Markets, 2025).

However, much of mainstream porn leaves out important elements like emotional intimacy, consent, using condoms, discussing sexually transmitted infection (STI) risks, and varying body types. It often includes objectification and degradation of women (cis and trans) and people of color, unrealistic behaviors, poor treatment, and poor financial reimbursement of the actors, as well as presents a distorted, unrealistic, frequently nonconsensual version of sexuality. Violent behaviors, such as choking, are represented as normative and even desired by most women, and there is research documenting the increased frequency of unwanted, nonconsensual choking, usually by cis men to cis women, in dating relationships (Herbenick et al., 2020).

Herbenick et al. (2021) found that half of college students who had been choked reported that they had never (21%) or only sometimes (32%) been asked for consent or if it was okay to be choked, prior to being choked. Rostad et al. found that "Violent pornography exposure was associated with all types of TDV [(teen dating violence)], though patterns differed by gender. Boys exposed to violent pornography were 2–3 times more likely to report sexual TDV perpetration and victimization and physical TDV victimization, while girls exposed to violent pornography were over 1.5 times more likely to perpetrate threatening TDV compared to their non-exposed counterparts. Comprehensive prevention strategies for TDV may consider the potential risks associated with exposure to violent pornography, particularly for boys, and provide an alternative source of education about healthy sexual behavior and relationships" (2019, Abstract).

Rebekkah Rennick, in a Tapestry presentation on "Digital Sexuality and Youth" (2021), noted that 89% of youth report the internet as their primary source of sexuality information and that "unwanted" exposures comprise 66% of youth exposure. Teaching our youth, our clients, and ourselves how to critique these images is becoming more and more essential for sexual health well-being.

Rennick espouses the Responsible Sex Ed Institute's (RSEI; affiliated with Planned Parenthood) *porn literacy* definition:

> [teaching] individuals to think about, analyze, and evaluate the media they choose to consume [plus surrounding] media, such as billboards and advertisements. Everything has a message, whether intentional or not. Knowing how, why, and for whom content was created can help [everyone] better understand what they see and hear and make healthy decisions. (RSEI Educator, 2019, para. 4)

Boston University's professor and researcher Emily F. Rothman, via the Boston Public Health Commission, created a curriculum to teach youth porn literacy called "Start Strong" and presents some of this information in her TED Talk "How Porn Changes the Way Teens Think About Sex" (Rothman, 2019). This TED Talk, as well as other resources on porn literacy and sex education programs like Our Whole Lives (OWL), can help clients and others gain more accurate information on sexuality in general.

The Gottman Institute, a facility famous for researching and developing science-based approaches to healing and changing problematic relationship problems, published an "An Open Letter to Porn: Pornography Poses a Serious Threat to Couple Intimacy and Relationship Harmony" on its website in 2016 (Gottman & Gottman, 2024). It is worth reading this post in its entirety as they do not outright condemn porn altogether, noting that when both members of a couple have an interest in viewing porn together, it can enhance communication about each person's likes and dislikes, and even increase the ratio of orgasms between people with vulvas and people with penises.

However, the Gottmans do acknowledge many potential detrimental impacts of porn: "A 2010 meta-analysis of several studies found an 'overall significant positive association between pornography use and attitudes supporting violence against women'" (Hald, et al., 2010, Abstract, as cited in Gottman & Gottman, 2024, Update).

Viewers can report lower self-esteem, inaccurate perception of relationship and sexuality information, possible decrease in intimacy between two people in a relationship (especially if one prefers engaging with porn versus a live human in the room), potential numbness to violence and degradation, and susceptibility to a *supernormal stimulus.*

"Supernormal stimuli are [all] around us" and include most things in advertising like "photoshopped" bodies, and even "junk food." The supernormal stimulus of porn can "lead to a lack of desire for sex with one's partner, [which usually is] a normal sex stimulus." Some people with penises who report heavy adolescent porn use with masturbation later can suffer from "erectile dysfunction" (Gottman & Gottman, 2024, Update).

The Gottmans conclude, "The frequent consumption of porn, especially coupled with masturbation (at least by men), can reduce the quality and quantity of sex in a committed relationship."

Some of my (S. Baird) clients have mentioned positive results from the Your Brain on Porn program (yourbrainonporn.com). Specifically, they reported noticing an improved sense of sexual health and daily functioning after 3 or 4 weeks of not using porn. This program may be helpful for clients who report a daily constant use that interferes with general life and sexual functioning, possibly due to overexposure to the "supernormal stimulus." This is not to say that a client or individual must refrain from porn viewing for the rest of their life. Helping a client become more in charge of what and how often they view pornography can dramatically increase their sense of self and bring their sexual health into better balance.

The Stop Enabling Sex Traffickers Act (SESTA) law passed in 2018 (Allow States and Victims to Fight Online Sex Trafficking Act of 2017, 2018), while initially positive in the sense that it hoped to limit sex trafficking and slavery, also limits consensually working and paid sex workers, and even educational sexual health internet content that can now be labeled "obscene." Ultimately, the legalities of what can be outlawed and what is acceptable have remained complicated by varying perceptions of what the "average person" considers okay or not okay. Another troubling aspect of the porn industry overall is the lack of regulations.

Sex-positive activists have defined some working elements of ethical pornography as well as the concept of porn literacy. Ethical pornography (also sometimes called "feminist" or "fair trade" pornography) includes fair payment of the filmmakers and workers; is made in a safe environment where everyone is of consenting age and is respected; shows real (not faked) sexual pleasure (especially for bodies with vulvas); is created for all viewers (including ciswomen); is 100% consensual in every way; and shows diversity across body type, age, race, sexuality, and ability.

Sex activists also highly encourage porn users to pay for their porn, ensuring that consenting sex workers get paid a fair wage for their work. A few places for adults to look for ethical porn include makelovenotporn.com, Bellesa.co (porn by women), Ifeelmyself.com (focus on female pleasure), and some reddit subthreads such as r/chickflixxx. Dan Savage hosts an annual porn film festival "for everyone" (humpfilmfest.com), and David Ley (2016) has published a book on how to find ethical porn.

There is also a burgeoning audio porn market, possibly even more ethically minded, as there are no physical depictions. Some good audio options include tryQuinn.com (helping people feel comfortable in their bodies) and Dipseastories.com (celebrating healthy sex).

Pornography and Psychotherapy

Indeed, if clients seek therapy for a self-reported so-called pornography *addiction*, then we can explore and potentially treat their unwanted behaviors (rephrasing them as *out of control*) through psychoeducation and psychotherapy (including EMDR targeting and processing, possibly via the Feeling State Addiction Protocol (Miller, 2010, 2012, 2021).

Some questions to ask our clients include assessing how disruptive it is to daily life (relationships, work, etc.). We can also ask about their preferred porn type and what it is doing for them. Some clients may prefer porn because masturbating to porn seems easier than engaging in partner sex, or that they enjoy the enthusiasm and eagerness often displayed. Others may report that with watching porn they do not have to worry about performance anxiety, contraception, STIs, or negotiating another partner's sexual interests (Klein, 2010). And still others may note feeling inadequate with partners, overwhelmed with life responsibilities, or tired of boring and monotonous sex (Klein, 2010).

Klein (2010) notes that the most common pathology regarding porn use is the secrecy, and that "rigidity around porn is rigidity." Certainly any kind of stressor that results in someone withdrawing from previously healthy and satisfying sexual relationships is worth exploring, and the individual may benefit from therapy versus simply maintaining porn use.

Indeed, the governing body of sexuality education and counseling, the American Association of Sexuality Educators, Counselors and Therapists (AASECT), issued a historic statement in 2016 asserting that

> AASECT recognizes that people may experience significant physical, psychological, spiritual and sexual health consequences related to their sexual urges, thoughts or behaviors. ... AASCET 1) does not find sufficient empirical evidence to support the classification of sex addiction or porn addiction as a mental health disorder, and 2) does not find the sexual addiction training, treatment methods and educational pedagogies to be adequately informed by accurate human sexuality knowledge. Therefore, it is the position of AASECT that linking problems related to sexual urges, thoughts or behaviors related to a porn/sexual addiction process cannot be advanced by AASEST as a standard of practice for sexuality education delivery, counseling or therapy. (n.d., para. 2)

Some clients may seek therapy because someone else exposed them to unwanted porn viewing. The EMDR therapy case composites (Cases 10.1 and 10.2 that follow) demonstrate how to process this type of trauma.

The more we all speak to our clients and each other about consent, healthy sexuality, positive relationships, and well-being, the less we will be satisfied by the more exploitative types of porn foisted on us. Hopefully our clients can develop a balanced approach to porn and/or erotic imagery, using porn literacy strategies to find content that is appealing, inclusive, realistic, consensual, safe, and arousing, if they so desire.

Pornography Exposure Case Studies

These case composite examples focus on the disturbances that can particularly develop in children after being exposed to pornography—a "sexualization" typically falling within the covert sexual abuse category if no touching occurred.

Case Study 10.1: Akari, Unmonitored Access to Porn During Childhood

Akari, a 20-year-old self-identified queer Asian cisfemale college student, majoring in art, sought EMDR therapy for recent "negative sexual experiences that brought back memories of sex-related images and porn from childhood." She reported concurring recent depressive moments and episodes, and feeling overall down and disinterested, especially related to sexual thoughts and activity. Akari also noted having unmonitored internet access around ages 10 and 11, googling sexuality-related topics, and stumbling upon pornography. She recalled intense shame around her discoveries, to the extent that she felt "broken," no longer "innocent and pure," and had "thrown her life away."

As we developed the EMDR timeline, we ascertained 10 EMDR targets, four of which are mentioned here:

1. Age 10—An older adult man pushing her against a wall at a visit to a grandparent in a nursing home, reaching to touch her
2. Age 10—Being caught late at night searching the internet

3. Age 11—Watching a satire video and being caught by surprise to learn what "rape" actually was
4. Age 18—A friend taking advantage of her being drunk to touch her sexually, against her consent

Akari's negative cognitions (NCs) for the early pornography incidents were "I'm impure, disgusting, damaged, a bad person, dumb, and/or broken" as well as "I have no control" (for the early and recent sexual assault). Her positive cognitions (PCs) included, "I'm normal, a good person." Regarding the sexual assaults, her PCs included, "It's not my fault, I have choices now, I'm allowed to make mistakes, I'm learning, I can say no."

Akari was able to fully process through her EMDR target timeline, eventually bypassing a couple of later targets as her adaptive healing increased. As we approached the end of the target list, she reported feeling more back "to normal" with improved interest in college, friends, and her art. She had started dating and noted that while she and her new partner were taking it slow, so far she was able to stay in the moment and enjoy physical touch and intimacy without any prior porn or assault images interfering. We also completed EMDR future templates on effectively "handling and enjoying" future sexual intimacy and activities (e.g., enjoying oral sex with her new partner).

Case Study 10.2: Martina, Child Exposed to Porn

Martina's mother brought her to EMDR therapy to process through prior sexual abuse from a caregiver's son. Martina, a female-identified Latina, currently age 9, was 5 years old when the 13-year-old son, David, of her biological father's girlfriend "kissed and touched her, and showed her porn." Her parents had been divorced since she was 2 years old. At age 5, Martina showed inappropriate knowledge about sex soon after the incidents with the boy. A case was opened, investigated, and the boy was found guilty. Her father disappeared shortly after. Four years later, Martina reported having "nightmares" and trouble hearing the words "sex," "penis" or other words with an "x" in them.

As Martina was very insightful and articulate, we developed a modified EMDR timeline of "yucky things" and were able to process through both the molestation from David (which included him wrapping his arms around her, preventing her from moving away from the porn on the computer screen) and the lingering vivid pornographic images she still remembered. Her NCs included, "I'm trapped and disgusting." Her PCs included, "I'm free, I can just be a kid, I'm fine as I am. Let adults deal with that stuff (sex)." Much psychoeducation, validation, and normalization of symptoms was provided as well. A few weeks later she reported no longer having nightmares or being bothered by the word "sex" or other words with an "x" in them.

SEX WORK

This section is included to help correct misinformation and terminology. Activists (sex activists, academics, etc.) no longer generally use the word *prostitute* to describe someone who receives money (or other valued items) for sex. Instead, the terms *sex work* or *sexual marketplace* are now the umbrella terms for any consenting adult engaging in the exchange of sexuality-related activities for money (making or appearing in pornography, stripping, providing sex for money, phone or web cam sex work, etc.). Certain activities under these umbrella terms are arbitrarily legal or illegal in different states and countries.

It is important to remain nonjudgmental and open if a client discloses a background of sex work, whether providing or receiving. *If* the client reports distress around sex work, *then* it can be helpful to obtain your client's consent and permission to inquire about the circumstances surrounding the distress, whether any coercion was involved, if your client was of age at the time, if there were any substances forced upon them, and how they perceive the events now.

People may choose to go into sex work for a variety of reasons, including positive reasons such as higher wages than other available jobs, and having their sexuality and defined boundaries work for them. Therefore, it is crucial that we do not impose our own values or beliefs. American feminist sex-positive activists have long regarded sex work similarly to how it is viewed in the Netherlands (where it is legal and regulated). Activists urge the establishment of parameters that protect the sex workers and make it safe for them to report any abusive behavior, versus forcing them into the shadows for fear of being criminally charged themselves (and potentially suffering more abuse at the hands of law enforcement; Chloe, 2018).

Many sex workers maintain intimate relationships with partners and have families, thereby experiencing both positive and negative elements in their intimate relationships, similar to those who are not sex workers.

Case Study 10.3: Liliana, Stripping to Pay for College

One EMDR and sex work case example is Liliana, a Latinx ciswoman college student who sought EMDR therapy for middle school and high school sexual assaults. At intake Liliana described a fairly typical college existence: juggling classes, friends, and a supportive boyfriend. After a few sessions Liliana disclosed that she earns her college tuition by stripping at a couple of strip clubs in the state. She noted making more than enough cash each weekend to pay for her private college tuition. She reported feeling empowered by using her sexuality in a way that was also furthering her education. She stated her boyfriend did not mind her stripper work, although he did not attend any of her shows.

Consistent with her referral and intake information, Liliana prioritized working on the preteen and teen sexual assaults she had experienced by older neighborhood kids and one older cousin who sometimes babysat her. She noted these memories were bothering her more and more, often interfering with her sexual interest in her boyfriend. Once we worked through these targets, she then determined that a couple of prior situations at work also bothered her. One occurred a year earlier and involved another staff member who became obsessed with her, eventually stalking her via text messaging and arranging to work the same shifts she did. Liliana had explicitly informed this person she was not interested in dating or a relationship. Eventually Liliana informed the management, who responded by scheduling the stalker on opposite days.

Liliana's EMDR targets for this situation included (a) telling the person to leave her alone (yet the person stayed in her physical space) and (b) seeing the harassing text messages on her phone. Liliana no longer worked at that particular club, nor had any recent contact with the stalker, at the time of processing these targets with EMDR therapy. She had found work at a different strip club managed by women, which felt safer to her. Once these targets were resolved, Liliana was able to process EMDR future templates on the possibility of running into the stalker again. Her positive cognition of "I have boundaries, choices, and can act" remained completely true throughout the future template. She also noted interest in sexual activity with her boyfriend returning. She continued to do stripper work as that was the highest paying hourly rate available to help her pay for college.

Case Study 10.4: Fred, Sex Video Work Preferred Over in Real Life (IRL)

Fred, a Black gay cisman working as an accountant, sought EMDR therapy for domestic violence (DV) targets that occurred in a prior relationship in his early twenties. He also had witnessed DV between his caregivers growing up. He was eventually interested in dating again, but felt quite nervous, as he did not want to fall into "that same rabbit hole." After a few sessions he disclosed enjoying sex cam work (performing and verbalizing sexual activities over live video with paying customers). This felt very safe, as the other person was not in the same room and therefore could not physically hurt him. He was also released of any possible emotional connection, as these customers were and remained strangers, further reducing any risk of abuse.

Once we worked through the EMDR DV-related targets, Fred pondered what it might be like to date again. After completing much boundary work and several EMDR future templates of meeting new people and asserting boundaries (based on the PCs of "I am strong, capable, and worthy of care and respect"), Fred eased into in-person dating. His sex video work slowly ebbed away as time with a new loving and respectful partner steadily increased.

SEX TRAFFICKING

Sex trafficking (enslaving a person for sexual purposes) is a different topic altogether and is considered a huge human rights issue with estimates between 12 and 27 million victims enslaved or forced into some kind of sexual activity a year. It is the second largest criminal industry in the world, at $32 billion a year. Sex trafficking, as it is defined under federal law, requires "force, fraud, and coercion"; sex work does not (Grant, 2018). The passing of FOSTA-SESTA in th United States in 2018, making it illegal to assist, facilitate, or support human trafficking, has created many difficulties for sex workers and inconsistencies in how sex work is legally considered.

Rather than resulting in high numbers of sex traffickers being indicted and charged, critics note that the law simply seems to allow more legal targeting of sex workers (Chloe, 2018). Activists talk about how "these bills not only do nothing to actually reduce sex trafficking, but they also create dangerous conditions for both sex trafficking victims and consenting sex workers" (Chloe, 2018, para. 7). This is because the ability to use the internet to advertise or screen sex work clients has been greatly hindered (as all parties, including the internet platform such as Craiglist, could be charged with sex trafficking), resulting in increased difficulty in screening clients (Chloe, 2018). Additionally, many sex workers who were able to operate independently due to internet screening and unrestricted access to harm-reduction information now use pimping services or solicit outdoors, which are much more dangerous scenarios. In fact, Chloe (2018) cites research that shows that when Craigslist introduced the Erotic Services section, violence against women had actually dropped by 17.4%.

In the case of a sex trafficking victim, there will most likely be traumatic memories and events associated with their enslavement, particularly as many victims are trafficked by foster homes, their caregivers and family members, or intimate partners (Chloe, 2018). Some of their trauma may be more related to a sense of betrayal from the groomer who enticed them into this path (similar to survivors of childhood incest, who sometimes report that the betrayal by the trusted person was worse than the actual acts). Not many folks (usually children or teenagers) simply "stumble" into trafficking. There is usually a process of getting to know the child, grooming, and attaining their trust, before moving into enslavement.

Case Study 10.5: A True Trafficking Story, Circa 2005, Written by M.L.

My story is based on my true experience. I met my ex-husband "M" after my college graduation through mutual friends and we had attended the same school. He was strong (a swimmer), smart, involved in the university's government, and enjoyed many of the same activities as I.

We were married for 28 years and lived in a suburb west of Boston and raised three amazing children. But during our youngest child's junior year in high school, I began noticing odd changes in M's behavior. I had a bachelor's degree in sociology/psychology and had some experience with abnormal behavior in work situations.

M had earned his MBA while we were married (Sloan School at MIT). A brilliant strategic planner in the high tech industry, he worked hard and often traveled. He struggled with alcohol, and once he even passed out from it. He went for counseling and stayed off alcohol for 15 years (so I thought). Over time M became more easily agitated at home and often yelled. He was verbally abusive. We all started to feel like we were walking on eggshells because we never knew what would set him off on a rage. He constantly checked his emails early in the morning before work on the family computer. We only had one and we kept it in plain sight in the family room. He would bring me a cup of coffee up to the bedroom as he rose before me. This would keep me upstairs getting ready for the morning. He became increasingly more anxious, and soon I didn't want the coffee ... I was nervous that he might put something in it.

I started to discover money missing out of our joint accounts. He hid the retirement plan stocks that were in both our names.

We owned two homes, including a home on Cape Cod where we spent summers. His mind seemed to be elsewhere a lot. He often missed returning my phone calls and once it happened regarding picking up our child from a summer camp out of state. I didn't believe his story or the reason why he didn't answer my calls, and therefore I drove to do the pickup.

He began taking plastic bags of food out of our refrigerator to bring to work. He had a great office building off of Route 128, with many food stores available, so that was odd.

One summer I had to have a mammogram at my local hospital, so I left the beach house and went to the appointment west of Boston. When I returned to our regular year-round house it smelled weird in the kitchen, like an intense burning smell, but it was not cigarettes or pot. As I went into the dining room, I noticed a paper bag full of empty beer cans on the floor and a videotape cassette on the table. I immediately felt that something was going on and grabbed the tape, put it in my pocketbook, and started to walk out the door. He surprised me by being in the kitchen. He knew I had come home and asked me if I saw a videotape on the table. I lied and continued to walk to the door, got in my car, and drove off with the tape.

A month later I returned home with the children and had access to a video player. I finally played the tape and viewed the contents. The tape revealed that he had an underage young teenage girl in the living room. She appeared naked underneath my bathrobe, dazed and confused, and could not speak English, suggesting she may have been an immigrant. There were lines of what appeared to be cocaine on a mirror on a leather hassock in front of her. M was asking her if she would like a vodka drink. She looked really afraid. I wondered what happened to her. If she were undocumented, no one would be missing her if something went wrong. He had taken her to our home! At nighttime no one would have noticed any activity, because the entrance from the garage was very private.

I then confided in my dad, saw my doctor, started seeing a therapist, meditated heavily, met with my lawyer, and consulted the police.

I found the password to his emails and was able to discover more evidence. M had tried to obtain a gun permit, but was denied by the state due to a juvenile offense on his record. I had no idea! He had porn photos on his emails, which were under several alias names. He had purchased a lot of batteries online (possibly to make crystal meth). The court did a long hair follicle test on him and it was positive for cocaine and crystal meth. I divorced him as soon as possible. As my lawyer had hopes he would smarten up and didn't want serious charges on his public record, he was not charged with trafficking or child porn. He had one prior arrest years earlier for drunk driving.

M was later arrested for not paying my court-ordered child support. To this day he still owes me over $350,000. He quit working and spent 6 months in jail. He was awarded SSDI [Social Security Disability Insurance] and the court lowered what he had to pay me monthly, but they did not dismiss the amount due.

He has never met our four grandchildren. Our children do not want any involvement with him.

His LinkedIn account looks like he is doing great.

This could easily have been anyone's neighbor. I have no idea how many people were in my home over the years or how many young girls he was grooming somewhere—or worse! When he was court ordered to move out, he asked for a certain kitchen knife and one of our trash barrels. That's all he wanted. I also gave him the bed.

Chilling ... You never really know what a person does all day long. I followed my instincts. I had to stay strong. I got my support from my circle, my God, my family, my running, and my art. Thankfully I had the training I needed and still need. I don't want this to happen to anyone ever again. Men (or anyone) can not just TAKE US.

"OUT OF CONTROL" SEXUAL BEHAVIORS

Much discussion has been made of the term *sexual addiction* over recent years, particularly in relation to prevalently available internet porn. The current sexual health thinking eschews the term of *addiction,* preferring *out of control* sexual behavior.

Additionally, the governing body of sexuality education and counseling, the American Association of Sexuality Educators, Counselors and Therapists (AASECT), issued a historic statement on sexual addiction in 2016 (see page 201 in Chapter 10).

Whether someone's sexual behavior is "out of control" is completely subjective. However, it is generally agreed that any behavior interfering regularly with daily functioning and relationships might meet criteria for "out of control."

For clients who present stating "I have an addiction," it is vital to truly assess to see if the behavior is as problematic and interfering as the client may describe. Indeed, some clients may cry with relief as they unburden themselves of what they deem as out of control (e.g., "excessive" porn viewing, multiple and frequent unsanctioned extramarital affairs, unwanted visits to strip clubs or sex workers, constant sexting) and are ready to receive any help necessary to get it "back under control."

However, these behaviors may be the result of deeper underlying problems such as relationship dissatisfaction/unhappiness/discord, or loneliness. Additionally, even as therapist and client work together to get the behavior more "under control," it is important to keep in mind that these behaviors may hold some erotic templates that are integral to the client. The goal is not necessarily to wholly eliminate the behavior (unlike heroin addiction). Depending on the circumstances and client, it may be more appropriate to uncover the useful and positive elements of the feeling states and related erotic templates, helping the client reshape their behavior toward something they themselves deem more healthy and helpful.

If the client and therapist determine that the client's life would greatly improve if the problematic behavior is changed, then Robert Miller's Feeling-State Addiction Protocol (FSAP) is an excellent tool for shifting intrusive/negative behavior patterns. Another tool (not included in this text) is A. J. Popky's (2010) DeTUR (Desensitization of Triggers and Urge Reprocessing) protocol. DeTUR is an adaptive information processing (AIP) model urge protocol to treat addictions and dysfunctional behaviors. Michael Hase's CravEx protocol (2009) can also help.

Case Study 10.6: Jerry Wants First-Time Sex, Every Time

By Robert Miller, PhD

Jerry, a White cisman, self-reported a "sex addiction" in which he had to have "first time" sex with a different ciswoman every time. Once he had sex with a woman, no matter how good the sexual experience, he still had to seek out another woman to satisfy this need. Jerry would cheat on his wife whenever she would go out of town, acting on his sexual urge. The last few years Jerry had started meeting with sex workers because it was easy for him to have "first time" sex.

Jerry's problematic sexual behaviors began in college when he was 20 years old. Jerry had wanted to have a relationship with a woman who, for over a year, had only wanted to be friends. Then they began a sexual relationship that lasted a few months. Because Jerry had been wanting to have sex with her for so long, the first time he had sex with her, it was "mind blowing." Jerry experienced an intense feeling of "acceptance" that he had wanted all his life but didn't get. The result was a Feeling-State memory linking the feeling of "acceptance" with a "first time" sexual encounter. From that point on, Jerry sought out women to experience the feeling of "acceptance" he had experienced when having "first time" sex.

Jerry's "first time" sex Feeling-State was treated by using the FSAP. The FSAP uses the eye movement protocol of EMDR to break the linkage between the feeling and behavior. In the first session, Jerry was able to identify the feeling of acceptance as the feeling he was seeking. The memory of the sexual experience with the college woman was targeted using eye movements to process the memory. After three sets of eye movements, the linkage between the feeling of acceptance and the behavior of "first time" sex was broken. Once his Feeling-State memory was processed, Jerry's desire for "first time" sex was eliminated.

In the next session, Jerry reported that not only did his desire cease regarding that sexual behavior, but processing the Feeling-State had had an impact in another area. Previously, whenever he was in the process of acting out his sexual urge, he would start by looking at pornography. However, after processing the Feeling-State in the previous session, pornography was no longer interesting to him. In other words, Jerry was only interested in the pornography because it was leading to the feeling of acceptance he would experience when he acted out his sexual urge. Without the feeling of "acceptance" as a goal for the sexual acting-out behavior, the pornography was no longer exciting. Jerry's current life had been "run" by his 20-year-old self. Releasing Jerry from the chains of the Feeling-State allowed Jerry to seek the feeling of acceptance in healthier ways.

Jerry's therapeutic experience of a quick breaking of the Feeling-State memory is not unusual. The challenge for processing the Feeling-State is the identification of the feeling linked with the behavior. Usually, the feelings linked with sexual behaviors are easy to identify. Once identified, the Feeling-State is easy to process. After Jerry's Feeling-State of "first time" sex was broken, therapy focused on his underlying problems from childhood regarding why he so intensely needed to feel accepted.

As a result of eliminating the Feeling-State, Jerry did not have to contend with a whack-a-mole problem when he stopped acting out. The whack-a-mole problem occurs when a person attempts to control behavior. Controlling behavior does not eliminate the need for the feeling linked with the behavior. The person will seek other means to experience the feeling. Only breaking the link between the feeling and behavior frees the person to seek the desired feeling in a healthy manner. Processing the Feeling-State prevents both the whack-a-mole problem and relapse caused by a Feeling-State memory.

For a more complete understanding of the concepts and practice of the FSAP, consult the book *The Feeling-State Theory and Protocols for Behavioral and Substance Addictions,* Third Edition (Miller, 2021).

SEX OFFENDERS

ASSESSING SEX OFFENDERS

My (S. Baird) first postgraduate work in 1999 was assessing male-identified sex offenders for psychopathy at the maximum security Bridgewater Treatment Center for Sexually Dangerous Persons (in Bridgewater, Massachusetts), as well as providing group treatment for female-identified sex offenders at MCI-Framingham (both facilities are prisons). As a brand new clinician I utilized the assessment resources and relapse prevention/cognitive behavior models available to me by the Justice Resource Institute, the organization responsible for providing treatment.

Most of the group therapy with the female-identified sex offenders (often convicted as accessories to a partner's crimes) involved treating the very high rates of sexual abuse they themselves had experienced as children, as well as victimization in adulthood by other adults (usually their coperpetrators who orchestrated the grooming and sexual abuse of their child victims). Looking back, I certainly wish I had been EMDR therapy trained at that time. EMDR therapy likely could have helped them process their own trauma history more effectively and efficiently. This healing, along with potentially more stable and symptom-free mental health, may have then increased their capacity to address their own criminal sexual offending behavior more authentically and insightfully.

As for working with the inmates at Bridgewater, a great many of their substantial files also noted a history of their own experiences of sexual or physical abuse during childhood, and/or high ACE scores. Obviously, the great majority of survivors of childhood sexual trauma grow up to become productive members of society, with many even going into the helping professions (versus harming others). However, this group of incarcerated individuals was caught and convicted of heinous sex offenses.

At the time there was a huge divide in how the corrections officers versus the treatment providers (psychiatrists, psychometrists like myself, psychotherapists, and clergy) viewed these inmates. The corrections officers would have happily executed the offenders, as severe as that sounds. The treatment providers believed in the goal of sentencing and rehabilitating. We believed in treating and reforming these individuals as best as possible as most of the convicted offenders experienced incredible victimization during their own childhoods.

As an aside, while much of the population at Bridgewater met the criteria for antisocial personality disorder (APD), about 20% of this particular inmate population at Bridgewater were rated as having severe APD (aka "psychopaths") via the Hare Psychopathy Checklist. Hence, their treatment typically involved behavior reform, close supervision, and relapse prevention.

DEFINITIONS AND STATISTICS

Adult rapists tend to reoffend across several violent crime categories, not just sexual assault, and assault out of "anger, hostility, and vindictiveness." They may have more social competence than child molesters, on average, but also have poor self-regulation, offense-supportive attitudes, negative peer influences, and intimacy issues (Simons, 2015). Acquaintance rapists are less violent than stranger rapists, using an opportunity to transgress a boundary (Simons, 2015). It is well known that many offenders are motivated by a desire to gain power and control over their victim. Many of the sex offenders of adults at Bridgewater had been charged against more than one victim.

According to the Race Against Abuse of Children Everywhere website (www.raace.org/statistics-information), the average serial child molester may have "400 victims" across their lifetime. Certainly at Bridgewater many of the inmates who committed child sexual abuse were charged with crimes against several known victims. It was impossible to know how many other victims were out there, unnamed.

The *DSM-5* (APA, 2013) makes a distinction between pedophilic and nonpedophilic child sexual abusers. For a diagnosis of pedophilia, an individual has recurrent, intense, and sexually arousing fantasies, urges, or behaviors directed toward a prepubescent child (generally 13 years of age or younger) over a period of at least 6 months. The individual will have acted on or been distressed by these urges; in addition, they must be at least 16 years old and at least 5 years older than the child victim.

Adult sexual abusers of children may engage in sexual abuse of children outside of their family (extrafamilial) and/or may sexually abuse children within their family (intrafamilial, aka incest). Although it is thought that adults who sexually abuse children may have difficulty maintaining adult sexual/romantic relationships, that is not always the case. There are other possible contributing factors, for example, the belief that sexual abuse of children is acceptable behavior, or opportunistic sexual abuse due to proximity of the victim and the ability to avoid detection. Intrafamilial abusers tend to have fewer victims (generally only those children that are easily accessible) and lower recidivism (Simons, 2015).

The treatment providers felt wholeheartedly that any sex offender capable of experiencing remorse and insight deserved to be treated for their own trauma histories, and deserved a chance to live as a healthy, functioning adult (including learning how to and having healthy sexual relationships with consenting adult partners, upon release from prison).

EYE MOVEMENT DESENSITIZATION AND REPROCESSING THERAPY WITH SEX OFFENDERS

There is some research in recent years that EMDR therapy with sex offenders can provide many positive treatment results (such as decreased recidivism), particularly as most sex offenders have higher levels of ACEs than the general population (Ricci & Clayton, 2016). If you are interested in working with this client population, I highly recommend consulting the article "EMDR With Sex Offenders: Using Offense Drivers to Guide Conceptualization and Treatment," (Ricci & Clayton, 2016). This article provides a summary of the EMDR therapy and sex offender research to that date, as well as a description of the authors' "offense drivers" model. They posit that "sexual offenses are propelled by *offense drivers* which may be implicitly held beliefs, vulnerability factors, maladaptive coping strategies, or any combination thereof that contribute to crossing the line between legal and illegal sexual behavior" (Ricci & Clayton, 2016, p. 110).

Another article described a case study of using EMDR therapy to treat an "adult male who had sexually offended against prepubescent children" (Wright & Warner, 2020, Abstract) The EMDR therapy was used to treat his own childhood sexual abuse, and took place over about a year (33 sessions). At the 3-year follow-up he reported a "reduction in the frequency and strength of sexual arousal to children," although that was not the actual direct focus of treatment (Wright & Warner, 2020, pp. 98–99).

A second case study used EMDR therapy to treat the cognitive distortions of a male sex offender who did not think his offending behavior was wrong (Ten Hoor, 2013). Although he had been sexually abused as a child, he initially did not perceive those experiences as negative, therefore justifying his adult abuse. Nine sessions of EMDR therapy resulted in eliminating these cognitive distortions, increasing openness and authenticity around continued group therapy treatment.

ENCOUNTERING CLIENTS WITH A BACKGROUND OF SEXUAL OFFENDING

Some of us will encounter clients in our offices that reveal a sex offense of some kind. Most disclosed offenses will likely have been committed in late childhood or young adulthood (this has been my experience with client disclosures). As therapists, we can still provide relief for their own trauma history in the form of trauma therapy, while working our way to their targets of offending behavior.

If a client discloses to you, possibly for their first time, desire or interest in engaging in sexually offending behavior (e.g., sexual assault or molestation, frottage, voyeurism), or discloses distant, prior offending (and if no one is in immediate or recent danger), take care not to alarm them with immediate discussions of turning themselves into the police. We may be presented with a first chance opportunity to help these clients begin to rework their neural networks, client willing, away from any potentially harmful, offending, and nonconsensual behaviors and dysfunctional "erotic templates" toward healthier, adaptive, and adult/consent-oriented behaviors.

If you chose to continue to work with this client, the process will likely begin with helping them identify and process their own childhood traumas—sexual or otherwise—with the goal of breaking through any denial. Once they have worked through their own trauma, as well as any disclosed past (or possible future) offending behaviors, referrals to sex offender treatment programs may then be the best course of action.

Unanticipated clients in this category may be very challenging for the general clinician, including sex therapists and/or trauma therapists. If you feel in over your head, immediately seek specialized consultation or coordinate a more appropriate referral for the client. Hopefully more studies and guidelines regarding perpetrators will continue to emerge, and any individual experiencing nonconsensual urges will have direct and speedy access to proficient treatment. This section is but a cursory introductory look into working with this small population, as we will most likely all encounter at least one client who will disclose some type of prior offending behavior.

Case Study 10.7: Joe, Soldier With Juvenile Conviction of Sex Offense

Joe, a 28-year-old heterosexual White cisman, sought therapy for a recent diminished interest in sex and arousal (trouble having and maintaining erections) with his wife (Clarissa), with whom he had a 6-year-old son named Leo. Joe was stationed at a local military base. During the intake, he was very forthcoming about a juvenile sex offense conviction. He disclosed that at age 14 he had molested a much younger female cousin. This incident was essentially immediately discovered, and he was arraigned, tried, and convicted as a minor with indecent sexual assault, serving probation and receiving counseling for the remainder of his youth.

In that period of youth counseling it was learned that he had been abused around the age of 6. This abuse was treated with talk therapy.

Upon further compassionate inquiry, it was determined that all of the sexual events of Joe's youth continued to hold disturbance, and some shame, for him. We made a timeline, and after much EMDR resourcing, including using the Developmental Needs Meeting Strategy (DNMS) Healing Circle to help him develop adult nurturing, protecting, and spiritual core selves, processed these events (the sexual victimization he received, then perpetrated) with EMDR therapy. His NC for the abuse he experienced was, "I'm vulnerable and powerless." His PC became, "I am safe and have choices." His NC for the abuse he perpetrated was, "I'm rotten, disgusting, and can't be trusted." His PC evolved into "I acknowledge and accept my crime, and am now living my life safely, healthfully, and respectful of others." We often called upon his adult nurturing and protector selves during EMDR processing, and as we progressed through the targets, his spiritual core self became more active, as well.

At one point we made the connection that Joe had been abused around the age of 6; his own victim was age 6 when he abused her, and now he himself had a child around the age of 6. He reported no sexual attraction to males, and that during the first 2 years of his marriage, he very much experienced sexual attraction to his wife. He had also been in other adult relationships prior to this marriage where he reported healthy consenting mutual sexual interest. Once his child was born, however, he noted a gradual decline in sexual interest. We surmised that the addition of the child in his life had slowly started pressing on his sexual brakes, for many of the same reasons this happens to nonoffending folks: lack of time and energy for consistent sensual connection with his wife.

Additionally, whereas Joe's sexual interest within his marriage had diminished slowly for a few years, his own child approaching the age of 6 (linking up of all these age 6 parallels) put a screeching halt (aka emergency sexual brake) on his interest in sex with his wife. We then used EMDR therapy (bringing in his Healing Circle often) to target and process two separate fears: (a) his fears that he would molest Leo, and (b) worries that others might molest Leo. Throughout our treatment he mentioned that he spoke openly to his wife about his EMDR therapy, having her full support. He was encouraged to engage in sensate focus with Clarissa and learn relaxation and mindfulness skills to stay in the moment. He was also given permission to explore his new erotic templates emerging post EMDR therapy. While he maintained no sexual interest in youths, he did notice a wish to be submissive to his wife. As she was open to this, they began to explore dominance and submission dynamics together.

After about a year of therapy, Joe discharged, feeling more in charge of his adult sexuality (and factors conducive for erections), more free from his past, hopeful about Leo's chances to experience a much better (and appropriately boundaried) life, and some burgeoning excitement for his own developing adult-oriented erotic templates.

VICARIOUS TRAUMA

This last section shares information relevant to ongoing clinical work with clients who have experienced violence and/or trauma (whether survivors or perpetrators). *Vicarious trauma* (VT) attempts to explain the cumulative effects of repeated exposure to trauma survivors. VT includes disruptive and painful psychological effects that can persist for months, or, if left untreated, for years.

Pearlman and Saakvitne, two of the original developers of this concept, state that VT is the "transformation in the therapist's inner experiences resulting from [the cumulative] empathic engagement with (survivor) clients and their traumatic material" (1995, p. 151). Or, "when we open our hearts to hear someone's story of devastation or betrayal, our cherished beliefs are challenged and we are changed" (Saakvitne et al., 1996, p. 25). VT can profoundly impact the therapist's world and self-view as well as their sense of meaning and identity (Pearlman & Saakvitne, 1995). Changes in core beliefs and relationship difficulties may develop, resulting in problems with security, trust, esteem, intimacy, and control. The therapist begins to question what is safe and what is not safe.

Briefly, these are common VT symptoms:

- *PTSD-like intrusive imagery*, including flashbacks, dreams, and intrusive thoughts that impact daily life (McCann & Pearlman, 1990).
- *physical symptoms*: sleep disturbance, somatic symptoms, sexual dysfunction, frequent illness, sensory alterations
- *psychological symptoms*: mood swings, aggression, cynicism, increased sensitivity to violence, social withdrawal, problems maintaining boundaries with clients, diminished self-capacities and ego resources

The antidote and best prevention strategy against VT is ongoing self-care, which will be addressed more in the final chapter.

SUMMARY

SV (including sexual assault, abuse, molestation, rape, harassment, FGM, etc.) continues to persist at alarmingly high rates, although rates have slightly decreased over the past few decades. Any kind of SV may result in diagnoses of PTSD or CPTSD. For clients seeking sex therapy who also have a history of trauma, it is usually important and more productive to treat the trauma first. Sex therapists may refer these clients for trauma-informed and focused therapy such as TF-CBT or EMDR therapy.

Sex work and sex workers have been criminally marginalized in our country through many laws, including the 2018 FOSTA-SESTA bills, making it more difficult for sex workers to remain autonomous and safely screen clients. While this bill is targeted toward sex trafficking, a global problem, it has not been shown to increase true sex trafficking arrests. Independent sex workers maintain relationships, marriages, and family life just like any other individual. They may seek therapy for disturbing events not at all related to their sex work. We must remain nonjudgmental and supportive, following their lead should they chose to disclose their sex work.

Survivors of sex trafficking will benefit from trauma-informed therapy to treat any traumatic symptoms resulting from their experience.

Pornography can both positively and negatively impact our clients' sexual health. Exploring this impact can greatly benefit our clients' sexual health and esteem.

Some clients may seek therapy stating they have a sex addiction. Modern sexual health frameworks urges clinicians to helps these clients reframe these behaviors as "out of control," and assist them in finding balance.

Treating sex offenders is very complicated. Convicted sex offenders also themselves generally have experienced being sexually abused as children. They ideally receive some kind of trauma and relapse prevention treatment in prison. Outpatient clients may disclose (for the first time) a history of sex offending. How we respond to this disclosure can greatly impact whether the client continues to seek services and therefore receives direct assistance to function healthfully and consensually. Offering therapy (particularly EMDR therapy) for any abuse they themselves experienced can help redirect any CETs related to the abuse. If there is imminent harm or danger, you may need to involve local or state agencies or authorities. When in any kind of doubt, seek consultation from someone who regularly treats sex offenders.

DISCUSSION QUESTIONS

- What are some reasons why sexual violence persists at high rates, despite the #metoo movement and other prevention efforts?
- What are some of the main symptoms people may report, relating to their experiences of trauma events and assaults?
- How have sex workers been negatively impacted by stereotypes and legislation?

- What are some differences between "mainstream" and ethical/feminist pornography, and which type is more likely to positively impact sexual health and pleasure?
- What type of events might be in the childhood history of someone convicted of sex offending?

LEARNING ACTIVITIES

CourseConnect

To access self-assessment questions and interactive, competency-based learning activities for this chapter, visit www.springerpub.com/courseconnect. See inside front cover and tear-out card for CourseConnect details.

ADDITIONAL RESOURCES

Additional resources are online and available at www.springerpub.com/courseconnect.

REFERENCES

Allow States and Victims to Fight Online Sex Trafficking Act of 2017, Pub. L. No. 115-164, 132 Stat. 1253 (2018).

American Association of Sexuality Educators, Counselors and Therapists. (n.d.). *AASECT position on sex addiction*. Retrieved February 20, 2025, from https://www.aasect.org/position-sex-addiction

American Association of Sexuality Educators, Counselors and Therapists. (2016, December 8). *AASECT position on sex addiction*. https://www.aasect.org/position-sex-addiction

American Psychiatric Association. (2013). *Diagnostic and statistical manual of mental disorders* (5th ed.). https://doi.org/10.1176/appi.books.9780890425596

Baird, S. (2023, Spring). Sexual trauma and sexual health: A brief introduction. *Go With That Magazine, 28*(2), 15–25. EMDR International Association.

Centers for Disease Control and Prevention. (n.d.). About the CDC–Kaiser ACE Study. Retrieved March 13, 2025, from https://www.cdc.gov/violenceprevention/aces/about.html

Centers for Disease Control and Prevention. (2024, January 23). *About sexual violence*. https://www.cdc.gov/sexual-violence/about

Chloe. (2018, July 19). *Offline shadows: How sex workers become marginalized victims of morality-based legislation*. Autrostraddle. https://www.autostraddle.com/offline-shadows-how-sex-workers-become-marginalized-victims-of-morality-based-legislation-426191

Courtois, C. A. (2004). Complex trauma, complex reactions: Assessment and treatment. *Psychotherapy: Theory, Research, Practice, and Training, 41*, 412–425. https://doi.org/10.1037/0033-3204.41.4.412

Ehlers, A., & Clark, D. M. (2000). A cognitive model of posttraumatic stress disorder. *Behaviour Research and Therapy, 38*, 319–345. https://doi.org/10.1016/s0005-7967(99)00123-0

Foa, E. B., Keane, T. M., Friedman, M. J., & Cohen, J. A. (Eds.). (2008). *Effective treatments for PTSD: Practice guidelines from the International Society for Traumatic Stress Studies* (2nd ed.). Guilford Press.

Gallagher, K. (2014, October). *Pandora's Box: Sex from A to Z in clinical work* [Presentation]. Brattleboro Retreat, Holyoke, Massachusetts.

Gottman, J., & Gottman, J. (2024, June 25). *An open letter on porn: Pornography poses a serious threat to couple intimacy and relationship harmony*. The Gottman Institute. https://www.gottman.com/blog/an-open-letter-on-porn

Grant, M. (2018, January 30). In 'anti-trafficking' New Orleans strip club raids, police make no trafficking arrest. *The Appeal*. https://theappeal.org/in-anti-trafficking-new-orleans-strip-club-raids-police-make-no-trafficking-arrests-a51f374b4e9

Hald, G. M., Malamuth, N. M., & Yuen, C. (2010). Pornography and attitudes supporting violence against women: Revisiting the relationship in nonexperimental studies. *Aggressive Behavior, 36*(1), 14–20. https://doi.org/10.1002/ab.20328

Hase, M. (2009). CravEx: An EMDR approach to treat substance abuse and addiction. In M. Luber (Ed.), *Eye movement desensitization and reprocessing (EMDR) scripted protocols: Special populations* (pp. 467–488). Springer Publishing Company.

Hase, M., Balmaceda, U., Ostacoli, L., Liebermann, P., & Hofmann, A. (2017). The AIP model of EMDR therapy and pathogenic memories. *Frontiers in Psychology, 21*, 1578. https://doi.org/10.3389/fpsyg.2017.01578

Herbenick, D., Fu, T.-C., Wright, P., Paul, B., Gradus, R., Bauer, J., Jones, R. (2020). Diverse sexual behaviors and pornography use: findings from a nationally representative probability survey of Americans aged 18 to 60 years. *The Journal of Sexual Medicine, 17*(4), 623–633. https://doi.org/10.1016/j.jsxm.2020.01.013

Herbenick, D., Patterson, C., Beckmeyer, J., Rosenstock Gonzalez, Y. R., Luetke, M., Guerra-Reyes, L., Eastman-Mueller, H., Svetina Valdivia, D., & Rosenberg, M. (2021). Diverse sexual behaviors in undergraduate students: Findings from a campus probability survey. *Journal of Sexual Medicine, 18*(6), 1024–1041. https://doi.org/10.1016/j.jsxm.2021.03.006

Herman, J. L. (1992). Complex PTSD: A syndrome in survivors of prolonged and repeated trauma. *Journal of Traumatic Stress, 3*, 377–391. https://doi.org/10.1002/jts.2490050305

Klein, M. (2010, April). *When sex gets complicated: Pornography, kink, cybersex, and other clinical challenges* [Workshop]. American Association of Sexuality Educators, Counselors and Therapists.

Kort, J. (n.d.). *Shades of play: Trauma reenactment versus trauma play.* Center for Relationship and Sexual Health. https://crsh.com/2018/09/14/shades-of-play-trauma-reenactment-versus-trauma-play

Lewis, R. W., Fugl-Meyer, K. S., Corona, G., Hayes, R. D., Laumann, E. O., Moreira, E. D. Jr., Rellini, A. H., & Segraves, R. T. (2010). Definitions/epidemiology/risk factors for sexual dysfunction. *The Journal of Sexual Medicine*, 7(4 Pt. 2), 1598–1607. https://doi.org/10.1111/j.1743-6109.2010.01778.x

Ley, D. (2016). *Ethical porn for dicks: A man's guide to responsible viewing pleasure.* ThreeL Media.

Maltz, W. (n.d.-a). *Relearning touch.* Retrieved September 15, 2021, from https://healthysex.com/booksdvdsposters/videos/relearning-touch

Maltz, W. (n.d.-b). *Partners in healing.* Retrieved September 15, 2021, from https://healthysex.com/booksdvdsposters/videos/partners-in-healing

Maltz, W. (2012). *The sexual healing journey: A guide for survivors of sexual abuse* (3rd ed.). William Morrow/HarperCollins.

Maltz, W., & Holman, B. (1987). *Incest and sexuality: A guide to understanding and healing.* Lexington Books.

McCann, I. L., & Pearlman, L. A. (1990). Vicarious traumatization: A framework for understanding the psychological effects of working with victims. *Journal of Traumatic Stress, 3*(1), 131–149. https://link.springer.com/article/10.1007/BF00975140

Meriwether, E., & Rosenstock, K. (Executive Producers). (2025). *Dying for sex* [TV series]. 20th Television.

Miller, R. M. (2010). The feeling-state theory of impulse-control disorders and the impulse-control protocol. *Traumatology, 16*(3), 2–10. https://doi.org/10.1177/1534765610365912

Miller, R. M. (2012). Treatment of behavioral addictions utilizing the feeling-state addiction protocol: A multiple baseline study. *Journal of EMDR Practice and Research, 6*(4), 159–169. https://doi.org/10.1891/1933-3196.6.4.159

Miller, R. M. (2021). *The feeling-state theory and protocols for behavioral and substance addictions* (3rd ed.). ImTT Press.

Morin, J. (1996). *The erotic mind: Unlocking the inner sources of passion and fulfillment.* Harper Perennial.

Neumann, D. A., Houskamp, B. M., Pollock, V. E., & Briere, J. (1996). The long-term sequelae of childhood sexual abuse in women: A meta-analytic review. *Child Maltreatment, 1*(1), 6–16. https://doi.org/10.1177/1077559596001001002

Office of Public Affairs. (2023, February 6). *Justice Department and federal partners recognize Zero Tolerance Day for female genital mutilation* [Press Release 23-142]. U.S. Department of Justice. https://www.justice.gov/archives/opa/pr/justice-department-and-federal-partners-recognize-zero-tolerance-day-female-genital

Pearlman, L. A., & Saakvitne, K. W. (1995). *Trauma and the therapist: Countertransference and vicarious traumatization in psychotherapy with incest survivors.* W. W. Norton.

Popky, A. J. (2010). The desensitization of triggers and urge reprocessing (DeTUR) protocol. In M. Luber (Ed.), *Eye movement desensitization and reprocessing (EMDR) scripted protocols: Special populations* (pp. 489–511). Springer Publishing Company.

Porges, S. (2011). *The polyvagal theory: Neurophysiological foundations of emotions, attachment, communication, and self-regulation*. W. W. Norton.

Psychology Tools. (n.d.-a). *What is EMDR?* https://www.psychologytools.com/resource/what-is-emdr

Psychology Tools. (n.d.-b). *What is trauma-focused cognitive behavioral therapy (TF-CBT)*? https://www.psychologytools.com/resource/what-is-tf-cbt

Rennick, R. (2021). *Digital sexuality and youth* [Webinar]. Tapestry.

Research and Markets. (2025). *Online adult entertainment market by content type, monetization models, interactive type, age group, end-user: Global forecast to 2030*. 360iResearch. https://www.researchandmarkets.com/reports/6033005/online-adult-entertainment-market-content-type

Ricci, R., & Clayton, C. (2016). EMDR with sex offenders: Using offense drivers to guide conceptualization and treatment. *Journal of EMDR Practice and Research, 10*(2), 104–118. http://doi.org/10.1891/1933-3196.10.2.104

Rostad, W. L., Gittins-Stone, D., Huntington, C., Rizzo, C. J., Pearlman, D., & Orchowski, L. (2019). The association between exposure to violent pornography and teen dating violence in grade 10 high school students. *Archives of Sexual Behavior, 48*(7), 2137–2147. https://doi.org/10.1007/s10508-019-1435-4

Rothman, E. F. (2019, September 4). *How porn changes the way teens think about sex* [Video]. TED Conferences. https://www.ted.com/talks/emily_f_rothman_how_porn_changes_the_way_teens_think_about_sex

RSEI Educator. (2019, August 26). *Teaching porn literacy to youth*. Responsible Sex Education Institute. https://responsiblesexedinstitute.org/rsei-blog/teaching-porn-literacy-to-youth

Saakvitne, K. W., Pearlman, L. A., & Traumatic Stress Inst, Ctr for Adult & Adolescent Psychotherapy. (1996). *Transforming the pain: A workbook on vicarious traumatization*. W. W. Norton.

Shapiro, F. (2001). *Eye movement desensitization and reprocessing: Basic principles, protocols, and procedures* (2nd ed.). Guilford Press.

Shapiro, F. (2018). *Eye movement desensitization and reprocessing (EMDR) therapy: Basic principles, protocols, and procedures* (3rd ed.). Guilford Press.

Simons, D. (2015). *Adult sex offender typologies*. SOMAPI Research Brief. https://smart.ojp.gov/sites/g/files/xyckuh231/files/media/document/adultsexoffendertypologies.pdf

Solomon, R. M., & Shapiro, F. (2008). EMDR and the adaptive information processing model: Potential mechanisms of change. *Journal of EMDR Practice and Research, 2*(4), 315–325.

Steinem, G. (1977). Pornography–Not sex but the obscene use of power. *Ms. Magazine, VIII*(1), 43–44.

Ten Hoor, N. M. (2013). Treating cognitive distortions with EMDR: A case study of a sex offender. *Interpersonal Journal of Forensic Mental Health, 12(2)*, 139–148. https://doi.org/10.1080/14999013.2013.791350

van der Hart, O., Nijenhuis, E., & Steele, K. (2006). *The haunted self: Structural dissociation and the treatment of chronic traumatization*. W. W. Norton.

World Health Organization. (2021). *International classification of diseases* (11th revision [ICD-11]). (Original work published 2019)

World Health Organization. (2025, January 31). *Female genital mutilation*. https://www.who.int/news-room/fact-sheets/detail/female-genital-mutilation

Wright, L. C., & Warner, A. (2020). EMDR treatment of childhood sexual abuse for a child molester: Self-reported changes in sexual arousal. *Journal of EMDR Practice and Research, 14*(2), 90–103. https://doi.org/10.1891/EMDR-D-19-00060

Yehuda, R., Lehrner, A., & Rosenbaum, T. Y. (2015). PTSD and sexual dysfunction in men and women. *The Journal of Sexual Medicine, 12*(5), 1107–1119. https://doi.org/10.1111/jsm.12856

III

Resources and Specific Populations

CHAPTER 11

Marginalized Populations and Sexual Health

Stephanie Baird

LEARNING OBJECTIVES

- Learn about sexual health concerns of physically marginalized (visible and invisible disabilities and marginilization) populations, illustrated with a case study.
- Learn about sexual health concerns and the sexual rights of intellectually marginalized populations (those with intellectual disabilities and/or developmental delays).
- Learn about sexual health concerns of neurodiverse populations.
- Learn essential sexual health information about *erotically* marginalized kink populations (e.g., kink/bondage, discipline or domination, sadism, and masochism), illustrated with case studies.
- Learn about fetish versus paraphilia, and potential clinical issues.

INTRODUCTION

"Marginalized communities are those excluded from mainstream social, economic, educational, and/or cultural life. Examples of marginalized populations include, but are not limited to, groups excluded due to race, gender identity, sexual orientation, age, physical ability, language, and/or immigration status. Marginalization occurs due to unequal power relationships between social groups" (Sevelius et al., 2020, p. 2009).

This chapter looks at a few specific marginalized communities. It would take several more volumes of this book to perform adequate justice with all the types of marginalized groups and individuals in this country (and abroad). For in-depth learning, please refer to the following books for professionals.

Exploring Sexuality and Disability: A Guide for Human Service Professionals (Kattari, 2023) is a very recent comprehensive book covering sexuality and disability for the following groups: queer/trans disabled folks; neurodivergent folks; and people with intellectual/developmental disabilities, deafness, blindness, chronic pain, chronic illness, physical size differences, and aging and disability issues, among others.

The Routledge Handbook of Disability and Sexuality (Shuttleworth & Mona, 2021) is another comprehensive book that examines the enduring challenges disabled individuals face in gaining sexual health access, including psychological, interpersonal, social, political, and cultural obstacles, as well as their ongoing fight for sexual rights and inclusion.

The *Ultimate Guide to Sex and Disability: For All of Us Who Live With Disability, Pain, and Chronic Illness* (Kaufman et al., 2007) is an excellent resource for clients and anyone living with a disability or pain, or in a relationship with a disabled or chronically ill person.

Mark Nickerson's book on *cultural competency* (2017) encourages cultural humility and expanding cultural competence for eye movement desensitization and reprocessing (EMDR) clinicians with many different groups, including BIPOC (Black, Indigenous, and People of Color) communities, refugees, immigrants, folks with addictions, and folks from the uniformed services, among other groups. I wholeheartedly endorse the excellent chapters in his book to increase awareness of different groups.

Marginalized groups are also addressed throughout this book and in other specific chapters. Chapter 5 entirely explores gender, including potential marginalization. Chapter 6 shares brief descriptions of the nine principles of clinical support by Constantinides et al. (2019). Chapter 10 provides information on people with LGBTQ sexual and affectional orientations, as well as non-monogamous individuals, groups that continue to be marginalized despite many advances like equal marriage and antidiscrimination laws.

The communities explored in this chapter are marginalized due to external characteristics (like having a visible prosthetic leg) or internal characteristics (such as an intellectual disability [ID]). Some are erotically marginalized due to sexual behaviors and identities. Clinicians and students reading this may find that they identify with a variety of marginalized groups. It is helpful to have a good awareness of one's owns identities.

PART A

BLACK, INDIGENOUS, AND PEOPLE OF COLOR COMMUNITIES AND SEXUAL HEALTH by Kristen Benson, PhD, LMHC

BIPOC individuals are still underrepresented in the helping professions, as both clinicians and clients (although numbers in both domains continue to increase). Given White dominant ideologies, they may also experience internalized racism (David et al., 2019). This section provides information regarding the treatment of BIPOC clients within a historically institutionally racist system, and is intended to encourage accountability practices for providers, with special attention to those who are generally not targets of racism (often White clinicians) and who also work with BIPOC clients.

To establish inclusive practices in efforts to work humbly and competently with BIPOC clients, providers must avoid the temptation to be "color blind." Racial color blindness is defined as having two dimensions: Color-evasion refers to the ideology that all people are equal and we do not see race; White superiority is diminished. In contrast, power-evasion refers to the belief that all people have the same opportunities; White privilege and institutional racism are denied (Neville et al., 2013). Attempting to treat all people equally does not reverse racial injustices (Williams et al., 2002) and does not allow therapists to examine intergenerational ancestral trauma that contributes to current hardships that BIPOC people experience.

BIPOC people have been sexually dehumanized throughout U.S. history by way of White supremist ideology and oppressive legislation. The most notable examples include the genocide of Indigenous People, enslavement of African People, expulsion of non-European immigrants, and Jim Crow laws which suppressed BIPOC people's sexual autonomy and contributed to ongoing racist sexual stereotypes (Gary-Smith et al., 2022). Primary examples include the adultification of Black girls, which hypersexualizes Black girls and perceives them as more adult and less innocent than White girls (Epstein et al., 2017), and the portrayal of Black men as having overdeveloped sexual organs and excessive sexual desire (Brandt, 1978).

Structural racism throughout history has contributed to economic, housing, educational, and health disparities for BIPOC people, who are less likely to receive preventative healthcare and also receive lower-quality care, leading to worse health outcomes compared to White people (Hostetter & Klein, 2018). For example, Black maternal mortality rates were 2.6 times the rate for White women in 2021 (Hoyert, 2023), Black and Latina women are less likely to receive contraceptive care and HPV vaccinations (Beroukhim et al., 2022), and sexually transmitted infections continue to be elevated for BIPOC youth and young people (Boutrin & Williams, 2021). This is further compounded by mistreatment by health providers; for example, a study found that BIPOC women experience up to 32.8% increased mistreatment in maternity care compared to 14.1% of White women; and White women with Black partners were twice as likely to report mistreatment than White women with White partners (Vedam et al., 2019).

Therefore, racial justice is central to the sexual health and rights of all people as structural and contextual factors shape sexual motivations and behaviors (Future of Sex Education Initiative, 2020), which are relevant to both sexual health education and sexual healthcare. Yet, sex education programs in the United States tend to promote racialized stereotypes, and many sex educators are unaware of how experiences of racism inform and impact BIPOC youth's sexual identity and experience (Gary-Smith et al., 2022). Sexual healthcare providers report that they receive minimal training explicit to racial/ethnic and LGBTQ+ health equity, which results in uncertainty of sexual health communication and care with minoritized patients (Noh et al., 2024).

Recent movements center antiracist sexuality in an effort to promote inclusive change. As such, the revision of the National Sex Education Standards (Future of Sex Education Initiative, 2020) integrates racial justice as a guiding principle and value, and Carole Clements's book, *Sex Positivity and White-Sex Supremacy: Ending Complicity in Black Body Erasure* (2024), promotes a racially just and embodied sexual ethic to highlight the relevance of Black sexuality. Healthcare provider organizations are acknowledging the impacts of racism and committing to change. The American College of Obstetricians and Gynecologists (ACOG, n.d.) issued a statement of their commitment to confronting explicit and implicit bias and racism in an effort to eliminate disparities, and signed onto a joint statement of collective action to address racism with 24 sexual and reproductive health organizations (ACOG, 2020). In addition, scholars and practitioners have called for examination of U.S. policies that contribute to racism within the healthcare system (ACOG, n.d.).

DIVERSITY, EQUITY, BELONGING, AND INCLUSION GUIDELINES

While we recognize BIPOC communities experience marginalization, oppression, and discrimination at disproportionate rates, we have purposely included intersectionality throughout this entire book to illustrate the constant interplay of race and culture with sexual health. Briefly, we describe here guidelines for greater inclusion and affirmation, as this positively impacts the provision of clinical care. *Diversity, equity, inclusion,* and *belonging* (DEIB) guidelines promote a more just and inclusive setting. Diversity reflects an aspiration to affirm and celebrate all identities and experiences. Equity refers to ensuring fair treatment and opportunities, which means that some people may need additional or different resources to access quality care. Inclusion focuses on engaging all participants, ensuring respectful, democratic, and equal participation. Belonging fosters connection, acceptance, and community support, as well as authentic expression of self.

INTERSECTIONALITY AND ANTIRACIST WORK

Providers must be aware of their positionality and actively engaged in accountability practices. This involves examining one's own race along with other aspects of identity and considering the ways they compound, resulting in social advantages or disadvantages. Kimberlé Crenshaw coined the term *intersectionality* to acknowledge the intersections of race, class, gender, and other categories of identity that overlap and intersect, which can produce further marginalization and discrimination (1989).

There are implications for sexual well-being based on how a person experiences themselves in relation to their social position or identities (Heredia & Rider, 2020), which include but are not limited to race, ethnicity, socioeconomic status (SES), gender, sexual orientation, ability, and immigration status (Bowleg, 2012). Therefore, a heterosexual Latino cisgender man with access to financial resources has a different social and interpersonal experience seeking sexual healthcare compared to a low-SES queer Muslim cisgender woman.

An intersectional public health framework acknowledges that multiple intersecting identities contribute to complex health disparities and recognizes how systems of privilege and oppression result in macrostructural-level social inequalities that maintain such disparities (Bowleg, 2012). For example, a transgender Black woman may face employment and housing discrimination, which can increase housing instability and decrease access to preventative healthcare. AntiBlack sentiments, heterosexism, and transphobia contribute to short- and long-term health outcomes (Thurston et al., 2024). Antiracist evidence-based comprehensive sex education is critical to improving health outcomes for young people, yet race is often omitted from sex education curricula (Massicotte, 2023).

Antiracist approaches are reflected in cultural humility, which is a framework where providers engage with clients from diverse backgrounds by focusing on critical self-examination of cultural biases and power dynamics rather than reliance on knowledge about multiculturalism (Mosher et al., 2017). Experiences of racism are believed and validated. Cultural humility requires healthcare and social service workers to recognize that they do not know a client's experiences and are willing to learn from clients and patients (Lekas et al., 2020). The shift to process-oriented cultural humility prioritizes a person-centered stance that equalizes the patient–provider partnership to improve quality of care (Julian et al., 2021; Lekas et al., 2020). For example, Owen et al. (2016) found that therapists who engaged in cultural humility had better treatment outcomes. Cultural humility can be especially helpful for White providers yet contribute to challenges for BIPOC providers; therefore, institutional policies, procedures, and resources must be in place to provide structural supports to BIPOC providers engaging in cultural humility practices, as they are at risk for burnout and high turnover rates (Moon & Sandage, 2019).

IMPORTANCE OF INCREASING ACCESS TO SEXUAL HEALTH

The World Health Organization defines sexual health as "fundamental to the overall health and well-being of individuals, couples and families, and to the social and economic development of communities and countries" (n.d., Overview). Structural barriers (Hostetter & Klein, 2018) and healthcare provider implicit biases toward historically marginalized groups lead to health inequities (Casanova-Perez et al., 2022), which compromises BIPOC quality of life. White colonization has perpetuated racist beliefs about Black and Brown bodies throughout history, which continues in sexual health education, research, and healthcare (Massicotte, 2023) and must change in order for BIPOC people to experience improved sexual health outcomes and overall well-being.

Addressing structural barriers that prevent BIPOC people from accessing sexual healthcare will help to achieve sexual health equity (Sutton et al., 2021). The *Joint Statement: Collective Action Addressing Racism* (ACOG, 2020) outlines actions to eliminate racial inequities, which require (a) collaboration with communities, providers, advocates, and scholars; (b) educating students and health and medical professionals about the role of the health community's history in racist oppression; (c) formally recognizing the abuse of enslaved women in the name of advancing science; (d) addressing racism in scholarship, research, and publication; (e) adopting policies and procedures that promote inclusive excellence; (f) caring for patients and community by recognizing the impact of racism, treating racism as an evidence-based risk factor, and training providers accordingly; and (g) advocating for public policies that eliminate racial inequities in the delivery of healthcare and healthcare outcomes, as well as policies that address systemic inequities outside of healthcare that contribute to poor health outcomes.

BIPOC access to sexual health through antiracist healthcare and sexual health education addresses health disparities and improved quality of life. Integrating cultural humility training in medical and public health training is necessary to improve the quality of care by providers, as well as to address sexual health access and improve BIPOC experiences of sexual healthcare (e.g., Lekas et al., 2020). Additionally, research shows that engaging disadvantaged communities in the design and implementation of public health interventions can reduce health inequities (O'Mara-Eves et al., 2015), which includes sexual health professions' training curriculum (Julian et al., 2021). A recent review of community engaged sexual and reproductive health literature found that interventions that encouraged community participation, consultation, and collaboration are likely to be accepted in the community and more sustainable (Tohit et al., 2024). Similarly, community-based participatory research that includes partnerships with racial and ethnic minority populations has resulted in culturally relevant sexual health intervention strategies that reduced sexual health inequities (McCuistian et al., 2023). Therefore, establishing partnerships and including BIPOC community members in the planning and governance of sexual health programming and services can lead to increased access and positive health outcomes.

Most notable is the impact of public policy on BIPOC access to public health. Policy-level interventions have the ability to address structural barriers and increase access to sexual health for BIPOC people (Sutton et al., 2021). Access to health insurance as addressed in federal laws such as the Affordable Care Act increases the likelihood of receiving family planning services such as contraception and preventative sexual healthcare such as mammograms and cervical cancer screenings (Stolp & Fox, 2015). As such, advocating for a comprehensive healthcare system will have a tremendously positive impact on BIPOC communities' access to sexual health care.

DISABILITY AND SEXUAL HEALTH

DISABILITY STATISTICS

According to the Centers for Disease Control and Prevention (CDC; Okoro et al., 2018), nearly one in four U.S. adults report a disability. Some writers define disability as a *bodymind* that operates differently from societal expectations and norms (Clare, 2017). Categories of disabilities in an ongoing survey of more than 400,000 adults each year include hearing, vision, cognition, mobility, self-care, and independent living (CDC, n.d.-a). More specifically, individuals may have central nervous system damage (e.g., cerebral palsy), musculoskeletal conditions (e.g., scoliosis), congenital disorders (e.g., cystic fibrosis, cleft lip, spinal bifida, club foot, seizures, etc.), medical conditions that may be lifelong or temporary (e.g., diabetes, asthma, cancer), or accident-related injuries such as wearing a back brace or using a cane or cast (Bruess & Schroeder, 2018). Some clients may be grappling with chronic pain and/or illness that interferes with daily activities. Many of these clients will make their way to our offices.

ABLEISM

Some clients readily recognize and name *ableism*: discrimination and social prejudice that devalue people with disabilities and/or people who are perceived to be disabled (Smith, n.d.). Other clients, especially newly disabled, are new to this term and may benefit from learning about this type of prejudice. Supportive therapy can help identify and process the few or many instances of discrimination and prejudice they may have encountered. Avoid using the term *differently abled*; this term is experienced as dismissive of people with disabilities.

VISIBLE DISABILITES

Some disabilities may be visible due to the person using a wheelchair or walker, having a service animal assisting with vision or other support, using sign language, having a different walking gait, having a differently appearing limb or a missing limb, and so on.

INVISIBLE DISABILITIES

Many disabilities may be invisible to some degree (i.e., asthma, hearing difficulties, chronic illness, chronic fatigue, fibromyalgia, immune disorders, or now "long-haul COVID"). Some of these clients have been living with their disability for their lifetime (e.g., type 1 diabetes, lifelong hearing impairment). Still other clients may have a newly acquired disability due to a recent disease, injury, or an aging complication (e.g., cardiovascular disease, hypertension, stroke, arthritis, and/or osteoporosis). With my apologies, the types of disabilities that can occur to all of us are numerous, and impossible to do justice here. Please continue to seek current information from trusted sources on sexuality and disability.

SOCIAL MODEL OF DISABILITY

The *social model of disability* views disability not as the impairment itself; rather, it is the result of a particular impairment's interactions with social and environmental barriers. Solutions to disablism (prejudice and discrimination against people with disabilities) include everyday equality strategies like ramps and structures for wheelchair accessibility, braille translations, closed captioning, assisted hearing technologies, Americans with Disabilities Act (ADA) light switches and door knobs, sensory modulation for neurodivergent folks, and using font and text that is easier to discern. While many activists (often White, heterosexual cisgender), have worked for decades on behalf of the disability rights movement, a more recent disability justice movement has arisen, predominantly created and led by queer and trans disabled people of color. Consult Kattari's comprehensive book on sexuality and disability (2023) for more in-depth exploration.

IMPACT ON SEXUAL HEALTH

Many illnesses and diseases can impact sexual health and functioning. For example, a cancer diagnosis and treatment can reduce desire and interest in sex. A majority of clients with chronic fatigue syndrome or fibromyalgia report difficulties with having an orgasm, vaginal irritation, and decreased interest in sex (Buehler, 2022). Diabetes can result in erectile dysfunction, low sexual interest, and delayed ejaculation. Diabetes can also correlate with vaginal dryness and uncomfortable intercourse; decreased blood flow to the clitoris and vulva can also occur more frequently (Buehler, 2021).

There are many myths and prejudices in play with how society tends to view the sexuality of people with disabilities. The most recent *Our Whole Lives (OWL)* sexuality education curriculum (Davis, 2019) lists these common myths and stereotypes: People living with disabilities and chronic conditions are not sexual (false), not desirable (false), and cannot have "real" sex (also false—sex includes innumerable kinds of erotic and sensual activities). And lastly, people living with disabilities and chronic illness are not sexually adventurous (false), or are "perverted" (false).

Every human being has the capacity to be sexual and enjoy sexuality, in whatever consenting form that takes. Every human body can experience some form of pleasure. People with disabilities, depending on the changes in how their body parts and organs work, may need to more creatively explore their bodies or learn to orgasm. They may need partners and/or devices (e.g., vibrators) to help them discern paths to pleasure if they have no sensations in their genitals. For example, they may experience "emotional orgasms" (more full body relaxation) versus traditional orgasms (Joannides, 2017). Encouraging exploration, knowledge acquisition, communication, and empowerment (as we do with temporarily able-bodied people) all remain great strategies for safe and pleasurable sexual health.

One excellent sex education resource that serves many populations well is the *Drawn to Sex* (Moen & Nolan, 2018, 2020) book series (which is also useful for individuals with IDs). The best gift we can give anyone, especially those frequently dismissed as nonsexual, is accurate, affirming, and empowering sex education.

Case Study 11.1: Terry Has Cerebral Palsy and Wants a Sexual Relationship

Terry, a 25-year-old graduate student, identifies as a White bisexual ciswoman. She was born 8 weeks prematurely with cerebral palsy, limiting her mobility and her use of her right hand and leg. She has a visible impairment with her gait and hand mobility. Her very supportive parents "mainstreamed" her in public school as her intellectual abilities matched and often exceeded those of the "mainstream" students.

Terry's reason for seeking therapy was that she "struggled to be vulnerable," yet was "tired of being alone" and urgently "wanted to be in a romantic and sexual relationship, yesterday." She reported a lack of experience with dating and intimacy, somewhat due to her academic focus for many years, but also due to fears that no one would want to date her. Additionally, she had experienced one unrequited love with a college peer, Alex. Although they had enjoyed emotional closeness, the peer sent mixed messages about engaging romantically. Ultimately nothing romantic or sexual transpired. At this point, Terry confessed she did not feel like a worthy sexual being.

During the intake, Terry shared many negative incidents related to her cerebral palsy, despite the good intentions of her parents and much of the community she grew up in. She reported bullying incidents in elementary school. One incident involved a peer calling her a "cripple"—the first time she heard that word. Another incident involved a teacher humiliating her by calling out her inability to tie her shoes. Fortunately, she had told her parents about this when she got home. Her parents complained to the school, resulting in the teacher being disciplined and Terry switched to a different class. She also reported two incidents at dances of not feeling desired in high school (compared to the "able-bodied" peers around her), and then several events related to the unrequited love with Alex. As Terry was open to the idea of EMDR therapy, we identified her timeline of disturbing targets and installed several resources (including a resource development and installation [RDI] that featured supportive friends, family, a beloved pet cat, Stephen Hawking, Franklin Delano Roosevelt, and Frida Kahlo).

As we processed through the timeline, her negative cognitions (NCs) tended to be, "I'm not worth anything, something is very wrong with me." Her positive cognitions (PCs) tended to be "I'm worthy, fine as I am, and deserve love and respect." Additional targets arose concerning coming out to herself and others as bisexual. One target included a college acquaintance snickering and implying that Terry did not get to be a sexual being due to her cerebral palsy. Her NC for this target was, "I'm worthless, nothing, a broken, sexless human." Her PC was, "I am worth a lot, I'm amazing as I am, I get to be sexual like everyone else." At last, Terry was beginning to see herself as a sexual being.

Once we successfully processed these targets, we then created and installed several future templates oriented toward building confidence around dating and sexual intimacy (including a template about feeling sexy and desirable). During this time, Terry asked out a fellow graduate student, Mary, who said yes. They began dating and Terry noted that as they increased their physical and sexual intimacy, she was able to keep her PC in mind of "I am worth a lot, I'm amazing as I am, I get to give and receive sexual pleasure like everyone else," quelling her fears of being undesirable. Months passed and their relationship solidified into a healthy, sexually vibrant bond. Terry discharged, feeling confident and joyful in her sexual, romantic, and relationship skills.

NEURODIVERSE POPULATIONS

Neurodiversity refers to the notion that neurological variations within the human population are normal. Neurodiverse groups include people with attention deficit hyperactivity disorder (ADHD) diagnoses, dyslexia (trouble with number and letter decoding), dyspraxia (having difficulties in planning and executing fine and gross motor operations), Tourette syndrome, epilepsy, and/or being on the autism spectrum. Some researchers are also including diagnoses of traumatic brain injury, posttraumatic stress disorder (PTSD), obsessive-compulsive disorder (OCD), depression and anxiety, and bipolar disorder as well, due to potential brain differences over time.

Estimates of neurodiversity in the general population are around 20% or higher, depending on how large the umbrella categorization (Doyle, 2020). It's important to understand that "just like fingerprints, each brain is unique" (unknown quote). Recent research, education, awareness, and advocacy, as detailed in books like *The Dyslexic Advantage* (Eide & Eide, 2023) and *Unmasking Autism* (Price, 2022), have been bringing awareness to the strengths and evolutionary benefits of neurodiversity. One emerging theory is that with around one-fifth of the population (or more) having some type of neurodivergence, this may actually be an essential evolutionary aspect. This particularly applies to the idea that humans engage with their world in *exploitative* and *exploratory* ways.

The word *neurodivergent* is used to describe the specific individual within the broader neurodiverse population. Some neurodivergent brains, particularly those with ADHD, may gravitate toward exploratory behaviors, that is, looking for and finding resources, finding new or unusual connections between various elements, developing original solutions, and seeing things differently (Eide & Eide, 2023; Price, 2022). Exploitative behaviors refer to the continued access and utilization of a resource (i.e., now that we have found a water source, we now develop a way to continuously access that water). And while exploitative actions and decisions may relate to predictable rewards (eating the same familiar lunch every day), exploratory behaviors result in more unpredictable rewards (cooking a new recipe could be extremely delicious, or a total dud). To illustrate this regarding sexuality, one client with ADHD mentioned their preference for more interactive kink sexual behaviors as the newness and variety helped focus them, whereas engaging in more predictable "vanilla" behaviors felt boring and allowed them to "stay in their head more." Anecdotally, many of my clients with ADHD or neurodivergence identify as a "role enactor" (enjoying more interaction during sex).

Autism, in particular, is a vast neurological spectrum that affects how people experience the world, particularly cognitively, emotionally, sensorily, and socially (Autism Self Advocacy Network, n.d.). Autistics also generally prefer *person-first* versus *identity-first* language—meaning, being referred to as *autistic* versus *person with autism*. However, have your client share their preferred identity language. Autistics tend to perceive and process the world *bottom up* versus *top down*, meaning they may pick up on many contributing micro details before they see and digest the macro picture (i.e., seeing the trees first, then noticing they are part of a forest). Many autistic brains may "take in about 40% more input than allistic (neurotypical) brains, therefore (may) get overstimulated more frequently and may need to regulate more frequently and/or differently than allistic people" (i.e., via "stimming"—repetitive behaviors that are self-soothing; VanVactor-Lee, 2024). "Sensory overwhelm can lead to meltdowns and shutdowns" (VanVactor-Lee, 2024). Many autistics are adopting the infinity symbol to represent the infinite variety of neurodivergence.

Some recent studies have shown that up to 70% of autistic people surveyed report nonheterosexuality (George & Stokes, 2018a, 2018b; Maggio et al., 2022; Weir et al., 2021) as well as higher rates of gender diversity and dysphoria (and less concern about the gender of their romantic partner; Dewinter et al., 2015). Research shows that autistics typically experience less sex education than their peers (to their detriment; Barnett & Maticka-Tyndale, 2015). For those in romantic and sexual relationships, practicing explicit communication such as "literal declaration" is helpful in maintaining intimacy (Barnett & Maticka-Tyndale, 2015), particularly as autistic folks tend to be direct and need clarity (VanVactor-Lee, 2024). I identify as neurodiverse and find that this resonates. From youth I have tended to verbalize specifically what I was willing to do or not do, and what I wanted from my partners (despite the overt socialization I received as a cisgender woman to keep quiet and not speak up about my own needs and desires). I find that literal declaration has been effective in carrying me successfully, consensually, and pleasurably through most sexual interactions.

There are eight sensory systems: olfactory (hearing), visual (sight), gustatory (taste), auditory (sound), tactile (touch), vestibular (balance), interoception (internal body signals), and proprioception (motor control, planning; Star Institute, n.d.). Neurodivergent individuals' "unique processing experiences" may include tactile, auditory, olfactory, and/or gustatory hypersensitivity or hyposensitivity, with preferences for firmer or lighter touch, as well as specific environmental aspects (Katz Kattari, 2024).

Chapter 4 in the book *Exploring Sexuality and Disability* ("Infinity and Rainbows: Supporting the Sexuality of Neurodivergent People"; Kattari, 2023) has excellent suggestions for ways to support neurodiverse folks in accessing positive sexual health and (desired) intimacy, whether for themselves and/or with others. Initial support may involve filling in the gaps regarding any lack of fact-based sex education and validating and affirming wherever they are at with their sexuality and interests (i.e., exploration of nonbinary gender, pursuit of similar gender sexual relationship, validation of asexuality and/or demisexuality, etc.). Ongoing support may involve helping neurodivergent people identify and name their sexual, affectional, and sensory interests and needs; practice ways to seek their identified needs; and advocate for themselves. Seemingly simple details like attending to body temperature, hygiene, odors, tactile comfort, and moisture (before, during, and after sex) may also facilitate more pleasurable and comfortable sexual interactions (VanVactor-Lee, 2024).

Just as temporarily abled and/or neurotypical individuals are considered and assumed to be sexual beings from the day they are born until they die, so, too, does this apply to individuals with any type of disability or neurodiversity (Bruess & Schroeder, 2018). Individuals with neurodiversity deserve and need sexuality education and counseling as much as the rest of their planetary companions. It is important to recognize these clients as individuals with sexual needs. We can help empower them (as we do with nonneurodivergent clients) to increase their accurate sexual health knowledge base so that they may more easily articulate any sexual goals.

Neurodiverse individuals may report self-esteem issues and lack of worthiness for romantic and sexual relationships. Supportive therapy (along with accurate sexual health psychoeducation), addressing any doubts, negative self-esteem, and/or prior diminishing incidents, and then developing and processing ideal future templates/rehearsals for romance and sexuality can help boost confidence in social and sexual abilities and desirability.

WORKING WITH PEOPLE WITH DISABILITIES: A PERSONAL AND PROFESSIONAL PERSPECTIVE by Jenny Wright, LMHC

Personal Background

As someone who has an obvious physical disability, a rare form of dwarfism, and some invisible disabilities, my younger years were spent avoiding seeing myself as disabled. When I watched shows with characters with dwarfism—*Willow*, *Simon Birch*, and a few others—though I related with the physical and emotional burdens the characters carried, I never quite saw myself as similar.

I came from a family who adapted to my disability easily, as my mother reports being happy to find out there was not a life-threatening reason that I was not growing. My mother strongly advocated for me in school, but at home I was just Jenny. There were no step stools or accommodations, I climbed counters to get what I needed. I was relieved of many tasks because my mother was concerned I would hurt myself, for example, climbing up onto the washer to use it. Also, back in the 1980s, resources and social media groups were not as easily accessible as they are now. I was infantilized as many people with disabilities are. Even now, people in my family say ableist statements such as, "I don't even see you as little."

I now understand the impact of ableism that continues to devalue me, and so many others, even now at 43 years old. I have more examples than I could ever share, but a poignant one was when I was a clinician working in early intervention providing in-home evaluation and therapy to infants and toddlers. At a home visit with my team to evaluate a toddler, the mother asked one of the other therapists if it was *Take Your Daughter to Work Day* to explain why I was there. As was observed in my upbringing, I handled this with positivity and grace. When we left, another therapist on the team was flabbergasted and strongly advocated for me and my credentials in the moment. In some ways I am used to this negative treatment. As people with disabilities are frequently not taken seriously, we often process our anger differently. Though I tend toward manifesting healthy anger, I have had shame to work through at various times in my life.

Disability Psychoeducation

The impact of having a disability on sexual health extends far greater than the surface level of disability. As those with disabilities are at increased risk for sexual violence, age-appropriate sexual education should start in school and at home from a young age. Properly naming body parts from the first year of life and teaching consent is crucial. Building on this topic, accommodations should be made for those who learn differently with various learning resources–books, videos, social stories, and so on. Amaze.org is an excellent resource that has good video shorts about sexual development of varying abilities and sexual orientations for teens and young adults.

For the disabled, sexual health is not often mentioned by doctors, therapists, and so on, and we are often left to figure it out for ourselves. Unless it affects our fertility, there is little information given. For those with disabilities such as brain injuries, chronic pain and health issues, autism, and varying physical disabilities, sexuality is impacted in many different ways.

Fundamentally, unless a disabled person identifies with a form of asexuality, we have the same varieties of sexual thoughts, desires, and actions as a nondisabled person. There may be implications to sexual enjoyment such as how the disability and/or medications may affect the body and mind. There may be certain sexual positions that are best, given a person's abilities. Emotionally we are like everyone else in that we can get insecure—sometimes more so if we have to explain our sexual differences to a partner. Low energy level (such as being interested in and enjoying sex) is a common theme among those with disabilities. Chronic health issues or sensory overload can impact one's interest in sexual activity from moment to moment.

Case Study 11.2: Eye Movement Desensitization and Reprocessing Therapy Helps Sarah (Diagnosed With Autism) Seek Romantic Relationships

Sarah sought therapy in her mid-twenties after a challenging transition to adulthood. She identified as a single, White, cisgender woman working full time in retail and living on her own. Sarah was diagnosed with autism as a child and needed low supports in and outside of school. Sarah considered herself close with her parents and also with a few good friends. During high school, after her first sexual experience, she became aversive to sex, avoiding it ever since. This was a major roadblock to a fulfilling relationship which Sarah desperately wanted.

Sarah also wanted to work on alexithymia (difficulty identifying what one is feeling) and attachment. We discussed the potential for EMDR therapy for various events in her life. If our work together needed more specialization, we agreed I would refer her to someone with that specialty.

We worked through much of her attachment and Sarah gained understanding about how autism and an emotionally shut down family affected her, both then and now. We worked on tools she could use to process and share her emotions more effectively. This included using the emotion wheel, noticing where this emotion might be felt in the body, sitting with this sensation for a moment, wondering if the feeling is familiar feeling, and learning ways to cope with the emotion (breathe, notice what feels okay in the body, look around the room visually and find an anchor).

During our work together, we identified several key moments in her childhood and various relationships which EMDR could help. Sarah had formative childhood moments such as her parents' (verbal) fights that often led to her having nightmares and dissociating, which made it difficult to function in school. She showed anxiety going to school and reported parental pressure for good grades. We first reprocessed those childhood events. Over the course of many months, this led to new insights and decreased body activation when thinking about these events. Sarah was more easily able to name emotions using the emotion wheel and did even better with a somatic list of what sensations she was feeling in her body.

Using DNMS Institute's *Resource Development Protocol* (developing an adult nurturer, adult protector, and adult spiritual self), we were able to develop various self-attachment figures as guideposts that she imagined protecting her during these challenging EMDR targets. After we successfully processed her childhood events we moved on to her first few dating relationships.

Sarah shared that she had overall "okay typical high school relationships," dating less than a year. During a steady relationship at 20 years old she engaged in sexual intercourse for the first time and instantly felt "numb and dissociated." This led her to stop engaging in sex as it felt "wrong to not know what I feel." We did EMDR therapy on these experiences, and with immense support (interweaves) and newfound skills gained earlier in therapy, she was able to process through these events to completion. Sarah made connections to parts of her upbringing that affected these later experiences, noticing some lifelong OCD-like tendencies with intrusive thoughts and avoidance themes.

After EMDR therapy, Sarah was able to establish a romantic relationship with much hard work and despite some autistic burnout. She came to understand herself better and her particular needs and how to advocate for them with her partner. Along with EMDR therapy working quite well to process some key moments in Sarah's life, she also gained better understanding of the lifelong process of navigating her disability. She recognizes that some times she may need more, or less, supports, and currently knows how to utilize her resources.

Conclusion

Regardless of a person's abilities, I offer accommodations to all of my clients for therapy (including the EMDR process). I send them resources we will be referencing so they can print them. I also share the screen with them if they prefer that. I offer visual scales to help clients gauge their rating scales. If clients cannot do an abstract exercise we adjust to make it more concrete (talking about it or bringing in a visual). Sherri Paulson, LCSW, has an excellent protocol to use with autistics and I find it crosses over to being useful for many people of various disabilities.

INTELLECTUALLY MARGINALIZED POPULATIONS by Traccie Hillion, MA, CAGS, LMHC, Melanie Peele, MA, MEd, LPC, and Stephanie Baird, MS, LMHC

Clients with IDs are a vital population to engage in sexual health education and psychotherapy, including trauma treatments as needed. IDs refer to "limits to a person's ability to learn at an expected level and function in daily life" (CDC, n.d.-b, para. 1). Some causes of IDs include Down syndrome, fetal alcohol syndrome, head injury or stroke, and/or birth defects (CDC, n.d.). Levels of ID can vary greatly, and individuals with IDs can have a more difficult time letting others know their wants and needs (CDC, n.d.).

Individuals with ID are more likely to experience traumatic events (Kildahl et al., 2020; Mevissen et al., 2016). Unpublished U.S. Department of Justice data show adults with ID are *seven times* more likely to be sexually assaulted than those without disabilities (Shapiro, 2018). Compounding their increased risk, individuals with ID are also less likely to receive appropriate sexual health education (Roden et al., 2020). Individuals with IDs are also more prone to develop PTSD after a traumatic experience (Kildahl et al., 2020; Mevissen et al., 2016). Given this greater vulnerability, increasing the focus on trauma resolution rather than simply behavior modification (Barol & Seubert, 2010) could greatly benefit individuals with IDs and improve their quality of life.

SEXUAL HEALTH RIGHTS

The Better Health Channel website on Cognitive Disability and Sexuality details sexual health rights for people with IDs. They state that people with IDs have the right to receive accurate and understandable sex education that affirms their right to have satisfying and pleasurable sexual lives. Sex education should be tailored to the individual, and cover "age-appropriate sexual issues that may be associated with their particular disability" (n.d., Sexuality Education).

The Better Health Channel also spells out that some people with IDs need assistance and support from family members and caregivers to explore sexuality and relationships. Support can include finding ways for them to have privacy, learning about private versus public behavior, utilizing appropriate contraception, learning how to give informed consents, and remaining free from sexual exploitation. Comprehensive, cognitively and developmentally appropriate, and recurring sex education can help people with IDs learn what is acceptable and unacceptable behavior from others and learn ways to resist, protest, and report inappropriate transgressions against them.

SOCIAL ROLE VALORIZATION THEORY

When considering sexual health empowerment (which may potentially include trauma treatment) with clients with ID, it can be helpful for clinicians to familiarize themselves with the historical and societal context in which those with IDs are marginalized.

As a part of his *social role valorization* theory, Wolf Wolfensberger (2013), world-renowned historian, advocate, and scholar in the field of disability, describes 18 *wounds* people with ID and other marginalized people face. These wounds are also referenced as the *social consequences of disability*. He identified them as:

1. Bodily impairment
2. Functional impairment
3. Relegated to low social status/social roles/deviancy
4. Rejected—disproportionately/relentlessly
5. Cast into one or more historic deviancy roles: sick/diseased, eternal child, object of ridicule, menace, pitiable, and burdens on society
6. Subjected to symbolic stigmatizing, "marking," "deviancy imaging," "branding"
7. Multiply jeopardized/scapegoated
8. Physically distanced: usually via segregation and also congregation
9. Absence or loss of natural, freely given relationships and substitution with artificial/purchased ones
10. Loss of control, autonomy, and freedom
11. Discontinuity with the physical environment and objects, "physical discontinuation"
12. Social and relationship discontinuity and even abandonment
13. Deindividualization, "mortification" reducing humanness
14. Involuntary material poverty, material/financial exploitation
15. Impoverishment of experience, especially that of the typical valued world
16. Exclusion from knowledge and participation in higher-order value systems (e.g., religion) that give meaning and direction to life and provide community
17. Having one's life "wasted"; mind-sets contributing to life wasting
18. Being the object of brutalization, killing thoughts, and death making

We will explore here more closely wounds 3, 4, 5, 8, 9, 10, and 15, and the potential impact on sexual health and autonomy, for people with ID. Though it could be argued that all the "wounding" experiences greatly impact one's sense of self and the development of psychosocial sexual identity, to review all wounding experiences would be beyond the scope of this book. For further reading, please consult Wolf Wolfensberger's 2013 book, *A Brief Introduction to Social Role Valorization: A High-Order Concept for Addressing the Plight of Societally Devalued People, and for Structuring Human Services.*

Considered a "hinge wound," being *relegated to low social status, and filling negative social roles (3),* functions much like a hinge of a door—that, once cast into negative social roles, opens up the likelihood for further wounding experiences. Specific to those with ID, the common negative roles people are subjected to are *sick/diseased, eternal child, object of ridicule, subhuman, menaces and burdens on society, and pitiable/charity cases (5).* In therapy, it is vitally important to consider the potential impact these forced negative roles might have on a person regarding their sense of self-worth, desirability, and their deserving of receiving and giving intimacy and pleasure. Additionally, many of these negative roles are established at birth or in early childhood, deepening the negative impact on the person, such that they themselves believe they deserve to be cast into such roles. Therefore, they may appear to embody some aspects of these roles, further compounding the complexity of addressing it in counseling. This circular process is known as *role expectancy.*

Once cast into a devalued role, having low social status, people with ID and other marginalized groups find themselves experiencing widescale *rejection (4),* both at the individual level and as classes or categories of people. Devalued people are systematically rejected by society as a whole, and individually, in some cases, even by their own family, neighbors, community, and by the workers in services that are supposed to assist them. This rejection is often experienced from infancy, if the ID is known at that time.

Many parents recount the time following the birth of their child with a disability/ID as a painful and lonely process. They describe seeing family and friends resisting holding their newborn, and avoiding looking or talking sweetly with them. The rejection and distancing grow as visits and calls become more infrequent. As this continues, both the individual and their family experience the pains of rejection and isolation and negative self-beliefs grow, furthering the divide.

Case Study 11.3: Theo Has Difficulty With Secure Romantic Relationships

Theo is a 24-year-old cisgender man with spastic quadriplegia and ID. In discussing his experiences of rejection and how deeply unlovable he felt, he explained how, in his infancy, his parents made the difficult decision to place him in a medical institution in Massachusetts, about 2 hours from their home. Theo remained at the institution during the week and was transported home on weekends and holidays. This continued until he turned 21, at which point he was moved into a small group home with one other man about his age. Recounting his time at the institution, Theo described the workers there as generally kind, but he always longed to be home with his parents and siblings. He felt that because of his disabilities he was difficult to love, was a burden on others, and that now, as a grown man, no one would or could ever love him.

During the time Theo was in romantic relationships, he struggled with feeling deeply insecure, and as a result would need constant reassurance from his love interest. The longer the relationship went on, the more his love grew, and the more insecure he became. As his insecurity deepened, the more desperately he demanded reassurance from his partner. In the end, this overwhelmed his partner and the relationship would come to an end. This pattern played out not only in his romantic relationship, but also in his friendships.

Distancing, via *segregation and congregation (8),* is another way the wound of rejection unfolds in the lives of people with ID (PWD). We need only to look at the recent historic treatment of PWD and the common practice of institutionalization, where large numbers of people with ID and other disabilities were warehoused, living in abominable conditions. For further information, read the free PDF *Christmas in Purgatory*: www.mn.gov/mnddc/parallels2/pdf/undated/Xmas-Purgatory.pdf.

In more current times, congregation and segregation of PWD are grouped together, separated from "valued people" and "valued settings," such as in group housing, enclave work places, day programs, segregated educational and recreational settings, and, in some cases, even in places of worship.

As an extension of segregation and congregation, there is an *absence or loss of natural, freely given relationships (9).* It is not uncommon upon meeting an adult with an ID to learn that their only "friends" are staff people who work in their group-home or day/work program. This phenomenon is so widely experienced that it is seen as both "normal" and "to be expected." However, to normalize these circumstances is to minimize its impact in the lives of PWD. The outcome is a life filled with "bought" relationships, fraught with the risk of discontinuity, such as when a staff person takes a new job, is laid-off, or moves away. The human service field is well known for its high turnover rates. It is a basic human need to experience enduring, freely given relationships; without such a relationship, heart-break, desperation, and loneliness are likely to prevail.

Case Study 11.4: Riley Was Institutionalized, Then Deinstitutionalized

In approximately 1958, Riley (diagnosed with ID) was 9 years old when his father told him they were taking a vacation. His father packed Riley's suitcase and delivered him to the Belchertown State School (BSS) in Belchertown, Massachusetts, where he would live the next 35 years of his life in one of the most deplorable state institutions.

Many years later, Riley often recalled that fateful summer day, saying how confused, frightened and sad he was, watching his father drive away from the dormitory building. He would never see his father or any other family member again.

A couple decades later, Riley was moved out of BSS as part of the statewide deinstitutionalization movement, which began in the 1970s. By the late 1980s, Riley lived alone in a comfortable apartment in a small city in western Massachusetts. He held a steady job at a small factory, and received help every week from a residential program for adults with disabilities for things like banking and general house upkeeping. He had a few friends, and a girlfriend, all of whom had been residents at the BSS.

Riley lived a quiet life and was well liked by his neighbors, and even though he was welcomed within his community, he gravitated to other people who had life experiences of institutionalization like he did. It took many years for Riley to acclimate to "community" living, outside the institution, and this remained a barrier to connecting with other people, finding it difficult to relate to people who had lives so drastically different from his own.

It was the support staff from Riley's residential service program who spent the most time with him and with whom he shared his stories and experiences of life in the institution. Many of the workers noticed how Riley kept to himself, despite his friendly demeanor and inviting sense of humor. It was especially noticeable during the holiday season when Riley spent time home alone. Many of the staff invited him to their family holiday celebrations, but he always declined. On one occasion, a staff person asked Riley why he wouldn't come to her home to share the holiday with her and her family. Riley said that although the offer sounded inviting, he needed to stay home in case his father was to call and invite him to celebrate with his own family. Riley knew, deep down, his father would not be calling, yet his profound longing kept him from being able to join in and connect with others.

At the untimely age of 52, Riley died alone in his apartment, while sitting in his easy-chair. The autopsy revealed a congenital heart condition, leading to a heart attack.

Born to choose, and having a "belief in one's ability to exert control over the environment and to produce desired results is essential for an individual's well being. It has been repeatedly argued that the perception of control is not only desirable, but it is likely a psychological and biological necessity" (Leotti et al., 2010). As such, having autonomy, agency, and freedom is considered foundational to having access to the "good things" in life, and contributing to one's sense of having a life worth living. In the lives of people with ID, *loss of control, autonomy, and freedom (10)* is a prevailing and wounding experience. Frequently other "able" people gain power over them and make decisions for them in nearly all domains of their lives, including their sexual life.

Having a life of lived learning through experience and participation is so basic a human need that to consider a life of *impoverishment of experience (15)*, especially that of the typically valued world, may be difficult for one to imagine. Yet this is often the case for people with ID. Rejection at the individual or societal scale, not being allowed or having access to opportunities of participation (particularly in settings where freely given relationships develop), all have a profound impact on forming (or being kept from forming) friendships and potential romantic partnerships.

"There exists a high degree of consensus about what the good things in life are" (Osburn, 2006, p. 4). Some major examples include "being accorded dignity, respect, acceptance; a sense of belonging; an education, and the development and exercise of one's capacities; a voice in the affairs of one's community and society; opportunities to participate; a decent material standard of living; a normative place to live; and opportunities for work and self support" (Osburn, 2006). For those who would like to improve matters related to sexual health empowerment in the lives of people with ID, it is important to understand their plight at both the individual and group/class perspective.

EYE MOVEMENT DESENSITIZATION AND REPROCESSING THERAPY WITH CLIENTS WITH INTELLECTUAL DISABILITIES

On the whole, the literature about the use of EMDR to treat those with mild to moderate IDs is supportive, showing consistent symptom reduction and acceptance by clients (Barrowcliff & Evans, 2015; Jowett et al., 2016; Keesler, 2020; Mevissen & de Jongh, 2010; Mevissen et al., 2012; Rodenburg et al., 2009; Smith et al., 2021). A small randomized controlled trial found EMDR effective and well-received by clients (Karatzias et al., 2019). Mevissen et al. (2012) also provide four case studies describing the successful use of EMDR with clients with severe IDs.

A few important considerations for the use of EMDR therapy with clients with IDs must be addressed. First, the definition of "trauma" for this population must be expanded by clinicians to better include the totality of their life experiences (Seubert, 2005), including systems-related violations as well as interpersonal ones. Second, clinicians must guard against misjudging PTSD symptoms as ID symptoms (Mevissen et al., 2016). Third, clients' possible limited expressive and receptive verbal capacity (Mevissen et al., 2016) may prove to be a barrier in the early phases of

EMDR, necessitating the involvement of caregivers. Fourth, the lack of appropriately adapted assessment and evaluation tools to measure the effectiveness of treatment (Mevissen & de Jongh, 2010) must be adapted for by clinicians. Many case study articles describe how clinicians have been creative in their assessment of symptom disturbance and improvement (Barrowcliff & Evans, 2015; Mevissen et al., 2011, 2012; Seubert, 2005).

While clients may find EMDR therapy different or more technical than other types of treatment to which they have been exposed (Unwin et al., 2019), EMDR therapy also offers unique benefits for use with clients with IDs. EMDR therapy does not require a high level of verbal expression, can be conducted with minimally verbal clients, and does not require homework outside of session (Mevissen et al., 2016). In addition, the use of visual and artistic modalities, such as picture cards and drawing, provide increased options for expressive communication (Dilly, 2014).

Yaskin and Seubert (2017) have a chapter on working with individuals with ID in Mark Nickerson's book *Cultural Competence and Healing Culturally Based Trauma With EMDR Therapy*. In this chapter, Yaskin and Seubert encourage EMDR therapists to "replace culturally [enforced] negative stereotypes [of people with ID as a "burden"] with a compassionate and humane understanding of people with ID as *individuals*" (2017, p. 247).

PART B

EROTICALLY MARGINALIZED POPULATIONS

INTRODUCTION

As you bring more sexual health concepts into your clinical practice, it is also helpful to be aware of erotically marginalized populations' behaviors, needs, and identities. Erotically marginalized "refers to people who are at risk of being ... oppressed both outside and inside ... clinical setting[s] due to their gender identities, sexual orientations, or sexual practices" (Constantinides et al., 2019, p. 1); that is, people at risk of oppression for not adhering to societally pressured norms of heterosexuality, monogamy, and other "straight" behaviors and identities.

As we have explored gender, sexual orientation, and nonmonogamy practices in previous chapters, here we will focus on sexual behaviors beyond "vanilla" activities (defined in the next section). While there are many books and articles that explore the world of kink in depth (see the References at the end of this chapter and the Additional Resources available at www.springerpub.com/courseconnect), this section provides some basic information around terminology.

The word *polysemicity* is helpful to keep in mind as you read through this section (and book). Polysemicity essentially means that another person's experiences may not mimic or duplicate your own experience, even if you both perform the exact same behavior (Klein, 2010). "Don't yuck my yum" (i.e., every person is entitled to their own preferences and interests regarding consenting adult sexual activities) is a useful catch phrase I learned at my sexual attitude reassessment class and can help our clients embrace and affirm their consensual sexual desires and interests.

DEFINITIONS

Kink is an umbrella term that covers any sexual, sensual, or erotic behavior not considered *vanilla*. Kink does not necessarily have to involve genital contact. Vanilla generally refers to nonkink/bondage identities and interactions (sexual activities like mutual masturbation, oral sex, and penis–vagina intercourse).

BDSM stands for bondage, discipline, domination, submission, sadism, and masochism.

Bondage can involve using physical restraints such as cuffs, rope, fabric, zip ties, and so on, to prevent or limit movements of a consenting person as well as psychological or verbal restraint (Moore et al., 2014). The purpose of bondage can include immobilizing the person, making the person "accessible" for others, and/or displaying the person. Any of these may be "intended to cause humiliation" (if desired by all consenting participants).

Discipline involves providing specific rules and/or punishments to a consenting person in order to exert agreed upon control over them (Moore et al., 2014). Punishment can involve physical (e.g., spanking or whipping) and/or emotional (e.g., verbal or nonverbal humiliation) actions.

Domination involves someone (consensually) assuming total power in a "scene, situation, or relationship." The names of dominants are typically spelled with a capital letter (Moore et al., 2014).

Submission involves an individual agreeing to be controlled or dominated by another individual. This power/control/authority could be granted for a single scene, or for an ongoing relationship. The names or designations of submissives are usually referred to with a lowercase letter (Moore et al., 2014). For example, donny granted Joe total domination.

Sadism involves the experience of sexual pleasure and/or excitation by the consensual giving of emotional and/or physical pain or force in a single or ongoing scene (Moore et al., 2014).

Masochism involves the experience of sexual pleasure and/or excitation by the consensual receiving of emotional and/or physical pain or force in a scene, and so forth (Moore et al., 2014).

When people hear the terms *kink* and *BDSM*, they may assume that only a small portion of the population practices these behaviors. However, a recent study (Joyal & Carpentier, 2017) found that actually about half of around 1,000 Canadian subjects studied have a desire for one or more kinky acts (e.g., voyeurism, fetishism, masochism), with about 40% of that sample having had engaged in such an act. There were no gender differences in this sample.

CONSENT IN KINK

An essential and vital concept in the BDSM or kink world is *consent*. "Consent is critical to the BDSM community as it separates kink from pathological or abusive behaviors" (Moore et al., 2014, p. 2). Consent is an agreement to engage in BDSM activity and has two major schools of thought within the community.

The first consent guidelines were *safe, safe, and consensual* (SSC). Some, however, prefer to define their consent as *risk-aware consensual kink* (RACK) to allow for going beyond the possibly limiting SSC if engaging in *edgeplay*, which is meant to challenge the conventional parameters of SSC.

Anyone engaging in these practices needs to be intimately familiar with consent, able to communicate their boundaries and limits, and be willing to dialogue with their partners about "responsibilities, expectations, and potential risks." Safe words or phrases need to be established and respected, often during the negotiation that precedes a scene (a period of play). "After a scene, it is encouraged and standard for the people in the scene to engage in *aftercare*, which is also discussed during the negotiation period, and may include eating to restore blood sugar, cuddling, being wrapped in a blanket, or spending a brief time alone" (Moore et al., 2014, p. 7). Purposeful and conscious BDSM behavior that involves any pain between consenting adults is meant to be performed with "caring intent" (Kort, 2018).

It is also important to note that many folks engage in kink or BDSM type behaviors (like spanking, blindfolding their partner, or role-playing), yet do not consider themselves part of the BDSM community or define themselves in that way. However, the same concepts of consent still apply to their interactions and behaviors with others.

Additionally, sexual sadism and masochism are only considered *Diagnostic and Statistical Manual of Mental Disorders* (5th ed.; *DSM-5;* American Psychiatric Association [APA], 2013) diagnosable conditions if the person practices these behaviors with nonconsenting individuals or if the client reports duress regarding their participation in these behaviors. Certainly, if someone discloses disturbance around wanting, performing, and/or receiving these behaviors, exploring the origins of any BDSM-related erotic templates and behaviors can be helpful, particularly if they also report a trauma history.

If clients are practicing their kink safely, sanely, and consensually, with the experience of pleasure and satisfaction, then the work may be around helping them reduce any unwanted shame and/or stigma regarding these desires and behaviors. This may involve identifying and processing past events related to kink/BDSM desires or scenes where they felt shame. For example, a client may report being shamed by asking a partner to tie them up and blindfold them. Once those prior events no longer cause disturbance, verbally rehearsing scenes and/or processing EMDR future templates of self-identified enthusiastic and desired participation in SSC activities may help the client move beyond any reported unwanted shame into joyful, confident, and empowered initiation and participation.

Lastly, I have had clients who requested therapy because a partner went beyond the agreed limits and boundaries of their negotiation, or a partner began enacting behaviors such as spanking, restraint, or even strangling, with no discussion, warning, or consent. EMDR therapy easily resolved this distress, allowing them to pursue their desired kink behavior freely and with pleasure.

Case Study 11.5: Leslie, Sadism Gone Too Far

Leslie, a late twenties Asian pansexual, demisexual gender nonconforming individual experienced an unwanted strangling attempt during sexual activity with their partner Josh. They were both in their early twenties. They had enjoyed mutually consenting sexual activity in their 5-month sexual relationship and added in bondage, dominance, and sadism activities such as being tied up and spanking. Josh had assumed the dominant role, with initial appropriate negotiation of consent and safe words, and Leslie noted enjoying this dynamic until one scene when Josh put his hands around their neck, while they were restrained, and began choking them. Leslie immediately verbalized their safe word, yet Josh did not stop. It escalated to Leslie fighting back, then suddenly blacking out.

Leslie left Josh's apartment that night, attempting to break up with him, but Josh began harassing them (texting Leslie videos and photos he had taken of them without their knowledge), culminating 3 weeks later in a sexual assault. Because of their initial agreed upon BDSM activities, Leslie felt ashamed and embarrassed to disclose the choking, harassment, and final sexual assault. Leslie eventually sought EMDR therapy, noticing "kink-aware" on the EMDR therapy profile. Once Leslie felt at ease with the EMDR therapist, Leslie was able to disclose these incidents.

After some resourcing, an EMDR timeline was formed, and the EMDR targets of the choking incident, harassment, and assault were processed over several sessions. Leslie's NCs were, "I have lost total control, my consent is gone." The PCs were, "I am truly consenting because I have fully negotiated my limits, and I can trust again."

Leslie then decided to press charges upon completing EMDR therapy, feeling more empowered. Leslie also reported meeting a new partner, Mary, for BDSM activities, who was well vetted by other BDSM community members. After some time getting to know her, Leslie was then able to continue exploring submission and masochism, giving full consent and enjoying ongoing safe, sane, and consensual communication and activities, which did not include choking.

Case Study 11.6: Derek, Boundary Crossed Submissive

Derek is a "mostly heterosexual-identified" professional Latino cisman in his early thirties. Over the course of a few months, Derek had become one of Nia's three submissives. Derek watched Nia, a dominant, gradually and methodically cross some of the boundaries and agreements with the other two submissives. Nia also began pushing some of Derek's boundaries (i.e., leaving him tied up for longer periods of time than agreed, requiring many days and weeks of grunge chore work with no reciprocal pleasurable contact). Nia rationalized this behavior by saying she was engaging in "edgeplay," working to ensure the submissives were getting "what they truly needed."

Derek eventually left the relationship, entering EMDR therapy due to PTSD symptoms of nightmares and interfering thoughts, mostly related to behaviors he witnessed her enact toward the other two submissives. He had tried to convince them to leave Nia's dominance, but both refused for a variety of reasons. This contributed to NCs of "I am helpless, my consent is gone. I have no control of any kind."

The EMDR timeline included earlier targets in grade school and with his family of origin where he reported difficulty speaking up for himself and others, eventually concluding with the Nia-related targets. Other NCs included, "I have no voice, I'm not worthy of speaking up." He emerged from EMDR therapy with a clearer sense of his boundaries in daily life as well as in kink/BDSM scenes. His PCs included, "I have choices, I am capable, I can speak up for myself and others, I choose when I consent to give." We also successfully completed EMDR future templates on seeing Nia at an upcoming kink/BDSM play event. Derek was able to install his PC of "I can speak up for myself and others" to a 7 (completely true) regarding this chance of running into her.

Case Study 11.7: Hannah, Childhood Sexual Abuse, Emotional Abuse, Eye Movement Desensitization and Reprocessing Therapy, PLISSIT Model, Parts Work, and Sexual and Kink Psychoeducation

By Nicole Cardarella-Gasper, MA, LPCC

The following example draws from multiple clients to demonstrate the intersection of using EMDR therapy and sexual and emotional trauma.

Hannah entered therapy with the goal of processing her childhood sexual abuse. This clinician suggested EMDR therapy to aid in reprocessing her trauma. Her perpetrator was her adoptive father. Hannah works full time as an optometrist. She identifies as a bisexual, cisgender woman in her early thirtiess. She is of Ethiopian descent and was adopted as an infant by a Caucasian couple (English & German heritage). She is not religious nor was she raised with any religion. Hannah is engaged to a cis, White, heterosexual man. She also reported low sexual desire due to her inability to orgasm, and an emotionally abusive ex-partner.

Hannah met the criteria for chronic PTSD and female orgasmic disorder. She reported hypervigilance, nightmares, sexual interaction avoidance, and negative beliefs about herself. She also reported not being able to orgasm with another person. She can only orgasm when masturbating. Together we decided to start EMDR therapy with the intention of treating her unprocessed trauma first, followed by treating the secondary/situational orgasm disorder. Hannah had met with a physician who determined that her inability to orgasm was not caused by any biological concerns.

Hannah's initial NCs were, "I am weak," "I am trapped," and "I am broken." As part of EMDR therapy Phase 2 preparation work, Hannah was provided psychoeducation about parts work. Hannah responded positively to identifying different parts of herself. She identified a childlike/young part that was "hurting the most." This indicated that we start with processing targets relating to childhood experiences of sexual abuse by her adoptive father. We reprocessed the abuse target memories and the corresponding negative belief of "I am broken." Hannah became unbothered by these memories and felt the courage to go "no contact" with her father.

We checked in with her "little part" and noticed that she felt less burdened by the past childhood abuse. However, we also noticed remaining sexual shame and fear.

We explored the sexual shame and discovered target and negative beliefs related to her sexual preferences. Hannah expressed interest in consensual nonconsent (CNC) sexual scenarios. Hannah reported feeling shame due to having been sexually abused, but wanted to explore CNC. With this information, I implemented the PLISSIT (Permission, Limited Information, Specific Suggestions, and Intensive Therapy) model. Hannah was given permission to be interested in and explore CNC and was provided psychoeducation about kink and safe kink practices. I suggested Hannah do research on CNC and affirmed her choice in continuing EMDR therapy.

We processed targets relating to "I am disgusting" and "Something is wrong with me." During reprocessing, Hannah connected the target of "Something is wrong with me" to more recent emotional abuse by an ex-partner. She felt "wrong" and ashamed for staying with him even though she knew he cheated on her. She was able to install the PC of "I was doing my best" and "I am growing."

Hannah also used her resourcing by taking her fiancé to a local sex store in order to prompt more open conversations about her sexual preferences with him. This led to a positive experience relating to sex. She reported feeling less shame and more safety when discussing sex with her fiancé. I helped Hannah install that positive experience into her positive neural network with bilateral stimulation (slow butterfly hug tapping on her own shoulders). Hannah went on to report that she was able to have an orgasm during a sexual encounter with her fiancé. At this point, Hannah no longer qualified for female secondary orgasmic disorder. She chose to continue EMDR therapy to reprocess adoption trauma.

ROUGH SEX/CHOKING

Peggy Orenstein (a prominent journalist and author who researches sexual behaviors among youth) wrote an opinion article for *The New York Times* (April 12, 2024) entitled "The Troubling Trend in Teenage Sex." In this article, Orenstein shares Dr. Herbenick's recent research on rough sex, particularly "sexual strangulation." In Dr. Herbenick's research of 5,000 anonymized college students, "nearly two-thirds of women" reported the experience of being choked "during sex (33% in their most recent encounter)." (Orenstein, 2024, para. 2). This statistic has rapidly risen in the past 4 years (possibly thanks to a feedback loop of choking having jumped from porn to mainstream media), with now 40% of women saying they were "between the ages 12 and 17 the first time (choking) happened" compared to the previously reported 25%.

Orenstein goes on to note that while she has observed how sexual trends can spread quickly, she has noticed a pattern: Basic sexual gratification activities (e.g., fellatio) tend to favor [(cis)] men. Pain or submissive-related activities, like choking, are generally directed toward [(cis)]women. And with this sexual trend, researchers are noticing that the chokers never or seldom ask permission or consent and that the "orgasm gap" favoring men has not changed. Many women, when asked, are reporting that they are scared of sexual strangulation happening to them.

Dr. Herbenick and Orenstein also note that some youth seem to be befuddled by the presence of choking—women think men want to do this (many men do not), and men think women want and expect them to do this (many women do not want this), but no one is explicitly discussing it.

While the immediate negative physical effects of choking (lightheadness, headaches, neck pain, ear ringing, loss of coordination) are temporary and seem to quickly resolve, "the true effects [of limiting blood flow] are silent, potentially not showing up for days, weeks, even years" (Orenstein, 2024, para. 19).

Possible permanent injuries include stroke and cognitive impairment, reduced cortical folding in the brain, widespread cortical thickening (inflammation associated with elevated risk of later-onset mental illness), a hemisphere imbalance (associated with mood disorders), "overwhelming anxiety, [and] sadness and loneliness, with the effect more pronounced as the [choking] incidence[s] rose: ... [O]xygen deprivation ... could be a contributing factor [to] soaring rates of depression and anxiety among young women" (Orenstein, 2024, paras. 20–21).

Orenstein goes on to note that "[n]onfatal strangulation ... has somehow been eroticized and made ... consensual enough .... Women's brains and bodies don't distinguish whether they are being harmed out of hate or out of love." (2024, para. 23)

As "many experienced kink/BDSM practitioners discourage choking, believing it to be too dangerous" (Orenstein, 2024, para. 7; and outright state that there are no fool-proof ways to "correctly" lightly choke someone during sexual activity), it is important for clinicians and educators to gain awareness of this trend and be ready to provide nonjudgmental and concerned responses, resources, information, and guidance. Providing information as to the inherent risks and dangers, including death, may not only save lives, but it may help bring more verbal consent into sexual interactions. This may lead to an awareness of tried and true sources of sexual pleasure for people with vulvas (e.g., clitoral stimulation coupled with a positive sexual context), as well as true mutuality and support for sexual enjoyment for all involved. Please refer to Orenstein's full groundbreaking article to better understand the burgeoning widespread occurrence and danger of choking and/or rough sex (Orenstein, 2024).

FETISHES AND PARAPHILIAS

Fetishes involve relying on "prop[s], body part[s], scene[s], or scenario[s] in order to get off sexually" (Joannides, 2017, pp. 494–495). This can occur in real life or fantasy. If this is done alone, or with a willing and consenting adult partner, then there is no reason to pathologize a particular fetish, especially if the person with the fetish can enjoy other types of sexual activity. However, problems can arise if the formerly willing partner no longer wants to engage with the fetish; begins to feel like the person is only interested in the fetish, not them; or the person with the fetish can only experience sexual arousal and/or orgasm with the fetish present.

If the fetish becomes indispensable for sexual arousal/orgasm, then the individual may be meeting criteria for a paraphilia. Again, if the consenting adults involved are happy with their paraphilia, treatment is likely unnecessary. However, if a client seeks therapy stating they feel alone and disconnected from the relationship, relying on their paraphilia to supply nondemanding acceptance, then the work may be in helping the client gain social skills and confidence to combat fear of closeness and reduce loneliness (Joannides, 2017). Any reports of anxiety, trauma, or distress around relationships with other humans may be good therapy targets to ultimately reduce fear of intimacy with others. Additional treatment can involve helping the client understand their core erotic templates or themes (CETs), finding ways to create new or additional CETs and sexually arousing scenarios (independent from the fetish), and/or approximating the fetish to more generic/universal sexual behaviors.

The *DSM-5* (APA, 2013) distinguishes between paraphilias and paraphiliac disorder. Paraphiliac disorder is when the paraphilia causes distress, interferes with the person's daily functioning, and/or harms (or potentially harms) self and/or other individuals. If your client reports a harmful or imminently harmful situation, you may need to take steps to prevent such harm through mandated reporting to local, state, or criminal agencies. Make sure you have gathered adequate information for your next step. Seek consultation with a specialist if you are in any doubt about what to do.

LIBERATION PSYCHOLOGY

As we conclude this chapter on working with marginalized, historically and systemically oppressed populations, we can learn some additional lessons from liberation-based clinical practices (LBCP) in our efforts to provide validation, education, treatment, equity, and access. LBCP evolved from the 1980s when the Jesuit priest Ignacio Martin-Baro (1986) advocated a shift in perspective away from biased scientific research methods and oppressive perspectives toward a framework where the experiences of the oppressed majority are valued and included.

LBCP has nine core tenets (Barton & Guzzo, 2020):

1. *Reorientation of Psychology*—deemphasize the experiences of the privileged and recenter experiences of oppressed people and indigenous knowledge.
2. *Recover Historical Memory* of those whom others have attempted to oppress and erase.
3. *Deconstruct Everyday Experiences* from the perspective of the oppressed.
4. *Denaturalization*—instead of normalizing the existence of discrimination, normalize equity and equality (p. 45; Torres Rivera, 2020).
5. *Problematization*—concretize the gap between actual daily existence experienced by oppressed peoples and their vision of a better life.
6. *Virtues of the People*—strengthen and support existing intergenerational resilience to help liberate.
7. *Conscientization*—raise consciousness of liberating potential.
8. *Power Dynamics*—address power dynamics that show up and have been reinforced in practice and research.
9. *Praxis* (when theory becomes practice)—envision a better future while considering the present reality.

Most of these tenets apply to developing a sense of empowered and positive sexuality, particularly when combined with the lenses of feminism, transfeminism, intersectionality, and queer theory. For instance, a client who arrives with the presenting problem of situational orgasmia (can only orgasm with clitoral stimulation) can be helped through LBCP by decentering a prior emphasis and importance of orgasm via penetrative intercourse (*reorientation of psychology*). Instead, the client's proven methods of orgasming via vibrator or manual clitoral stimulation can be validated, normalized, and centered in their ongoing sexual activity (*deconstructing everyday experience* and *normalizing equity*). This validation (*conscientization* and *problematization*), combined with assertive communication skills (addressing *power dynamics*), can embolden the client to seek equal experiences of pleasurable activity, thereby reducing the "orgasm gap" that is often seen between cisgender women and men (i.e., *praxis*: making theory into reality).

SUMMARY

Our clients come from different walks of life, many of them belonging visibly or invisibly in some way to *marginalized* or oppressed groups such as BIPOC individuals and communities which regularly encounter racism and racist systems, as well as people with physical, medical, neurodivergent, and/or intellectual disabilities. This chapter looks at historical inequities, discusses DEIB (diversity, equity, inclusion, belonging) principles, intersectionality, ableism, as well as the social role valorization theory and liberation psychology. Everyone deserves access, accurate information, and encouragement to obtain empowered sexual health.

Clients may disclose engaging in marginalized erotic practices such as kink and/or BDSM. Healthy kink/BDSM practice is "safe, sane, and consensual" or "risk aware consensual kink." For most kink/BDSM participants (which reflect the same percentage of trauma history as the general population), kink/BDSM is play, NOT trauma reenactment. Some clients may report experiencing negative kink/BDSM experiences, including experiences related to nonconsensual "rough sex" (including life-threatening "choking"). Therapy can help process those negative and/or non-consensual experiences, allowing clients to successfully re-engage with desired pleasure and life-affirming activities.

Fetishes involve the use of specific objects, body parts, role plays, and/or settings/environments to experience sexual arousal. If all adult parties consent, and enjoy the fetish, then there is no treatable concern. However, if an individual can only operate sexually via the fetish, and is concerned about this, then this may qualify as a paraphilia. A paraphilia rising to the level of a paraphiliac disorder involves considerable daily distress, impacts daily functioning, and/or harms (or potentially harms) self or others.

DISCUSSION QUESTIONS

- Why do sexual health barriers exist for marginalized populations and how do they prevent these populations from accessing and experiencing positive sexual health and experiences?
- What are some ways to circumvent and remove barriers of sexual health access for marginalized groups?
- What are some ways to help adults with IDs positively learn about, access, and experience their sexuality?
- What is your opinion regarding the rise of "choking/rough sex" among teens and young adults?
- How would you support a client who comes in disturbed or distressed by their participation in this (either as the choked or the choker)?
- How does the "choking" as researched by Dr. Herbenick differ from sanctioned and SSC/RACK kink/BDSM?

LEARNING ACTIVITIES

CourseConnect

To access self-assessment questions and interactive, competency-based learning activities for this chapter, visit www.springerpub.com/courseconnect. See inside front cover and tear-out card for CourseConnect details.

ADDITIONAL RESOURCES

Additional resources are online and available at www.springerpub.com/courseconnect.

REFERENCES

The American College of Obstetricians and Gynecologists. (n.d.). *Our commitment to changing the culture of medicine and eliminating racial disparities in women's health outcomes*. https://www.acog.org/about/our-commitment-to-changing-the-culture-of-medicine-and-eliminating-racial-disparities-in-womens-health-outcomes

American College of Obstetricians and Gynecologists. (2020, August 27). *Joint statement: Collective action addressing racism*. https://www.acog.org/news/news-articles/2020/08/joint-statement-obstetrics-and-gynecology-collective-action-addressing-racism

American Psychiatric Association. (2013). *Diagnostic and statistical manual of mental disorders* (5th ed.). https://doi.org/10.1176/appi.books.9780890425596

Autism Self Advocacy Network. (n.d.). *About autism*. https://autisticadvocacy.org/about-asan/about-autism

Barnett, J. P., & Maticka-Tyndale, E. (2015). Qualitative exploration of sexual experiences among adults on the autism spectrum: Implications for sex education. *Perspectives on Sexual and Reproductive Health*, 47(4), 171–179. https://doi.org/10.1363/47e5715

Barol, B. I., & Seubert, A. (2010). Stepping stones: EMDR treatment of individuals with intellectual and developmental disabilities and challenging behavior. *Journal of EMDR Practice and Research*, *4*(4), 156–169. https://doi.org/10.1891/1933-3196.4.4.156

Barrowcliff, A. L., & Evans, G. A. L. (2015). EMDR treatment for PTSD and intellectual disability: A case study. *Advances in Mental Health and Intellectual Disabilities, 9*(2), 90–98. https://doi.org/10.1108/AMHID-09-2014-0034

Beroukhim, G., Mahabamunuge, J., & Lubna, P. (2022). Racial disparities in access to reproductive health and fertility care in the United States. *Current Opinion in Obstetrics and Gynecology, 34*(3),138–146. https://doi.org/10.1097/GCO.0000000000000780

Better Health Channel. (n.d.). *Cognitive disability and sexuality.* Retrieved September 17, 2021, from https://www.betterhealth.vic.gov.au/health/ConditionsAndTreatments/intellectual-disability-and-sexuality

Boutrin, M. C., & Williams, D. R. (2021). What racism has to do with it: Understanding and reducing sexually transmitted diseases in youth of color. *Healthcare (Basel), 9*(6), 673. https://doi.org/10.3390/healthcare9060673

Bowleg, L. (2012). The problem with the phrase women and minorities: Intersectionality—an important theoretical framework for public health. *American Journal of Public Health, 102*(7), 1267–1273. https://doi.org/10.2105/AJPH.2012.300750

Brandt, A. M. (1978). Racism and research: The case of the Tuskegee syphilis study. *The Hastings Center Report, 8*(6), 21–29. https://doi.org/10.2307/3561468

Bruess, C. E., & Schroeder, E. (2018). *Sexuality education: Theory and practice* (7th ed.). ETR.

Buehler, S. (2022). *What every mental health professional needs to know about sex* (3rd ed.). Springer Publishing Company.

Burton, M., & Guzzo, R. (2020). Liberation psychology: Origins and development. In L. Comas-Díaz & E. Torres Rivera (Eds.), *Liberation psychology: Theory, method, practice, and social justice* (pp. 17–40). American Psychological Association. https://doi.org/10.1037/0000198-002

Casanova-Perez, R., Apodaca, C., Bascom, E., Mohanraj, D., Lane, C., Vidyarthi, D., Beneteau, E., Sabin, J., Pratt, W., Weibel, N., & Hartzler, A.L. (2022). Broken down by bias: Healthcare biases experienced by BIPOC and LGBTQ+ patients. *AMIA Annual Symposium Proceedings Archive, 2021*, 275–284. https://pmc.ncbi.nlm.nih.gov/articles/PMC8861755

Centers for Disease Control and Prevention. (n.d.-a). *Behavioral Risk Factor Surveillance System: History* [Fact sheet]. https://www.cdc.gov/brfss/factsheets/pdf/brfss-history.pdf

Centers for Disease Control and Prevention. (n.d.-b). *Facts about intellectual disability in children.* https://www.cdc.gov/ncbddd/actearly/pdf/parents_pdfs/intellectualdisability.pdf

Clare, E. (2017). *Brilliant imperfection: Grappling with cure.* Duke University.

Clements, C. (2024). *Sex positivity and White-sex supremacy: Ending complicity in Black body erasure.* Routledge/Taylor & Francis Group.

Constantinides, D. M., Sennott, S. L., & Chandler, D. (2019). *Sex therapy with erotically marginalized clients: Nine principles of clinical support.* Routledge.

Crenshaw, K. (1989). *Demarginalizing the intersection of race and sex.* University of Chicago Legal Forum.

David, E. J. R., Schroeder, T. M., & Fernandez, J. (2019). Internalized racism: A systematic review of the psychological literature on racism's most insidious consequence. *Journal of Social Issues, 75*(4), 1057–1086. https://doi.org/10.1111/josi.12350

Davis, M. (2019). *Our Whole Lives: Sexuality education for older adults.* Unitarian Universalist Association and United Church of Christ.

Dewinter, J., De Graaf, H., & Begeer, S. (2017). Sexual orientation, gender identity, and romantic relationships in adolescents and adults with autism spectrum disorder. *Journal of Autism and Developmental Disorders, 47*(9), 2927–2934. https://doi.org/10.1007/s10803-017-3199-9

Dilly, R. (2014). Eye movement desensitisation and reprocessing in the treatment of trauma with mild intellectual disabilities: A case study. *Advances in Mental Health and Intellectual Disabilities, 8*(1), 63–71. https://doi.org/10.1108/AMHID-06-2013-0036

Doyle, N. (2020). Neurodiversity at work: A biopsychosocial model and the impact on working adults. *British Medical Bulletin, 135*(1), 108–125. https://doi.org/10.1093/bmb/ldaa021

Eide, B., & Eide, F. (2023). *The dyslexic advantage (revised and updated): Unlocking the hidden potential of the dyslexic brain.* Plume.

Epstein, R., Blake, J., & González, T. (2017). *Girlhood interrupted: The erasure of Black girls' childhood.* Available at SSRN 3000695

Future of Sex Education Initiative. (2020). *National sex education standards: Core content and skills, K-12* (2nd ed.). https://siecus.org/wp-content/uploads/2020/03/NSES-2020-2.pdf

Gary-Smith, M., Alves, C. L., Harley, C., & Doyle, G. D. (2022). *Sex, race, and politics in the U.S.: A call to action to address racial justice in sexuality education*. SIECUS: Sex Ed for Social Change.

George, R., & Stokes, M. A. (2018a). Gender identity and sexual orientation in autism spectrum disorder. *Autism: The International Journal of Research and Practice, 22*(8), 970–982. https://doi.org/10.1177/1362361317714587

George, R., & Stokes, M. A. (2018b). Sexual orientation in autism spectrum disorder. *Autism Research, 11*(1), 133–141. https://doi.org/10.1002/aur.1892

Heredia, D., & Rider, G. N. (2020). Intersectionality in sex therapy: Opportunities for promoting sexual wellness among queer people of color. *Current Sexual Health Reports, 12*, 195–201. https://doi.org/10.1007/s11930-020-00270-8

Hostetter, M., & Klein, S. (2018). *In focus: Reducing racial disparities in health care by confronting racism*. Commonwealth Fund. https://doi.org/10.26099/1hjp-ct50

Hoyert, D. L. (2023). Maternal mortality rates in the United States, 2021. *NCHS Health E-Stats*. https://doi.org/10.15620/cdc:124678

Joannides, P. (2017). *Guide to getting it on: Unzipped. V.9.0.* Goofy Foot Press.

Jowett, S., Karatzias, T., Brown, M., Grieve, A., Paterson, D., & Walley, R. (2016). Eye movement desensitization and reprocessing (EMDR) for *DSM-5* posttraumatic stress disorder (PTSD) in adults with intellectual disabilities: A case study review. *Psychological Trauma: Theory, Research, Practice, and Policy, 8*(6), 709–719. https://doi.org/10.1037/tra0000101

Joyal, C. C., & Carpentier, J. (2017). The prevalence of paraphilic interests and behaviors in the general population: A provincial survey. *The Journal of Sex Research, 54*(2), 161–171. https://doi.org/10.1080/00224499.2016.1139034

Julian, Z., Mengesha, B., McLemore, M. R., & Steinauer, J. (2021). Community-engaged curriculum development in sexual and reproductive health equity: Structures and self. *Obstetrics & Gynecology, 137*(4), 723–727. https://doi.org/10.1097/AOG.0000000000004324

Karatzias, T., Brown, M., Taggart, L., Truesdale, M., Sirisena, C., Walley, R., Mason-Roberts, S., Bradley, A., & Paterson, D. (2019). A mixed methods, randomized controlled feasibility trial of eye movement desensitization and reprocessing (EMDR) plus standard care (SC) versus SC alone for *DSM-5* posttraumatic stress disorder (PTSD) in adults with intellectual disabilities. *Journal of Applied Research in Intellectual Disabilities, 32*(4), 806–818. https://doi.org/10.1111/jar.12570

Katz Kattari, S. (Ed.). (2024). *Exploring sexuality and disability: A guide for human service professionals*. Routledge.

Kaufman, M., Silverberg, C., & Odette F. (2007). *Ultimate guide to sex and disability: For all of us who live with disability, pain, and chronic illness*. Cleis Press.

Keesler, J. M. (2020). Trauma-specific treatment for individuals with intellectual and developmental disabilities: A review of the literature from 2008 to 2018. *Journal of Policy and Practice in Intellectual Disabilities, 17*(4), 332–345. https://doi.org/10.1111/jppi.12347

Kildahl, A. N., Oddli, H. W., & Helverschou, S. B. (2020). Potentially traumatic experiences and behavioural symptoms in adults with autism and intellectual disability referred for psychiatric assessment. *Research in Developmental Disabilities, 107*, 107388. https://doi.org/10.1016/j.ridd.2020.103788

Klein, M. (2010, April). *When sex gets complicated: Pornography, kink, cybersex, and other clinical challenges* [workshop]. American Association of Sexuality Educators, Counselors and Therapists.

Kort, J. (2018). *The trauma survivor and sexual health: How therapists can help*. Presentation. The Brattleboro Retreat.

Lekas, H. M., Pahl, K., & Fuller Lewis, C. (2020). Rethinking cultural competence: Shifting to cultural humility. *Health Services Insights, 13*, 1178632920970580. https://doi.org/10.1177/1178632920970580

Leotti, l. A., Iyengar, S. S., & Ochsner, K. N. (2010). *Born to choose: The origins and value of the need for control*. https://doi.org/10.1016/j.tics.2010.08.001

Maggio, M. G., Calatozzo, P., Cerasa, A., Pioggia, G., Quartarone, A., & Calabrò, R. S. (2022). Sex and sexuality in autism spectrum disorders: A scoping review on a neglected but fundamental issue. *Brain Sciences, 12*(11), 1427. https://doi.org/10.3390/brainsci12111427

Martín-Baró, I. (1986). Hacia una psicología de la liberación [Towards a psychology of liberation]. *Boletin de Psicología, 22*, 1–11.

Massicotte, L. M. (2023). Implementing anti-racist strategies in the evidence-based sexuality education classroom. *American Journal of Sexuality Education, 18*(1), 149–169. https://doi.org/10.1080/15546128.2022.2076758

McCuistian, C., Peteet, B., Burlew, K., & Jacquez, F. (2023). Sexual health interventions for racial/ethnic minorities using community-based participatory research: A systematic review. *Health Education & Behavior, 50*(1), 107–120. https://doi.org/10.1177/10901981211008378

Mevissen, L., & de Jongh, A. (2010). PTSD and its treatment in people with intellectual disabilities: A review of the literature. *Clinical Psychology Review, 30*(3), 308–316. https://doi.org/10.1016/j.cpr.2009.12.005

Mevissen, L., Didden, R., & de Jongh, A. (2016). Assessment and treatment of PTSD in people with intellectual disabilities. In C. Martin, V. Preedy, & V. Patel (Eds.), *Comprehensive guide to post-traumatic stress disorder* (pp. 1–15). Springer Nature. https://doi.org/10.1007/978-3-319-08359-9_95

Mevissen, L., Lievegoed, R., & de Jongh, A. (2011). EMDR treatment in people with mild ID and PTSD: 4 cases. *Psychiatric Quarterly, 82*(1), 43–57. https://doi.org/10.1007/s11126-010-9147-x

Mevissen, L., Lievegoed, R., Seubert, A., & de Jongh, A. (2012). Treatment of PTSD in people with severe intellectual disabilities: A case series. *Developmental Neurorehabilitation, 15*(3), 223–232. https://doi.org/10.3109/17518423.2011.654283

Moen, E., & Nolan, M. (2018). *Drawn to sex, volume 1: The basics.* Erika Moen Comics and Illustration.

Moen, E., & Nolan, M. (2020). *Drawn to sex, volume 2: Our bodies and health.* Erika Moen Comics and Illustration.

Moon, S. H., & Sandage, S. J. (2019). Cultural humility for people of color: Critique of current theory and practice. *Journal of Psychology and Theology, 47*(2), 76–86. https://doi.org/10.1177/0091647119842407

Moore, L., Pincus, T., & Rodemaker, D. (2014). *What professionals need to know about BDSM* [Pamphlet]. https://counselingbdsmclients.wordpress.com/wp-content/uploads/2016/03/what_professionals_need_to_know_about_bdsm_1.pdf

Mosher, D. K., Hook, J. N., Captari, L. E., Davis, D. E., DeBlaere, C., & Owen, J. (2017). Cultural humility: A therapeutic framework for engaging diverse clients. *Practice Innovations (Washington, D.C.), 2*(4), 221–233. https://doi.org/10.1037/pri0000055

Neville, H. A., Awad, G. H., Brooks, J. E., Flores, M. P., & Bluemel, J. (2013). Color-blind racial ideology: Theory, training, and measurement implications in psychology. *The American Psychologist, 68*(6), 455–466. https://doi.org/10.1037/a0033282

Nickerson, M. (2017). *Cultural competence and healing culturally based trauma with EMDR therapy.* Springer Publishing Company.

Noh, M., Hughto, J. M. W., Austin, S. B., Goldman, R. E., Potter, J., & Agénor, M. (2024). Promoting equitable sexual health communication among patients with minoritized racial/ethnic, sexual orientation, and gender identities: Strategies, challenges, and opportunities. *Social Science & Medicine, 344*, 116634. https://doi.org/10.1016/j.socscimed.2024.116634

Okoro, C. A., Hollis, N. D., Cyrus, A. C., & Griffin-Blake, S. (2018). Prevalence of disabilities and health care access by disability status and type among adults–United States, 2016. *Morbidity and Mortality Weekly Report, 67*(32), 882–887. http://doi.org/10.15585/mmwr.mm6732a3

O'Mara-Eves, A., Brunton, G., Oliver, S., Kavanagh, J., Jamal, F., & Thomas, J. (2015). The effectiveness of community engagement in public health interventions for disadvantaged groups: A meta-analysis. *BMC Public Health, 15*, 129. https://doi.org/10.1186/s12889-015-1352-y

Orenstein, P. (2024, April 12). The troubling trend in teenage sex. *The New York Times.* https://www.nytimes.com/2024/04/12/opinion/choking-teen-sex-brain-damage.html#

Osburn, J. (2006). An overview of social role valorization theory. *Social Role Valorization Journal, 1*(1), 4–13. https://socialrolevalorization.com/wp-content/uploads/2019/03/srv_theory_joe_osburn.pdf

Owen, J., Tao, K. W., Drinane, J. M., Hook, J., Davis, D. E., & Kune, N. F. (2016). Client perceptions of therapists' multicultural orientation: Cultural (missed) opportunities and cultural humility. *Professional Psychology, Research and Practice, 47*(1), 30–37. https://doi.org/10.1037/pro0000046

Price, D. (2020). *Unmasking autism: Discovering the new faces of neurodiversity.* Harmony Books.

Roden, R. C., Schmidt, E. K., & Holland-Hall, C. (2020). Sexual health education for adolescents and young adults with intellectual and developmental disabilities: Recommendations for accessible sexual and reproductive health information. *The Lancet Child and Adolescent Health, 4*(9), 699–708. https://doi.org/10.1016/S2352-4642(20)30098-5

Rodenburg, R., Benjamin, A., de Roos, C., Meijer, A. M., & Jan Stams, G. (2009). Efficacy of EMDR in children: A meta-analysis. *Clinical Psychology Review, 29*(7), 599–606. https://doi.org/10.1016/j.cpr.2009.06.008

Seubert, A. (2005). EMDR with clients with mental disability. In R. Shapiro (Ed.), *EMDR solutions: Pathways to healing* (pp. 293–311). W. W. Norton.

Sevelius, J. M., Gutierrez-Mock, L., Zamudio-Haas, S., McCree, B., Ngo, A., Jackson, A., Clynes, C., Venegas, L., Salinas, A., Herrera, C., Stein, E., Operario, D., & Gamarel, K. (2020). Research with marginalized communities: Challenges to continuity during the COVID-19 pandemic. *AIDS and Behavior, 24*(7), 2009–2012. https://doi.org/10.1007/s10461-020-02920-3

Shapiro, J. (2018, January 8). The sexual assault epidemic no one talks about. *NPR.* https://www.npr.org/2018/01/08/570224090/the-sexual-assault-epidemic-no-one-talks-about

Shuttleworth, R., & Mona, L. (Eds.). (2021). *The Routledge handbook of disability and sexuality.* Routledge.

Smith, A. N., Laugharne, R., Oak, K., & Shankar, R. (2021). Eye movement desensitisation and reprocessing therapy for people with intellectual disability in the treatment of emotional trauma and post traumatic stress disorder: A scoping review. *Journal of Mental Health Research in Intellectual Disabilities, 14*(3), 237–284. https://doi.org/10.1080/19315864.2021.1929596

Smith, Leah (n.d.). *#Ableism* [Blog post]. Center for Disability Rights. https://cdrnys.org/blog/uncategorized/ableism/

Star Institute (n.d.). *Star pyramid* [Handout]. https://sensoryhealth.org/sites/default/files/file-attachments/STAR_Pyramid_03.pdf

Stolp, H., & Fox, J. (2015). Increasing receipt of women's preventive services. *Journal of Women's Health, 24*(11), 875–881. https://doi.org/10.1089/jwh.2015.5552

Sutton, M. Y., Anachebe, N. F., Lee, R., & Skanes, H. (2021). Racial and ethnic disparities in reproductive health services and outcomes. *Obstetrics & Gynecology, 137*(2), 225–233. https://doi.org/10.1097/AOG.0000000000004224

Thurston, I. B., Fix, R. L., & Getzoff Testa, E. (2024). Anti-racism, heterosexism, and transphobia: Strategies for adolescent health promotion post-coronavirus disease 2019. *Pediatric Clinics of North America, 71*(4), 745–760. https://doi.org/10.1016/j.pcl.2024.04.008

Tohit, N. F. M., Rashid, S. A. Z. A., Fakuradzi, W. F. S. W. A., Zaidi, N. A. A., & Haque, M. (2024). Exploring pathways from community involvement to empowerment in sexual and reproductive health: A public health perspective. *Advances in Human Biology, 14*(4), 296–307. https://doi.org/10.4103/aihb.aihb_112_24

Torres Rivera, E. (2020). Concepts of liberation psychology. In L. Comas-Díaz & E. Torres Rivera (Eds.), *Liberation psychology: Theory, method, practice, and social justice* (pp. 41–51). American Psychological Association. https://doi.org/10.1037/0000198-003

Unwin, G., Willcott, S., Hendrickson, S., & Kroese, B. S. (2019). Eye movement desensitization and reprocessing for adults with intellectual disabilities: Process issues from an acceptability study. *Journal of Applied Research in Intellectual Disabilities, 32*(3), 635–647. https://doi.org/10.1111/jar.12557

VanVactor-Lee, S. (2024). *Intimacy and autism workshop* [Webinar]. Intimacy Professionals Association.

Vedam, S., Stoll, K., Taiwo, T. K., Rubashkin, N., Cheyney, M., Strauss, N., McLemore, M., Cadena, M., Nethery, E., Rushton, E., Schummers, L., Declercq, E., & GVtM-US Steering Council. (2019). The Giving Voice to Mothers study: Inequity and mistreatment during pregnancy and childbirth in the United States. *Reproductive Health, 16*(1), 77. https://doi.org/10.1186/s12978-019-0729-2

Weir, E., Allison, C., & Baron-Cohen, S. (2021). The sexual health, orientation, and activity of autistic adolescents and adults. *Autism Research, 14*(11), 2342–2354. https://doi.org/10.1002/aur.2604

Williams, M. T., Faber, S. C., & Duniya, C. (2022). Being an anti-racist clinician. *The Cognitive Behaviour Therapist, 15,* e19. https://doi.org/10.1017/S1754470X22000162

Wolfensberger, W. P. (1996). Reply to John O'Brien's "Nobody outruns the trickster: A brief note on the meaning of the word 'valorization.'" *SRV/VRS: The International Social Role Valorization Journal, 2*(1), 16–20.

Wolfensberger, W. P. (2013). *A brief introduction to social role valorization: A high-order concept for addressing the plight of societally devalued people, and for structuring human services* (4th ed.). Valor Press.

World Health Organization. (n.d.). *Sexual health*. Retrieved June 15, 2025, from https://www.who.int/health-topics/sexual-health#tab=tab_1

Yaskin, J., & Seubert, A. (2017). Left out and behind: EMDR and the cultural constriction of intellectual disability. In M. Nickerson (Ed.), *Cultural competence and healing culturally based trauma with EMDR therapy* (pp. 247–260). Springer Publishing Company.

CHAPTER 12

Aging Sexual Health

Ashley L. Mader

LEARNING OBJECTIVES

- Describe the current aging population and research on aging and sexuality.
- List common concerns and changes that affect the sexuality of aging cisgendered women.
- List common concerns and changes that affect the sexuality of aging cisgendered men.
- List common concerns and changes that affect the sexuality and well-being of LGBTQ individuals.
- Describe the social influences on sexuality and aging (loss of a partner, ageism, myths, etc.).
- Describe what healthcare professionals know about sexuality and aging and how they can better serve and communicate with the aging population about sexuality.

INTRODUCTION

As of 2018, there were 52 million adults that were 65 years and older. In 2024, the number of Baby Boomers was around 70.09 million people. Baby Boomers are individuals born between 1946 and 1964 (after World War II; Korhonen, 2024).

The Silent Generation are those adults born between 1928 and 1945 during the Great Depression and during World War II. There are an estimated 23 million people in this generation (Howe, 2014). In 2024, 18% of Americans were over the age of 65 (Schaeffer, 2024). The last time there was this high of a percentage of people past the age of 65 was during the Black Death, around 1350. This may come as a surprise given the death toll of the plague; however, it did not affect older adults as much (Minois, 1989).

A BRIEF HISTORY OF AGING

With modern medicine, people can now live well past 65 years of age; yet this was not always the case. Between the years of 1650 and 1850, older adults accounted for about 2% of the population. Because of this, older adults were highly regarded and deemed very wise. If one lived to an old age, one was most likely of a higher socioeconomic status. There were very few poor older adults, and if there were poor older adults they were thought to be a tax burden to society and looked down upon (Fleming et al., 2003).

The shift in how older adults were viewed began around the time of the American Revolution. Before the Revolution, powdered wigs were worn to give the impression of being aged and wise. Many older adults did not save for retirement, thus becoming a financial burden to their family. Aging became more of a disease rather than looked at in fascination (Fleming et al., 2003). In some cultures, such as in Greek, Native American, Korean, and Chinese cultures, aging is still revered (Huffpost, 2017).

AGING ADULT SEXUALITY EXPERIENCES

The Baby Boomers tend to have more liberal attitudes toward sexuality and be more satisfied with their sex lives than the Silent Generation. This may be due to Boomers growing up during the sexual revolution. Each subsequent generation seems to have more openness about sex (Beckman et al., 2008).

Many assume that advanced age negatively affects sexual quality of life. Although there is a change in the frequency of sex, the number of partners, and older adults' perceived control over sexual aspects of their lives, many older adults report a higher level of sexual quality of life than younger adults. In older adults, the quality of sex appears much more important than quantity of sex. Older men tend to have a higher level of sexual quality of life than women (Forbes et al., 2017). Women are often widowed and live 6 to 8 years longer than men, which may account for the lower level of sexual quality of life (Murphy et al., 2018).

Sexual frequency among older adults may decrease. This is mostly due to lack of a partner. However, even among partnered women, the frequency of sex is less than that of men. Other contributing factors to the decrease in sexual activity are health related such as heart conditions, physical limitations, and sexual dysfunctions. Lifestyle and health factors have a major impact on the sexual functioning of older adults. High cholesterol, diabetes, hypertension, and other heart conditions may cause sexual dysfunction. Medications that are used to treat these conditions may also cause sexual dysfunction. It is very important that helping professionals rule out medical problems when a person comes to them with a sexual dysfunction. Sometimes a sexual dysfunction, such as erectile dysfunction (ED) or pain during intercourse, is a sign that there is an underlying medical condition (Lindau et al., 2007).

SEXUALLY TRANSMITTED INFECTIONS

Sexually transmitted infections (STIs) are on the rise in the senior population. Half of the people currently living with HIV/AIDS are over 50 years old. STIs such as chlamydia, gonorrhea, syphilis, human papillomavirus (HPV), and herpes are also being diagnosed at a higher rate than they were previously. There are several reasons for this uptick in STI rates among older adults. There are more divorces in middle age; thus, people may enter the dating world online and potentially have more partners than before. Older adults often do not think they are at risk for STIs. When they were young adults, there was not as much focus on STIs and HIV/AIDS did not exist before the 1980s. The major prevention concern was an accidental pregnancy, not STIs. Given that older adults do not have to worry about pregnancy, they may not use protection.

Older adults today are also generally more sexually active than they were as adults in the 1990s. With the invention of Viagra and other erectile enhancement drugs, older adults are able to continue engaging in sexual activity. Lastly, medical professionals often misdiagnose STIs in older adults as "afflictions of old age." They may not ask if the patient is sexually active, therefore disregarding the possibility of an STI (Benjamin Rose Institute on Aging, 2019).

Older adults may be very distressed by an STI diagnosis. Psychotherapy (including eye movement desensitization and reprocessing [EMDR] therapy) can help reduce or eliminate any distress or shame.

CHANGES IN AGING WOMEN'S SEXUAL HEALTH

MENOPAUSE

What is menopause? Menopause is simply when the menstrual cycle ends (determined when a year passes with no menstruation). The average age of menopause is 52 years old; however, some may experience it years earlier or later. Alongside the cessation of the menstrual cycle, individuals may experience hot flashes and vaginal changes during menopause. Though hot flashes may be uncomfortable, they generally do not impact sexuality. A hot flash can be defined as a sudden wave of heat that may cause severe sweating and/or temperature discomfort.

Some people experience vaginal changes such as dryness or the thinning of the walls of the vagina or vaginal atrophy. Vaginal dryness can range from minimal discomfort to severe discomfort. This can have an impact on the experience of sexuality. Individuals may experience pain during penetration; therefore, more planning may be needed before engaging in sexual activity. Hydrating and over-the-counter water-based lubricants have proved helpful for vaginal dryness. In contrast, douches, perfumed sprays or toilet paper, and antihistamines may irritate the vulva and vagina more (Doress-Worters & Siegal, 1994).

Like other parts of the body, the vagina may become weaker if not engaged. There is relevance to the idea of "If you don't use it you lose it" (Vaden, as quoted in Taylor, 2019, "Self"). Though the vaginal canal is not exactly a muscle, it is made up of elastic tissue that is connected to the pelvic floor, which is a muscle. According to the Memorial Sloan Kettering Cancer Center (2018), it may be helpful to strengthen the pelvic floor with pelvic floor exercises, such as Kegels. Moreover, more penetrative sexual activity may result in less vaginal atrophy (Taylor, 2019).

According to the North American Menopause Society (NAMS, 2020), women may experience orgasm changes as they age. Orgasms may become shorter in duration and the clitoris may become less sensitive. Sexual desire can both increase and decrease over time. Many women say the reason they are not engaging in partnered sexual activity is because of the lack of a partner, not necessarily the lack of desire (Mader, 2014). Although some women report a lack of sexual desire as they get older, some aging women experience an increase in desire. Pregnancy fears have finally terminated, which is physically and mentally freeing for some, thus increasing sexual interest and activity (Rogers, 2019).

Hormone Replacement Therapy

Some women may opt for hormone replacement therapy (HRT). HRT is a medication that replaces the estrogen that the body loses during menopause. It can make menopause more comfortable, decrease hot flashes, and help vaginal discomfort. Some studies also show that it can prevent bone loss and fractures in postmenopausal individuals (Mayo Clinic, 2020).

Not everyone is a good candidate for HRT. Certain medical histories, such as heart disease, hypertension, liver disease, certain cancers, and blood clots, may not be suited for HRT (Mayo Clinic, 2020). There has been research on HRT and how it can increase the risk of both breast and endometrial cancer. Some people who experience only vaginal discomfort may opt for estrogen cream and avoid pills. There can be drawbacks or side effects to taking HRT, such as a recurrence of vaginal bleeding. Others have reported side effects, such as nausea, weight gain, bloating, and depression. It is important to weigh both the risks and benefits of HRT (Doress-Worters & Siegal, 1994).

Avoid completely medicalizing menopause. Certainly, there are times that medical treatment is needed, but menopause is also a naturally occurring process that people have experienced for millennia. Having open and candid conversations about the menopause process with both peers and helping professionals should not be underestimated (Doress-Worters & Siegal, 1994).

If individuals report distress around menopausal symptoms, unpleasant sexual experiences due to aging-related changes, or other loss or change in sexual functioning, psychoeducation and therapy may help reduce or eliminate this emotional distress.

Something to Consider: Cultural Differences

Not every culture treats or experiences menopause the same. Mayan women, for example, are excited for menopause; they eat a diet high in carbohydrates, with very little consumption of meat or dairy, and report no hot flashes. In contrast, Greek women have a diet similar to the women in the United States, have more anxiety about menopause, and also experience hot flashes. Japanese women report taking more herbal supplements and having fewer hot flashes. Cultures that have more ageism and medicalization around menopause may make the experience worse for women (Doress-Worters & Siegal, 1994).

Black women often experience heavier bleeding, which is often overlooked by healthcare providers or not treated appropriately. Black women also have a higher rate of hysterectomies than White women. It is not known whether those are absolutely necessary. They also experience a higher rate of symptoms with uterine leiomyomas or fibroid tumors than White women (85% vs. 63%, respectively; Weiss et al., 2009). Before 1996 women of color were underrepresented in menopause research. The Study of Women's Health Across the Nation started surveying women's experiences of menopause and have found that both Black and Hispanic women experience menopause 2 years earlier than White women (Velez, 2020).

HYSTERECTOMIES AND OOPHORECTOMIES

A hysterectomy is the removal of the uterus and an oophorectomy is the removal of the ovaries. As people age through menopause, their risk for uterine and ovarian cancers increases; therefore, Pap smears and pelvic exams remain extremely important. Hysterectomies and oophorectomies are often performed when the person has cancer or another life-threatening illness. Conversely, some of the gynecological issues that plagued female-bodied individuals premenopause may be alleviated after menopause (Doress-Worters & Siegal, 1994). However, many of these procedures are performed electively, rather than for life-threatening conditions. It is estimated that one in five hysterectomies are unnecessary (Whiteman, 2015).

It is a common belief that after menopause and the childbearing years female-bodied people do not need their reproductive organs. However, the uterus and ovaries have a purpose after menopause. Ovaries can continue to function long after the uterus is removed through a hysterectomy (Doress-Worters & Siegal, 1994). Both a hysterectomy and oophorectomy can cause a drop in hormones, which is often related to loss of sexual desire and vaginal dryness (Whiteman, 2015).

Even if the ovaries are left in place and the uterus is removed, an entire system is disturbed, which includes the vagina, ovaries, clitoris, cervix, and blood and nerve supplies. The uterus is cut out, leaving the connective tissues and nerves to heal and scar. Though some health professionals report that these procedures do not affect sexual functioning, many patients report decreases in sexual desire, less powerful orgasms, vaginal pain, and dryness (Doress-Worters & Siegal, 1994).

If there are problems with lubrication, estrogen creams can be inserted in the vagina to help increase comfortable and pleasurable vaginal–penis intercourse. However, Medicare alone does not pay for these medications. One would need to enroll in a Medicare Advantage plan for these types of medications to be covered (Malzone, 2024). There have been some recent improvements in Medicare's covering of medications related to menopause. Medicare Part D now covers drugs that treat severe dyspareunia (Andrews, 2019). For many individuals in distress, it is hard to navigate the ins and outs of Medicare and what it covers.

Case Study 12.1: Katie Grieves Her Hysterectomy

Katie is a 67-year-old woman who had a hysterectomy 15 years ago. It was a surgery she was told that she needed and that nothing would change about her sex life, except eliminating the possibility of pregnancy. When asked about how it affected her, she reported that it not only affected her orgasms, but also how she felt about being a woman. As an educator herself, she researched sex after a hysterectomy and learned how sexual satisfaction was measured most often by the frequency of sex, rather than someone's actual sexual response. While she remained functionally able to engage in sex, the quality of her experience dramatically diminished. "I said back then that the woman that I was died on the operating table. I had to evolve into a different person in many ways after that" (Mader, 2014, p. 83).

Psychotherapy (including EMDR therapy) could potentially help Katie grieve through these orgasmic and gender-identity changes. In this case, the earliest instances of orgasm change could be targeted and processed. The death of "the woman that I was" might potentially be another EMDR target or the focus of grief counseling. Psychoeducation and focused sex therapy might help Katie discover new ways of experiencing and increasing sexual response and pleasure.

Case Study 12.2: A Partner's Perspective on Hysterectomy

Frank is a 65-year-old man whose wife had uterine cancer. They had a very active sex life up until her cancer treatment necessitated a hysterectomy. In their sexual routine she would have an orgasm, and then he would have one. Once she had the hysterectomy, her lubrication decreased, which was discussed before the surgery. However, she would have severe pain right before her orgasm. He did not want to see her in pain, so he pretended to have an orgasm or avoided sex altogether (Mader, 2014).

EMDR therapy could target Frank's distress regarding his wife's pain. She may also benefit from sex therapy and/or EMDR therapy, particularly utilizing pain protocols to decrease pain. They may both benefit from EMDR future templates oriented toward finding new ways to be intimate and experience pleasure, or enhancing their advocacy skills with medical professionals as they search for ways to reduce or eliminate her pain.

Yes, some hysterectomies and oophorectomies can be life-saving and beneficial; however, it is extremely imperative that people weigh both the pros and cons of these surgeries, and do their own research for their own bodies.

BODY IMAGE

Changes in hormones and metabolism may affect aging bodies. The physical signs of aging that any gender may experience include weight gain, graying hair, thinning hair, loss of skin elasticity, loss of hearing and/or sight, and physical limitations. Any or all of these can have an effect on one's body image. A negative body image is also correlated with lower sexual desire (Quinn-Nilas et al., 2016). In an extremely youth-focused culture, it is hard to find aging bodies to compare oneself against. Body image issues can also include physical limitations, making certain activities more difficult than they once were. Many find it helpful to talk through the process (Hofmeier et al., 2017).

Psychotherapy, sex therapy, and/or EMDR therapy can help reduce or eliminate individuals' distress and/or focus on negative body image. An EMDR timeline of distressing targets can be developed based on specific dislikes. A positive cognition (PC) to work toward can include "I'm fine as I am," "My aging body is normal and attractive/beautiful/handsome," and "I'm still worth something."

CHANGES IN AGING MEN'S SEXUALITY

ERECTIONS

Erections start changing around the age of 40. This does not mean ED, but erections may change in firmness or frequency. Given there is not much information communicated about the changes that happen as one ages, men often become anxious thinking it is the beginning of ED, when it is a normal sign of aging. Because of this anxiety, some men end up with ED due to anxiety, rather than actual physical causes (Rienzo, 1985).

What actually constitutes ED? ED is essentially the inability to hold an erection long enough for satisfying sexual activity (Urology Care Foundation, 2018). ED becomes more prevalent as one ages. About 40% of men experience some kind of ED in their 40s, and by the age of 70, 70% of men are affected (Lakin & Wood, 2018). There are some factors that put older men at risk for ED, such as diabetes, high cholesterol, hypertension, low testosterone, obesity, and certain medications (Danoff, 2015).

Case Study 12.3: Hugh's Nervous Penis

Hugh, a 70-year-old healthy man, came to treatment for his ED. He was extremely healthy with no underlying health conditions or medications that would contribute to his ED. The only health condition of historical significance was Peyronie disease from 10 years ago, which had caused him tremendous pain when having intercourse, but was treated in its early stages.

Hugh at times used erectile enhancement drugs, but they did not always work. After taking a detailed sexual history and through numerous sex therapy sessions, it was revealed that Hugh had anxiety around lasting long enough to please his partner, and worried that he may never have sex again, which he linked to the prior Peyronie disease. The more Hugh worked on reducing his anxiety, the more he was able to have successful intercourse both with and without the help of erectile enhancement drugs.

Along with talk and sex therapy, EMDR therapy targeted Hugh's prior Peyronie disease experiences, his anxiety around "lasting long enough," and his worry that he may "never have sex again." PCs developed included "I'm fine as I am," "I am lovable no matter how I perform," and "I am capable and can handle what comes my way."

Treatment for Erectile Dysfunction

ED can be very troublesome to men. As stated, some ED is psychological and psychotherapy may be able to help. For biological ED there are numerous medications; Viagra, Levitra, Cialis, Staxyn, and Stendra are the most common among phosphodiesterase-5 (PDE-5) inhibitors. They all work in similar ways; they relax the muscles in the penis so that when the penis becomes aroused the arteries in the penis become wider, allowing the penis to fill with blood and the veins to expand. The blood is trapped for a period of time, thus leading to an erection. It should be noted that if a person without ED uses these drugs for sexual performance, the drugs do not behave in the same way (Danoff, 2015).

Other more invasive treatments of ED are surgical implants with a vacuum device (Danoff, 2015). With the invention of PDE-5 inhibitors, this is not as common. Injectables are also used for ED treatment. The more recent treatment is when prostaglandin-E1 (PGE-1) is directly injected into the shaft of the penis. Injectables are used when other medications have been tried but failed; however, the idea of inserting something into the penis is generally not a pleasant thought for many. There are also medications (such as Muse) that can be inserted in the tip of the penis through a urethral suppository. New technology has brought other treatments as well, such as low-intensity extracorporeal shock wave and stem cell injection therapy, which has the potential to repair damage of the corpora cavernosa (Wang et al., 2023). It is extremely important for an individual to talk to their doctor to decide what treatment is right for them (Danoff, 2015).

Are Erections a Privilege?

Many Americans over the age of 65 use Medicare as their healthcare benefits. However, Viagra, Cialis, and other drugs for ED are not paid for under Medicare. A nongeneric version of Viagra may cost approximately $60 per pill, whereas a generic version may be about $35 a pill. Nevertheless, many sexual enhancement medications are still not covered by Medicare Part D, and many individuals cannot afford to pay out of pocket for these types of treatments, leaving them impotent, sad, frustrated, and in pain (Andrews, 2019).

CHANGES IN SEXUAL DESIRE

Changes in sexual desire are common among aging men. Many older men report they do not desire sex as much as they did when they were younger. As with most people, many problems with sexual desire have psychological underpinnings. However, lower testosterone may cause low sexual desire. If the change in sexual desire is rapid, it is important to consult with one's physician to see what could be the potential cause. It may be related to medication or another underlying health condition (Nippoldt, 2020).

EJACULATION CHANGES

Ejaculation may also change with aging. Delayed (slow) or retrograde ejaculation may happen. Retrograde ejaculation is when ejaculate reverses back into the bladder rather than coming through the penis. There is no cause for concern; the semen will make its way out during urination (Danoff, 2015). Diabetes, spinal cord injury, multiple sclerosis, and certain medications are all related to retarded ejaculation. Medications such as antidepressants are especially linked to this condition (Villines, 2017).

Case Study 12.4: Will Cannot Ejaculate

Will (age 68) and Barbara (age 66) had been dating for 6 months. Will had been diagnosed with Parkinson disease 2 years ago and was able to control some of the physical decline by diet, exercise, and physical therapy. When they began engaging in sexual intercourse, Will was unable to ejaculate. He could maintain an erection, but he had no ejaculation. Barbara was saddened by this because she wanted her partner to enjoy sex as much as she did. Sexual intercourse eventually became emotionally painful for Barbara because of Will not being able to ejaculate. They decided to consult a sex therapist. When the sex therapist was taking a history, she found out that Will was taking citalopram, an antidepressant. Will said that he felt he did not need to take it anymore and that he was on a low dose. After consulting with his primary care physician, Will stopped taking the medication and his ejaculation returned. Both he and Barbara were much happier in their sexual relationship with each other.

BENIGN PROSTATE HYPERTROPHY

Benign prostate hypertrophy (BPH), or "enlarged prostate" as it is commonly known, affects about half of men over 50. It is not life-threatening, but may be very uncomfortable. Signs of BPH are decreased urine flow, difficulty fully eliminating the bladder, and weak urine flow. The prostate surrounds the neck of the bladder and may become larger with aging. This in turn can cause a change in urine flow. If the BPH is severe enough, a prostatectomy (full or partial removal of the prostate gland) may be recommended. It should be noted that, although this may sound scary, when done for a benign disease, it is not related to ED. Medication is a non invasive way to treat BPH. Older medications such as Proscar may lower the patient's sexual desire. New medications such as Avodart have minimal side effects. It is vitally important for an individual to talk to their primary care doctor and/or urologist about potential medications and side effects (Danoff, 2015).

BODY IMAGE

It is often thought that only women struggle with body image as they age. However, men, and other genders, may also struggle with their aging bodies and appearance. Some men report the loss of their hair and physical capabilities, which may be troublesome to them. As one gets older, body image does not only concern how the body looks, but also the physical functioning of the body. Losses of hearing, sight, and/or movement may make one feel like their body is betraying them. This is true for any body. Certain previous enjoyable hobbies may be more difficult; for example, arthritis in one's hands may prevent a person from sewing, knitting, or playing the piano. Losses of sight and hearing may cause people not to feel as independent. Common activities such as driving may be less available. This can be an adjustment for the older adult (Jankowski et al., 2014).

Case Study 12.5: Jack and His Aging Body

Jack is a 65-year-old Black man who has struggled with some ED due to medication issues. When asked about how he felt about his body and how it relates to his aging, he spoke about what it is like to look in the mirror and see his reflection. He sees his thinning hair and weight gain, and these changes diminish how he feels about himself. He views himself differently now and knows that he has changed, which also negatively impacts how he feels about himself sexually (Mader, 2014).

Psychotherapy and EMDR therapy can target these various negative self-perceptions, working toward the PCs of "I am fine as I am," "I'm worthy and deserve sexual pleasure like any other body."

LGBTQ+ AGING

Along with what has been mentioned previously about the changes that happen when one ages, LGBTQ+ elders face different challenges as they age. About 5% of the 65 and older people reside in nursing homes. By 2030, the last of the Baby Boomers will have reached 65 years old and this population will make up one-fifth of the total population. It is estimated that there are 1.5 million LGBTQ+ adults over the age of 65 in the United States. Many of them will rely on assisted living and nursing homes to take care of them in their old age. LGBTQ+ older adults are more likely to be single and childless as they age compared to their heterosexual peers. Some LGBTQ+ older adults have come out of straight marriages and then come out as LGBTQ, which may have caused a strain on their family relationships, leaving them more isolated (Bouton et al., 2023).

The experience varies among older adults. Lesbians and people of color are more likely to struggle economically than White gay men. Older bisexual individuals may experience more social isolation and depression (LGBT Movement Advancement Project [MAP] & Services and Advocacy for Gay, Lesbian, Bisexual and Transgender Elders [SAGE], 2010).

Only 50% of LGBTQ+ older adults who reside in nursing homes or assisted living feel comfortable being out about their sexual orientation. There have been cases of mistreatment in long-term care facilities by homophobic staff. Same-sex partners have been separated in the living situations as well (LGBT MAP & SAGE, 2010).

There is a light at the end of the tunnel, however. In certain cities, LGBTQ+ assisted living, long-term care facilities, and retirement communities are being created. Legislation, such as the SB 219—A Bill of Rights for LGBTQ+ elders—was passed in 2017 in California. Though change is being made, there is still much room for improvement (California Legislature, 2017).

INTERSEX AGING

More is known about intersexed individuals than there was in the past. However, given the evolution of treatment, older folks are still left in the dark on how to navigate medical care. Moreover, given the more invasive treatments of the past, there is less known on how older intersexed people age and the issues that may arise. Older intersexed individuals are at an increased risk of discrimination by healthcare providers. Many healthcare providers do not have experience in treating intersexed patients. The lack of knowledge of intersex variations also leads to not offering appropriate care for patients. Before the 1990s, many of the interventions were surgical and the long-term effects of these surgeries were unknown. The most common surgeries involved the removal of the penis or the clitoris. This not only led to physical problems, but also affected the mental health of the individual. It is essential for medical professionals to recognize the variability in bodies to ensure individuals get appropriate care (OII Europe, n.d.).

TRANSGENDER AGING

Some transgender older folks face an increasing likelihood of going back into the closet and not having their health needs met, such as an interruption of their hormone treatments for gender affirmation (Bouton et al., 2023). However, some individuals choose to come out later in life rather than when they were younger. Transgender individuals faced a much bigger stigma in the past than they do now, although transphobia still exists as evidenced by the increase of anti-trans legislation bills introduced throughout the country. As of June 2024, 43 states have introduced 602 anti-trans legislation bills, with 42 bills having passed (221 failed)—the others are still active.

Many individuals chose to stay in the closet, but with more mainstream acceptance and representation, such as Caitlyn Jenner, some folks have decided it is time to come out and be visible. In midlife, individuals may be more aware of the time they have left, want to live their lives as authentically as possible, and thus decide to transition (Fabbre, 2014).

There is a widely held fear among aging transgender individuals that if they become dependent or have to reside in a nursing home that their genders will not be affirmed, or they will not receive proper care. Furthermore, there is a concern of violence and sexual abuse in nursing homes. Not affording proper care can leave some more vulnerable to violence and abuse in nursing homes, as not all nursing homes and facilities are educated or competent in transgender care and issues. These transgender folks may be concerned that, for the first time in a long while, they will be outed. They may have lived in their gender for decades and may have never come out to certain people. Unfortunately, this leaves many transgender individuals vulnerable to depression and suicide. Some create "end of life plans" in case they reach the point where they can no longer take care of themselves (Witten, 2013).

Case Study 12.6: The Impact of April's Transition

Patrick (age 63) and Johanna (age 57) originally sought couples therapy to work through some infidelity issues. Patrick had always had a desire for BDSM (bondage, dominance, sadism, masochism) and would pay dominatrixes to engage in the behavior. Johanna was trying to accept this as she wanted their marriage to work. In one session, Patrick shared he really enjoyed wearing women's clothes and he became alive when he wore them. He always thought it was a kink behavior, but realized it has been something more. Soon, Patrick came out as a transwoman and changed her name to April. April very much wanted to stay married to Johanna, but Johanna was not attracted to women and they ended up divorcing.

April had difficulty coming out to her family. Her daughter, a teenager, was not comfortable with this and insisted that April present as male when she would visit her. April, not wanting to lose connection with her daughter, obliged, but it was painful to do so. April lost complete contact with her adult son. Though April is much happier and has created a wonderful LGBTQ community, she still struggles with the loss of some family contact and having to present as male at times.

April certainly can benefit from EMDR therapy, targeting these very sad instances of abandonment and invalidation by her family members. An EMDR future template might help strengthen her ability to explain and assert a refusal to appear male to her daughter. April could work toward these PCs: "I'm fine as I am," "I can be myself and be loved," and "I do the best I can." Her family members, if open to family therapy, could also greatly benefit from exploring and reducing their potential anger, sadness, and disappointment at losing a "man" as their father. Therapy could help April's daughter come to terms with, accept, and affirm April's transition.

Case Study 12.7: Staying in the Closet

Robert is a 70-year-old man. He has been married to his wife for 45 years. He is very active in his church as well as his senior center. He volunteered to be a part of a dissertation research study focusing on the experiences of older adults' sexuality as they age. He found the research both interesting and important. Throughout the interview, the researcher felt like Robert was holding something back. It was not until the end of the interview when the researcher asked, "Do you know anyone who is lesbian or gay who may want to participate in the research study?" Robert let out a giant sigh and said that he had same-gender sexual relations throughout his marriage. He admitted he knew it was wrong to cheat, but he got much more emotional and sexual satisfaction from men than he ever did from his wife. He admitted to the researcher he had never told anyone else about this and the researcher was the first person he told. He had no intentions of ever leaving his marriage (Mader, 2014, p. 95).

If Robert did choose to explore his same-gender history, therapy could help him identify and reduce any distress about potentially identifying as gay and leaving his marriage so that he may eventually more authentically pursue emotional and sexual satisfaction. In addition, EMDR therapy could help install PCs of "I have choices, I can handle big changes, I deserve to openly pursue what I want."

SOCIAL INFLUENCE ON SEXUALITY AND AGING

AGEISM

Ageism is discrimination based on one's age. It usually pertains to older adults rather than younger folks. Unlike other prejudices, racists are not going to wake up and find themselves with a different skin color. Someone who is anti-Semitic is not going to wake up and find themselves Jewish. However, if we are lucky, we will all one day grow old. "The most unproductive prejudice is one directed against a group you're going to join" (Dailey, 1981, p. 312).

It is not just younger people who hold ageist attitudes. Older adults also can have internalized ageism, which can be particularly harmful, especially in terms of sexuality. These views are usually developed when one is young, then carried to old age. Consider something as simple as going to the grocery store and looking at the magazines in the check-out line. What do you see? Usually, it is a younger person gracing the cover. The ads in the magazine often directly promote how one can look younger. Even when shopping for a birthday card one will find negative stereotypes, albeit humorous, depicting aging.

Seeing these images on a regular basis may be detrimental in how an older adult feels about themselves. Dr. Dennis Dailey (1981) refers to this phenomenon as the "laughter curtain." The laughter curtain is one way that people manage their feelings with uncomfortable life topics. This is just as detrimental to older adults as is silence. Having a helping professional or a family member laugh at the sexuality of an older adult causes shame. This in turn may become a self-fulfilling prophecy for many older adults. If people believe that older adults are asexual, older adults may very well shut down this part of their lives.

Internalized stereotypes and/or internalized ageism begins at a very young age and continues across the life span. Negative depictions of aging in the media, and different stories heard when one is young, affect how people feel about aging and older adults. It is easy for children to feel removed from the experiences of older adults because they are not yet in that stage of life. Given that our society is very youth focused, in some ways young adults benefit from this ageism, which exacerbates the stereotype (Levy, 2009).

Stereotypes on sexuality and aging are profound. Older women in the media are depicted as the sweet grandmotherly types or very unkempt, eccentric women. If they are depicted as sexual, "the cougar" stereotype is often presented. Older men in the media who have interest in sex are thought of as sex obsessed, hence the "dirty old man" stereotype, or they are the grouchy curmudgeons yelling at children to "get off their lawn" (Walz, 2002).

As of 2020, there has been a refreshing turnaround on how older adult sexuality is depicted in mainstream media. TV shows such as *Grace and Frankie* and movies like *Book Club* show older women and men enjoying sex well into their later years. Even with these advances there continues to be a need for improvement so that the negative stereotypes are no longer perpetuated.

Stereotypes can also negatively impact older adults' health. Older adults may not seek the medical treatment they need because of the idea that "it's just old age." By accepting these stereotypes, older folks may not take care of themselves in the ways that are needed (Levy, 2009). This is especially true when it comes to sexuality. Often older adults do not talk to their healthcare providers about sexuality due to embarrassment or the notion that this is "just a normal" aging process. Conversely, healthcare professionals do not address sexuality with their older patients because of this ageism and general embarrassment (Gore-Gorszewska, 2020).

Case Study 12.8: Cathy, Minimized Vaginal Dryness

Cathy, a 68-year-old woman on dialysis, went to her primary care doctor for a check up. She brought up a sexual concern of vaginal dryness, which is a common side effect from dialysis. The doctor became very uneasy and replied, "That's what gynecologists are for." Cathy's concern was never addressed. Due to her doctor's discomfort, she never brought it up to her gynecologist, either. This example makes it clear how lack of communication hinders older adults from the treatment that they need (Mader, 2014, p.110).

LOSS OF A PARTNER

Many older adults experience loss of a partner. The World Health Organization (WHO) has found that women tend to outlive men; thus, they are more likely to be widowed, living 6 to 8 years longer than men (WHO, 2024). This leaves many individuals alone for the first time in a long while and without a sexual partner. Many older adults would like to find some sort of companionship, and others are happy with friends and family (Mader, 2014). Finding a companion may prove to be difficult for some. Being out of the dating world for a long time, as well as internalized stereotypes, may prevent older adults from finding the companionship that they so desire. One of the main reasons older adults report not being sexual is because they do not have a partner (Parker-Pope, 2019).

FAMILY INFLUENCE

Even when older adults choose to date and enter a new relationship, it is not always smooth sailing. Family and especially adult children can be very critical about their aging parents being in a new relationship. This may be due to a plethora of reasons, such as the adult child's own ageism, their grief around the loss of the other parent, and/or fear of financial loss or loss of inheritance (Hughes & Fredenburg, 2020).

It is difficult for children of any age to think of their parents as sexual beings. Sexuality is not often a conversation topic in families, so it can be a big surprise to adult children when their parents want to engage in new relationships. This may be even a bigger problem if an aging parent in a nursing home begins a relationship. As difficult as it may be, adult children should not infantilize their aging parents and need to realize that people are sexual from the day they are born to the day they die. Although it may be hard to conceptualize depending on one's age, it is important to think about how one would want to be treated in a similar situation, and, even more specifically, how these aging adults would like to be treated. These aging parents had a life before their children and they can continue having one after their children are grown (Love & Harmony, 2010).

Older adults' sexuality is frequently infantilized, especially in nursing homes. Once they are in a nursing home, they often do not have automatic rights to sexual expression. Instead, their rights are left up to their families and the staff. The families may have to give permission for their loved one to engage in sexual behavior. In turn, the older resident may feel shameful about their very natural sexual behavior. In some cases, nursing home staff are more accepting of intimacy between two residents if those residents are married to each other. However, that same privilege is not always allowed to single older adults. While autonomy of older adults is generally promoted and advertised by nursing homes, sexuality is often not included in that autonomy (Doll, 2013).

Sexual contact in nursing homes can sometimes be considered an ethical dilemma. In 2014, Henry Rayhons (age 78), a state legislator from Iowa, was arrested for a third-degree felony sexual abuse after engaging in sexual acts with his wife, who was diagnosed with Alzheimer disease, in a nursing home. This was after the nursing home staff stated that Mrs. Rayhons was unable to consent to sex. Consent and dementia can be difficult to figure out. Some dementia researchers believe that consent may happen through facial expressions and body language. Intimacy is often very beneficial to dementia patients. While the family may be upset by sexual activities of their relative with dementia, many nursing homes are also caught in an ethical quandary. Most nursing homes do not have a sexual health policy that addresses these issues. Moreover, most nursing staff historically have not considered older adults as sexual. Fortunately, more people are researching consent and dementia, and more nursing homes are getting trained on how to manage the sexual rights of their patients (Belluck, 2015).

The Hebrew Home Nursing Home located in the Bronx, New York, created a sexual rights policy for their residents in 1995. Families are informed of this policy at the beginning of their family member's stay. Staff are trained to look for cues of consent as well as knocking before entering a resident's room. They are also trained to ask residents certain questions regarding sex and consent (Belluck, 2015).

Case Study 12.9: Ethel and George's Relationship in a Nursing Home

Ethel is a widowed, 94-year-old woman residing in a nursing home. She has lived there for the past 4 years. In the past few months she has sparked a relationship with George, a 96-year-old widower. The nursing home staff sees how happy the relationship makes them and allows them privacy to engage in intimacy. George's daughter came to visit and became irate that her father was in a relationship. She forbade her father to see Ethel and had the nursing home staff move George to another part of the nursing home. Soon after the move George died. Ethel wanted to go to the funeral, but the family had the police there to escort Ethel away from the funeral and forbade her to be there. Ethel became extremely depressed.

Ethel may also be experiencing some traumatic responses to how George's family handled their relationship, as well as grief and/or self-blame over his death. Grief and/or EMDR therapy could help reduce and eliminate any distress she continues to experience from their cruel treatment.

HEALTHCARE PROVIDERS AND AGING SEXUAL HEALTH

Older adults account for a substantial number of patients that seek care from different healthcare providers such as primary care doctors, physical therapists, and social workers. Although there is a significant number of older adults receiving care, healthcare professionals do not usually have formal training in gerontology, and there is even less training on gerontology and sexuality. In one study, it was found that psychology students had a better understanding of older adult sexuality than medical students did. It was also found that the more exposure and interest in the aging population a person had, the more open minded that person would be regarding older adult sexuality (Snyder & Zweig, 2010).

Even if a helping professional has knowledge about older adult sexuality, it does not necessarily mean that they have positive attitudes about it. It was found that the older the helping professional was, the less permissive their attitude (Langer-Most & Langer, 2010). This may be due to internalized ageism discussed previously in the chapter.

In a web-based survey of 3,000 self-identified women, 40% said that they did not seek help for sexual functioning. Fifty-four percent did seek help; however, they did not rank their experience with the helping professional high. Communication may be difficult for older adults, especially those socialized as women, in regard to sexuality. Older women may be conflict avoidant and want to remain neutral in their relationships, so sexual concerns may not be communicated. This lack of communication may impede the relationship between the helping professional and the older adult; thus, older adults may not receive the help they need (Laumann et al., 2005).

If older adults do communicate with their healthcare provider about sexuality, it is most often their primary care doctor. This may be because they do not realize there are specialists available to help them. Even still, older adults are often reluctant to bring up sexuality with their helping professionals because they perceive that the professional has a negative attitude about sex. Furthermore, many older adults have adopted the "that ship has sailed" mentality and do not bring up concerns (Gott & Hinchliff, 2003).

Mental health professionals do not fare much better in the comfort of addressing sexuality and aging. Sexual histories are often taken with new patients coming into a mental health setting. Mental health professionals often omit taking a sexual history with their older clients because they deem it inappropriate. In one study, psychiatrists were given two different scenarios about sexuality—one with a middle-aged adult and another with an older adult—and were asked what they would do. Most of them chose to refer the middle-aged adult to a sexual health professional and the older adult to community-based care (Bouman & Arcelus, 2001).

Older adults who prioritize their sexuality are more likely to shop around for a helping professional who is comfortable with the topic. Moreover, some doctors have aged along with their patients and there may be a comfort already established; thus, they may bring up the topic of sexuality more. Comfort and a good bedside manner are both imperative with communicating with older adults about sexuality and aging (Mader, 2014).

The good news is sexuality and gerontology knowledge can be taught and helping professionals can become more comfortable with the topic. Students who study more sexuality topics are more comfortable and are more likely to bring up the topic with their clients. Not communicating about sexuality may lead to misdiagnosis, such as mistaking HIV/AIDS for a disease of older age. This is extremely detrimental for older adults. In line with the vision for and purpose of this book, all helping professionals benefit from sexuality education (Verrastro et al., 2020).

Case Study 12.10: Alfred and Rebecca Persist in Seeking Helpful Care

Alfred is a 68-year-old White male who was diagnosed with Parkinson disease. He was divorced for several years when he met Rebecca (67). Both fell in love and decided to get married. Alfred and Rebecca came in for sex therapy because Alfred was not able to maintain an erection. He went to his primary care doctor to ask for guidance. His doctor informed him that due to his age and Parkinson that this would be something that he would "just need to accept." Both Alfred and Rebecca were very distraught by this. They then, on their own, sought the help of a sex therapist. Upon a further dive into Alfred's sexual history and medical history, it came to light that he was prescribed a selective serotonin reuptake inhibitor (SSRI) when he was diagnosed with Parkinson disease. He said that he didn't think he needed the antidepressant anymore, so with his doctor's guidance he went off it. After that, he was able to maintain an erection and didn't need to remain in sex therapy.

EYE MOVEMENT DESENSITIZATION AND REPROCESSING THERAPY AND AGING SEXUALITY

As illustrated throughout this chapter, just like with younger populations, EMDR therapy may be an excellent treatment modality to assist in identifying, targeting, and processing the many emotional and mental disturbances that may accompany aging and changing relationships. Hopefully all individuals get to experience aging, and hopefully everyone can turn to a trained EMDR therapist when the time comes to help us make peace with body changes and body image, differently functioning (or surgically removed) reproductive/generative organs, changing erectile organs, loss of partners, and any poor responses from family and/or healthcare professionals.

Case Study 12.11: Irene's Marriage "Slump"

This final EMDR therapy case study is contributed by Sandra Stephenson Murphy, LICSW (EMDR Certified Clinician), to further illustrate how EMDR Therapy may be of use and benefit aging adults.

Irene sought treatment to have support during the transition for her upcoming retirement. She is a 63-year-old White ciswoman who has been a school guidance counselor for 36 years. Irene is worried that much of her identity and social life has been through her career and reports that her current marriage of 23 years has been in a "slump." Irene describes her husband as a recovering alcoholic, about 2.5 years sober, kind and caring, and "would do anything for me." Yet Irene also describes her husband as "boring and sedentary," and has already been retired for 10 years. Irene also describes a lack of intimacy, both emotionally and sexually (no sexual activity for the past 2-plus years). Her husband shows sexual interest periodically, yet Irene describes herself as feeling irritable by his overtures due to her perception of a lack of emotional connection. "I'm just not into the sex because of that."

Through extensive history taking, three targets were identified:

1. Earliest/Touchstone memory: Irene's mother told Irene as she began puberty (age 10 or 11) that if she ever had sex and became pregnant before marriage she would "kill herself." Her mother was a devout Catholic and Irene is a practicing Catholic. An early link between sex, sexual urges, and causing pain to her mother was established. To this day, Irene reported hearing those words in her head at the stirring of any sexual interest.
2. During her first marriage, Irene's previous husband had an affair with her close friend. Even after the affair was discovered, and they both wanted to "save" their marriage by going to couples counseling, the husband continued the affair. They eventually divorced and Irene describes the entire experience as devastating. She felt suicidal and ashamed at the time. She currently worries about running

into her husband and her ex-friend, who is now his wife, in the community or at social events.

3. Irene wants sexual intimacy with her husband yet struggles with the lack of trust. Three years ago when her husband was drinking, Irene threatened to end the marriage if he continued to drink. He supposedly stopped drinking and began participating in Alcoholics Anonymous. A friend then told Irene that she saw her husband buying alcohol at a package store. Irene said she "flipped out" and described this as a betrayal similar to her first husband's affair. Since that time he has stopped drinking, yet Irene has also stopped having sex.

All three targets were successfully processed to a zero SUD (subjective unit of distress)

Three EMDR future templates were identified and processed:

1. Envision having a healthy relationship with sex free from guilt and shame. Her PC is, "I deserve a fulfilling and pleasurable sexual life."
2. Imagine running into her ex-husband and his partner, feeling strong and confident, and seeing them as smaller. Her PC is, "I am worthy, capable, and can handle it."
3. Envision sexual intimacy with her husband that feels "safe and sexy" for her. Her PC is, "I can safely trust and enjoy sex again."

Irene reported the return of quality and frequency of sexual intimacy with her husband, noting that their communication has improved greatly, resulting in greater emotional intimacy, safety, and trust as well. She reported enjoying the sexual intimacy, and mentioned that for the first time she experienced sex and orgasms without any resulting pain, "Catholic" guilt, shame, or hearing her mother's voice in her head. Irene also stated that her husband was now interested in EMDR therapy to look at his previous drinking as a possible escape or avoidance of intimacy.

SUMMARY

This chapter shared information about the current aging population and their sexual behaviors, exploring in detail female-, male-, and transgender-specific aging, and what each group may generally encounter as they age. Social influences such as ageism, family relations, grief, myths, and stereotypes about aging and sexuality were also addressed. The chapter also considered the aging needs and barriers of LGBTQ+ folks. Finally, the chapter emphasized the importance of communicating sexual health topics, questions, and concerns with helping professionals, so that all older adults can continue to have enriching lives.

DISCUSSION QUESTIONS

1. How do social influences like ageism, myths, and stereotypes impact the sexual health and well-being of older adults, and what strategies can be used to combat these issues?
2. How do the aging experiences differ between female, male, intersexed, and transgender individuals, and what implications does this have for providing inclusive and comprehensive care for all older adults?
3. Why is it important for older adults to communicate their sexual health concerns with healthcare providers, and what steps can professionals take to foster open dialogue?

LEARNING ACTIVITIES

CourseConnect

To access self-assessment questions and interactive, competency-based learning activities for this chapter, visit www.springerpub.com/courseconnect. See inside front cover and tear-out card for CourseConnect details.

ADDITIONAL RESOURCES

Additional resources are online and available at www.springerpub.com/courseconnect.

REFERENCES

Andrews, M. (2019, February 19). The high cost of sex: Insurers don't often pay for drugs to treat problems. *Kaiser Health News*. https://khn.org/news/the-high-cost-of-sex-insurers-often-dont-pay-for-drugs-to-treat-problems

Beckman, N., Waern, M., Gustafson, D., & Skoog, I. (2008). Secular trends in self reported sexual activity and satisfaction in Swedish 70 year olds: Cross sectional survey of four populations, 1971–2001. *British Medical Journal, 337*(7662), a279. https://doi.org/10.1136/bmj.a279

Belluck, P. (2015, April 15). Sex, dementia, and a husband on trial at age 78. *New York Times*. https://www.nytimes.com/2015/04/14/health/sex-dementia-and-a-husband-henry-rayhons-on-trial-at-age-78.html

Benjamin Rose Institute on Aging. (2019, June 12). *Sexually transmitted diseases in older adults*. https://www.benrose.org/-/resource-library/health-and-wellness-services/sexually-transmitted-diseases-in-older-adults

Bouman, W. P., & Arcelus, J. (2001). Are psychiatrist guilty of 'ageism' when it comes to taking a sexual history? *International Journal of Geriatric Psychiatry, 16*(1), 27–31. https://doi.org/10.1002/1099-1166(200101)16:1<27::AID-GPS267>3.3.CO;2-J

Bouton, L. J. A., Brush, A. M., & Meyer, I. H. (2023, January). *LGBT adults aged 50 and older in the US during the COVID-19 pandemic* [Report]. The Williams Institute, UCLA School of Law. https://williamsinstitute.law.ucla.edu/wp-content/uploads/LGBT-Older-Adults-Jan-2023.pdf

Burry, M. (2018, August 1). How your vagina changes in your 30s, 40s and beyond. *Health*. https://www.health.com/condition/sexual-health/vagina-healthy-aging

California Legislature. (2017). Senate Bill 219: Lesbian, Gay, Bisexual, and Transgender Long-Term Care Facility Residents' Bill of Rights (Chapter 483, Statutes of 2017). Retrieved from https://leginfo.legislature.ca.gov/faces/billNavClient.xhtml?bill_id=201720180SB219

Dailey, D. M. (1981). Sexual expression and aging. In F. J. Berghorn, D. E. Schafer, & Associates (Eds.), *The dynamics of aging* (pp. 311–330). Westview Press.

Danoff, D. (2015). *The ultimate guide to male sexual health: How to stay vital at any age*. Beyond Words.

Doll, G. M. (2013, July). Sexuality in nursing homes: Practice and policy. *Journal of Gerontological Nursing, 39*(7), 30–37. https://doi.org/10.3928/00989134-20130418-01

Doress-Worters, P. B., & Siegal, D. L. (1994). *The new ourselves, growing older: Women aging with knowledge and power*. Simon & Schuster.

Fabbre, V. D. (2014). Gender transitions in later life: The significance of time in queer aging. *Journal of Gerontological Social Work, 57*(2–4), 161–175. https://doi.org/10.1080/01634372.2013.855287

Fleming, K. C., Evans, J. M., & Chutka, D. S. (2003). A cultural and economic history of older age in America. *Mayo Clinic Proceedings, 78*(7), 914–921. https://doi.org/10.4065/78.7.914

Forbes, M. K., Eaton, N. R., & Krueger, R. F. (2017). Sexual quality of life and aging: A prospective study of a nationally representative sample. *Journal Sex Research, 54*(2), 137–148. https://doi.org/10.1080/00224499.2016.1233315

Gore-Gorszewska, G. (2020). "Why not ask the doctor?" Barriers in help-seeking for sexual problems among older adults in Poland. *International Journal of Public Health, 65*(8), 1507–1515. https://doi.org/10.1007/s00038-020-01472-6

Gott, M., & Hinchliff, S. (2003). Barriers to seeking treatment for sexual problems in primary care: A qualitative study with older people. *Family Practice, 20*(6), 690–695. https://doi.org/10.1093/fampra/cmg612

Hofmeier, S. M., Runfola, C. D., Sala, M., Gagne, D. A., Brownley, K. A., & Bulik, C. M. (2017). Body image, aging, and identity in women over 50: The Gender and Body Image (GABI) study. *Journal of Women & Aging, 29*(1), 3–14. https://doi.org/10.1080/08952841.2015.1065140

Howe, N. (2014, August 13). The Silent Generation "The lucky few" (part 3 of 7). *Forbes*. https://www.forbes.com/sites/neilhowe/2014/08/13/the-silent-generation-the-lucky-few-part-3-of-7

Huffpost. (2017, December 6). *7 cultures that celebrate aging and respect their elders*. https://www.huffpost.com/entry/what-other-cultures-can-teach_n_4834228

Hughes, C., & Fredenburg, B. (2020, July 24). How to help your adult children adjust to dating. *Divorced Moms.com*. https://divorcedmoms.com/how-to-help-your-adult-children-adjust-to-you-dating

Jankowski, G. S., Diedrichs, P. C., Williamson, H., Christopher, G., & Harcourt, D. (2014, April 28). Looking age-appropriate while growing old gracefully: A qualitative study of ageing and body image among older adults. *Journal of Health Psychology, 21*(4), 550–561. https://doi.org/10.1177/1359105314531468

Korhonen, V. (2024, August 6). *Population of the United States by generation 2023*. Statista. https://www.statista.com/statistics/797321/us-population-by-generation

Lakin, M., & Wood, H. (2018, June). *Erectile dysfunction*. Cleveland Clinic: Center for Continuing Education. http://www.clevelandclinicmeded.com/medicalpubs/diseasemanagement/endocrinology/erectile-dysfunction

Langer-Most, O., & Langer, N. (2010). Aging and sexuality: How much do gynecologists know and care? *Journal of Women and Aging, 22*(4), 283–289. https://doi.org/10.1080/08952841.2010.518882

Laumann, E., Nicolosi, A., Glasser, D., Paik, A., Gingell, C., Moreira, E., & Wang, T. (2005). Sexual problems among women and men aged 40–80 years: Prevalence and correlates identified in the global study of sexual attitudes and behaviors. *International Journal of Impotence Research, 17*(1), 39–57. https://doi.org/10.1038/sj.ijir.3901250

Levy, B. (2009). Stereotype embodiment. *Current Directions in Psychological Science, 18*(6), 332–336. https://doi.org/10.1111/j.1467-8721.2009.01662.x

LGBT Movement Advancement Project, & Services and Advocacy for Gay, Lesbian, Bisexual and Transgender Elders. (2010, March). *Improving the lives of LGBT older adults* [Report]. https://www.lgbtmap.org/file/improving-the-lives-of-lgbt-older-adults.pdf

Lindau, S. T., Schumm, L. P., Laumann, E. O., Levinson, W., O'Muircheartaigh, C. A., & Waite, L. J. (2007). A study of sexuality and health among older adults in the United States. *New England Journal of Medicine, 357*(8), 764–774. https://doi.org/10.1056/NEJMoa067423

Love & Harmony. (2010, January 20). Senior dating and dealing with adult children. *Eharmony*. https://www.eharmony.com/dating-advice/dating-tips/senior-dating-and-dealing-with-adult-children

Mader, A. L. (2014). *Older adult experiences of their sexuality: A phenomenological inquiry* [unpublished doctoral dissertation]. Widener University.

Malzone, M. (2024, December 5). *Does Medicare cover HRT?* SingleCare. https://www.singlecare.com/blog/does-medicare-cover-hormone-replacement-therapy

Mayo Clinic. (2020, June 9). *Hormone therapy: Is it right for you?* https://www.mayoclinic.org/diseases-conditions/menopause/in-depth/hormone-therapy/art-20046372

Memorial Sloan Kettering Cancer Center. (2018, December 18). *Pelvic floor muscle (Kegel) exercises for women to improve sexual health*. https://www.mskcc.org/cancer-care/patient-education/pelvic-floor-muscle-kegel-exercises-women-improve-sexual-health

Minois, G. (1989). *History of old age: From antiquity to the Renaissance*. University of Chicago Press.

Murphy, S. L., Xu, J., Kochanek, K. D., & Arias, E. (2018, November). *Mortality in the United States, 2017*. Centers for Disease Control and Pevention. https://www.cdc.gov/nchs/products/databriefs/db328.htm

Nippoldt, T. B. (2020, April 14). *Is the loss of sex drive normal as men get older*? Mayo Clinic. https://www.mayoclinic.org/healthy-lifestyle/sexual-health/expert-answers/loss-of-sex-drive/faq-20058237

North American Menopause Society. (2020). *Decreased response and pleasure*. https://www.menopause.org/for-women/sexual-health-menopause-online/sexual-problems-at-midlife/decreased-response-and-pleasure

OII Europe. (n.d.). *Elderly intersex people.* Author. https://www.oiieurope.org/elderly-intersex-people/#:~:text=Intersex%20seniors%20face%20a%20number,have%20had%20negative%20lifelong%20consequences

Parker-Pope, T. (2019, July 30). Why a woman's sex life declines after menopause (Hint: sometimes it's her partner). *The New York Times.* https://www.nytimes.com/2019/07/30/well/live/menopause-sex-decline-partner-husband-wife.html

Quinn-Nilas, C., Benson, L., Milhausen, R. R., Buchholz, A. C., & Goncalves, M. (2016). The relationship between body image and domains of sexual functioning among heterosexual, emerging adult women. *Sexual Medicine, 4*(3), e182–e189. https://doi.org/10.1016/j.esxm.2016.02.004

Rienzo, B. A. (1985). The impact of aging on human sexuality. *Journal of School Health, 55*(2), 66–68. https://doi.org/10.1111/j.1746-1561.1985.tb04081.x

Rogers, P. (2019, October 23). Sex and aging. *Healthline.* https://www.healthline.com/health/healthy-sex-and-aging#takeaway

Schaeffer, K. (2024, January 9). *U.S. centenarian population is projected to quadruple over the next 30 years.* Pew Research Center. https://www.pewresearch.org/short-reads/2024/01/09/us-centenarian-population-is-projected-to-quadruple-over-the-next-30-years/#:~:text=There%20are%20currently%20roughly%2062,estimated%2023%25%20of%20the%20population

Snyder, R. J., & Zweig, R. A. (2010). Medical and psychology students' knowledge and attitudes regarding aging and sexuality. *Gerontology & Geriatrics Education, 31*(3), 235–255. https://doi.org/10.1080/02701960.2010.503132

Taylor, E. (2019, March 8). *How to keep your vagina healthy in your 20s, 30s, 40s, and 50s.* Healthline. https://www.healthline.com/health/womens-health/vagina-changes-20s-30s-40s-50s

Urology Care Foundation. (2018). *What is erectile dysfunction?* https://www.urologyhealth.org/urology-a-z/e/erectile-dysfunction-(ed)

Velez, A. (2020, May 18). Menopause is different for women of color. *Endocrine Web.* https://www.endocrineweb.com/menopause-different-women-color#:~:text=the%20research%20in%20SWAN%20shows,transition%20than%20white%20women%20do

Verrastro, V., Saladino, V., Petruccelli, F., & Eleuteri, S. (2020). Medical and health care professionals' sexuality education: State of the art and recommendations. *International Journal of Environmental Research and Public Health, 17*(7), 2186. https://doi.org/10.3390/ijerph17072186

Villines, Z. (2017, December 16). What you should know about retrograde ejaculation. *Medical News Today.* https://www.medicalnewstoday.com/articles/320332

Walz, T. (2002). Crones, dirty old men, sexy seniors: Representations of the sexuality of the older persons. *Journal of Aging and Identity, 7*(2), 99–112. https://doi.org/10.1023/A:1015487101438

Wang, C. M., Wu, B. R., Xiang, P., Xiao, J., & Hu, X. C. (2023). Management of male erectile dysfunction: From the past to the future. *Frontiers in Endocrinology, 14*, 1148834. https://doi.org/10.3389/fendo.2023.1148834

Weiss, G., Noorhasan, D., Schott, L. L., Powell, L., Randolph, Jr., J. F., & Johnston, J. M. (2009). Racial differences in women who have a hysterectomy for benign conditions. *Women's Health Issues, 19*(3), 202–210. https://www.ncbi.nlm.nih.gov/pmc/articles/PMC3786579

Whiteman, H. (2015, January 11). Almost 1 in 5 hysterectomies are 'unnecessary,' study finds. *Medical News Today.* https://www.medicalnewstoday.com/articles/287736

Witten, T. (2013). It's not all darkness: Robustness, resilience, and successful transgender aging. *LGBT Health, 1*(1), 24–33. https://doi.org/10.1089/lgbt.2013.0017

World Health Organization. (2024, August 2). *Life expectancy at birth (years).* https://data.who.int/indicators/i/A21CFC2/90E2E48

CHAPTER 13

Sexual Health Resources for Clinicians and Clients

Stephanie Baird

LEARNING OBJECTIVES

- Learn about the importance of ongoing clinician self-care practices to continuously battle societal erotophobia;
- Help manage potential work-related stress, burnout, and vicarious trauma; and enable a long and productive career helping clients (many of whom bring trauma histories to therapy).
- Learn about current sexual health related websites, podcasts, television shows, videos, and books for professionals and clients.
- Learn about educational and training programs available for further professional learning.
- Learn about a short list of valuable assessment tools to administer to clients for sexuality-related concerns.

INTRODUCTION

This final chapter begins with a section on burnout (BO) and vicarious trauma (VT) prevention efforts, self-care practices, and sex-positive activism. Additionally, pages and pages of sexuality-related resources such as websites, podcasts, books, and educational programs are enumerated with descriptions for particularly helpful resources. Lastly, a few sexual health helpful assessment tools are listed.

This chapter (and book) is not meant to be an exhaustive sexual health resource or take the place of continued sexual health education. My hope is that this book validates and encourages clinicians, psychotherapists, and future sex counselors, educators and therapists, to embrace positive sexual health as an important and essential ongoing part of life both for oneself, as a trusted professional, and for clients seeking care. May this book encourage ongoing exploration, acquisition, and sharing of knowledge, helping to demystify sexuality, counteract erotophobia, and encourage sexual well-being and empowerment for all.

SELF-CARE PRACTICES FOR THE CLINICIAN

Counteracting constant erotophobia (from society, and potentially from colleagues, friends, family, and clients) is difficult and ongoing work. Engaging with clinical material (the problems our clients present to us) as a professional occupation can also be fatiguing, frustrating, and sometimes even demoralizing. Clients who also have histories of trauma (sexual or otherwise) bring the additional potentiality of VT into our lives.

BURNOUT DEFINED

BO is "a syndrome of emotional exhaustion, depersonalization, and reduced personal accomplishment that can occur among individuals who do people-work of some kind" (Maslach, 1982, p. 98). BO results from continual exposure to interpersonal demands that may come from many kinds of angry or distressed individuals, and is not limited to traumatic material and trauma survivors.

Physical symptoms may include exhaustion/fatigue, headaches, and insomnia. Emotional/psychological and/or internalized distress may surface as feelings of ineffectiveness or hopelessness, lack of motivation/lack of enthusiasm, anger, frustration, depression and paranoia. Externalized distress may take the form of cynicism, frustration, or blame, and may include behaviors such as isolation and substance use (Freudenberger, 1974).

VICARIOUS TRAUMA

In Chapter 10, VT was discussed as the cumulative psychological impact on therapists from exposure to clients' trauma. VT can lead to changes in core beliefs, identity, and safety, along with posttraumatic stress disorder (PTSD) type symptoms such as intrusive distressing imagery, physical issues, mood swings, and difficulties maintaining boundaries. If untreated, these effects can persist and disrupt both personal and professional life.

ADDRESSING STRESS, BURNOUT, AND VICARIOUS TRAUMA

Overall methods to address ongoing stress, BO, and potential VT include (Saakvitne & Pearlman, 1996):

- ***Self-care*** (basic care of one's self, maintaining work-life balance, setting boundaries, and seeking connection with others)
- ***Nurturing activities*** (provide oneself with comfort and psychological gentleness) such as pursuing interests/hobbies (e.g., take a new craft class) and opportunities to relax (e.g., massage, yoga, meditation, sound baths)
- Occasional ***escape*** (e.g., vacations, travel, reading, video games, TV and movies), which can provide relief or distraction and assist in attaining psychological space from one's work

Vicarious Trauma Intervention

Clinicians can transform the despair of erotophobia and VT by a) creating meaning in their work (understanding the positive rippled effect of something simple like providing corrective psychoeducation), b) challenge their own (if increasing) negative beliefs and assumptions, and c) participate in community-building activities such as self-care events, vigils against violence, and so on.

To specifically address VT it can be helpful to keep these easy to remember ABC's in mind: *Awareness* (of symptoms developing), *Balance* (work/life), *Connection* (with others doing similar work).

Stress, Burnout, and Vicarious Trauma Interventions

Professional Interventions

Helpful professional interventions to reduce stress and prevent BO and VT include:

- Effective supervision or consultation regarding difficult or challenging clients and clinical dilemmas and presentations
- Establishing balance between the various aspects of one's job (i.e. patient work, teaching, research, or writing)
- Self-care routines at work (e.g., tea, taking walks, taking an actual lunch break, peer support)
- Establishing a warm and supportive collegial social environment

Helpful organizational interventions to reduce stress and prevent burnout include:

- Ensuring clinicians have the tools and support they need
- Providing adequate pay/compensation/health insurance/time off

- Providing adequate office space or telehealth modifications
- Formal avenues established for providers to address vicarious traumatization as necessary

Personal Interventions

Personal interventions and strategies that can reduce stress and prevent BO and VT may include:

- Regular leisure activities (reading, puzzles, games)
- Regular physical movement (yoga, etc.)
- Psychotherapy for oneself (including eye movement desensitization and reprocessing (EMDR) therapy, etc.)
- Attention to medical and physical health
- News/social media/cell phone balance (take wifi and tech/internet breaks as necessary)
- Turning off work notifications (email, texts) on cell phones; closing out work emails on computers
- Consistently nurturing all of one's self (emotional, spiritual, sexual, interpersonal, creative, etc.)
- Trying out new sexual health developments and information in one's own life. If one is considering recommending a website, for instance, or new adult sex toy, perhaps splurge the time and money to try it for oneself; consider taking a class on BDSM (bondage, domination, sadism and masochism).
- Building a community of like-minded sex-positive practitioners and activists
- Sex-positive activism in the form of writing newspaper columns or op eds, blogs, or producing short educational videos for social media

"The most important (self-care) strategy in your personal life is to have one. Your personal life must be a priority, which is another way of saying that you must be a priority" (Saakvitne & Pearlman, 1996, p. 83).

SEX AND PLEASURE ACTIVISM

Now that we are at the end of this book, it may be obvious that any kind of positive engagement with sexual health, sexuality, sex education/information, and open (affirming and curious) dialogues with self, clients, and society at large constitutes sex and pleasure activism. Any time we recommend a truly helpful, nonjudgemental, and expansive book, we are engaging in sex and pleasure activism. Any time we ask our clients about the quality of their intimate lives, we are engaging in sex and pleasure activism. Any time we read new books, articles, or attend workshops and presentations on positive sexual health topics, we are engaging in sex and pleasure activism.

While the lineage of positive sex activism traces back to Betty Dodson, Shere Hite, and Susie Bright, among other writers, a recent and influential book is Black biracial feminist adrienne maree brown's book *Pleasure Activism: The Politics of Feeling Good.*

> Pleasure is a feeling of happy satisfaction and enjoyment. Activism consists of efforts to promote, impede, or direct social, political, economic or environmental reform or stasis with the desire to make improvements in society. Pleasure activism is the work we do to reclaim our whole, happy, and satisfiable selves from the impacts, delusions, and limitations of oppression and/or supremacy. Pleasure activism asserts that we all need and deserve pleasure and that our social structures must reflect this. (2019, p. 13)

brown makes a distinction between pleasure activism and "generating and indulging in excess," noting that "because most of us are so repressed, our fantasies go to extremes to counterbalance all that contained longing. Pleasure activism is about learning what it means to … generate … an abundance from which we can all have enough" (2019, p. 15).

brown's book is sorted into six sections, the first titled "Who Taught You to Feel Good?," with others titled "Radical Sex," "A Circle of Sex," and "Pleasure as Political Practice." Throughout the book she offers questions to consider, references to radical thinkers, pleasure exercises, and advice towards pleasure liberation.

One of the first "homework" suggestions is to write up one's "pleasure activism lineage," consider who "politicized your experiences of body, identity, sensation, and feeling good," and then express gratitude to them, living or dead.

As both prose and poetry is needed to address our society's pleasure deficit, here is a small section of brown's poem *Sex Ed.:*

Touch yourself early and often
Learn your body before you share your body
Use mirrors to learn how beautiful you are
Let yes come from every part of you before you share you (2019, p. 113)

brown then goes on to spell out "five tangible tools of a pleasure activist." Here is a brief summary of these tools:

1. *Self-love* (a.k.a. masturbation): "an orgasm a day keeps the doctor away." She explicitly states what I and many sex educators and trauma therapists observe: that the active encouragement of masturbation—and the resulting improved capability to communicate what feels good—would likely result in "less sexual trauma, assault, patriarchy, misogyny, and general awkwardness."
2. *Orgasmic meditation*: brown describes a practice she learned in San Francisco where she spent 15 minutes each morning for a few months "stroking the upper left quadrant of the clitoris." An orgasm is not necessary to engage in this practice, despite the title. brown noted that this practice made her day easier and more joyful. This practice apparently was originally designed to be partnered and to only focus on vulva/clitoris areas. Folks with penises could likely discover a similar practice to connect to themselves.
3. *Self-pornography*: brown details her process of taking pictures of herself, including every inch of her skin, beginning with her face—in order to truly understand her moods, expressions, and so on—and then filming herself masturbating. These images were only for herself, and increased her sense of power, personal agency, and knowledge of herself, particularly in a culture where so much pornography features white individuals.
4. *Developing erotic awareness*: brown also calls this quality "staying curious." This step is about finding an openness to learning about one's relationship to one's sexuality, one's lovers' sexuality, and the variety available to us all.
5. *Talking about sex*: Much harder than it sounds, the goal is to continuously converse with oneself, one's partners, one's friends, and perhaps even one's family members—in developmentally appropriate ways—about the realities of sex. Anytime we do this, we fight erotophobia.

Any or all of these activist steps and recommendations may help guide one's personal, clinical, and even societal work through the helping professions.

RESOURCES FOR CLINICIANS AND CLIENTS

SEXUAL HEALTH WEBSITES, TELEVISION, PODCASTS, AND VIDEO RESOURCES

Useful videos and podcasts have been popping up on YouTube, Vimeo, and other media and educational forums. Our younger clients also prefer information viewed through social media platforms such as Instagram or TikTok. It can be very helpful to share a link with a client struggling over a particular issue. Clients may have validating and/or normalizing "aha" moments from this psychoeducation; however, we may need to evaluate the material posted in social media websites for accuracy and to confirm sex-positive messaging.

Anatomical and Physiological Genital Information

These videos illustrate the anatomy and pathways of some sexual organs:

- BioDigital Human: www.biodigital.com
- Betty Dodson, The Internal Clitoris: http://videosift.com/video/Anatomy-of-the-Clitoris

- Gender-Inclusive Biology: www.genderinclusivebiology.com
- Human Physiology - Functional Anatomy of the Male Reproductive System: www.youtube.com/watch?v=v22CjFYizi0
- Foreskin anatomy: www.youtube.com/watch?v=foqXU8vwBHY
- Unwanted arousal: www.youtube.com/watch?v=L-q-tSHo9Ho; this TED Talk beautifully explains "The Truth About Unwanted Arousal" (Emily Nagoski)

Many survivors of sexual violence report signs of physiological arousal during the assault (vaginal lubrication, erections, orgasms, etc.). These are automatic physiological reactions to sexual stimulation and have no correlation with whether the survivor wanted that sexual interaction.

Sexual Consent

Consent is a basic sexual health right and has gained much more attention since the #metoo movement.

Consent: It's as Simple as Tea (www.youtube.com/watch?v=QDhKM8qWWBM): This video uses the metaphor of making someone tea to help explain consent.

Understanding Consent - FRIES (www.youtube.com/watch?v=pgydDscVnVQ): This video describes enthusiastic consent and its five elements (freely given, reversible, informed, enthusiastic, specific), helping to promote empowered and pleasurable sex.

Sex Educational Websites for Kids and Teens

Amaze.org: This site has many age-appropriate videos and short lessons for kids. Their mission: "AMAZE envisions a world that recognizes child and adolescent sexual development as natural and healthy, a world in which young people everywhere are supported and affirmed and the adults in their lives communicate openly and honestly with them about puberty, reproduction, relationships, sex and sexuality."

Scarleteen.com ("sex ed for the real world"): This is a treasure trove of age-appropriate content for teen "progressive, inclusive sexuality and relationships education, information and support organization and digital clearinghouse" info. A quick glance at their homepage netted these topics "gender, sexual identity, disability, abuse, sexual politics," and quarantine-relevant articles on "How to Actually Date Yourself!" and "Self-Care and Social Distance."

Planned Parenthood (www.plannedparenthood.org/learn/teens): Age-appropriate information related to teen sexuality and relationships

Go Ask Alice! (https://goaskalice.columbia.edu): Health website for kids, with expert information, including sexual health

Real Talk: Stories by Teens (https://myhealthed.org/product): Health and sex ed for teens; mobile app available on Apple IOS

Sex Educational Websites for Adults

Omgyes.com: Disclosure: This is a pay site with a one-time fee ($49 at last check) for Season 1, which includes "[p]ractical techniques to enhance clitoral pleasure [with over] 60 short videos, 12 touchable simulations, and dozens of infographics." No matter at what "sexpert" level your client might be, if they are interested in female-bodied pleasure, they will learn something new. Their practical pleasure techniques include "layering, hinting, signaling, surprise, orbiting, multiples, edging," and so on. Their information is research and science derived, and they state that the one-time fee contributes to ongoing research.

Sexsmartfilms.com: "Promoting sexual literacy" educational films about sex and sex therapy (subscription based)

A Woman's Touch (www.sexualityresources.com): Educational web resource by Ellen Barnard with excellent holistic sexual health information for all genders, including natural vaginal renewal for menopausal individuals

Aging and Sexual Health

American Psychological Association: *Aging and Human Sexuality Resource Guide* (bit.ly/2PkoDW2)

National Institute on Aging: *Sexuality and Intimacy in Older Adults* (bit.ly/2P8gcgF)

Our Better Half podcast (www.ourbetterhalf.net): This podcast has been produced since around 2010 and focuses on sex over the age of 50, with most episodes interviewing someone prominent in the field of sexuality.

SAGE (sageusa.org): Country's oldest and largest organization dedicated to improving lives of LGBTQ+ older adults, offering services, support, and resources for LGBT older adults and their caregivers.

Pelvic, Vulvar, and Urology Resources

American Physical Therapy Association (apta.org): Clients can search this website of physical therapists to locate a pelvic floor specialist in their area.

Endometriosis Association (endometriosisassn.org): Myths and facts about endometriosis

Interstitial Cystitis Association (ichelp.org)

National Vulvodynia Association (nva.org): Information on vulvar health.

PCOS Support - Overcome Your PCOS Symptoms (pcoschallenge.org)

Urology Care Foundation (urologyhealth.org): Includes information on erectile dysfunction and other urological conditions.

Voices for PFD (www.voicesforpfd.org): Educates patients and caregivers about pelvic floor disorders.

Sexual Health Experts and Activists (Websites)

Thankfully the field of sex-positive educators, commentators, and creators continues to expand since the Kinsey's initial foray back in the 1950s. This is a very short list of my favorite activists/educators not mentioned elsewhere.

Susie Bright: Susie has been promoting sex-positive living since the early 1980s and was one of the first prominent bisexual activist/educators to be referred to as a "sex-positive feminist." She has written many books, delivered lectures across the country, appeared in films, maintains a weekly podcast, and is referred to by many as a "national treasure." You can locate her books on Amazon or other book sites.

Betty Dodson (DodsonandRoss.com): Website and videos on bodysex, orgasm instruction, and so on. Although Betty Dodson is now deceased, her work carries on.

Emily Nagoski, PhD (www.emilynagoski.com): Sexologist and scientist behind several books, including the New York Times bestselling book *Come as You Are*.

Carol Queen (carolqueen.com): Carol is a writer, speaker, educator, and activist, with a doctorate in sexology. She is an organizer in the lesbian/gay and international bisexual community, with many published books on sex, activism, and porn.

Tristan Taormino (tristantaormino.com): Tristan, sex educator, write, media maker, and consultant, believes that everyone deserves sex education that is informed by inclusivity, pleasure, consent, accessibility for all, and that is, trauma-aware.

Sexual Health Podcasts

The Authentic Sex (Juliette Allen): Empowering information to transform your sex life; www.juliet-allen.com/podcast-authentic-sex

Brown Girls Do It Too (Poppy and Rubina): Conversations about sex from a South Asian woman's lens; www.bbc.co.uk/programmes/p08k5cp0

Call Her Daddy (Alex Cooper): Unfiltered conversations about women's rights, relationships & mental health; www.callherdaddy.com

Risk! (Kevin Allison): Participants tell stories they never thought they would share; www.risk-show.com

Savage Love (Dan Savage): This is a long-running sex advice podcast by the well-known Dan Savage. savagelovecast.com

Sex With Emily (Dr. Emily Morse): Nonjudgmental sex advice; sexwithemily.com/listen

Smart Sex, Smart Love (Dr. Joe Kort): podcast with expert guests. Kort has written books for therapists on working with LGBTQ clients, as well as self-help books for gay men; joekort.com/podcast

Science Vs (Wendy Zuckerman): Has several sex-related, science checking podcasts, including podcasts on orgasms, squirting, the G-spot, etc.

Speaking of Sex with the Pleasure Mechanics (Charlotte Mia Rose and Chris Maxwell Rose): Explicit yet soulful conversations about sex and sexuality; www.pleasuremechanics.com/speaking-of-sex-podcast

The Pleasure Positive Podcast (Katie, Lindsey and Madison): Wealth of information on their website; podtail.com/en/podcast/clit-talk

Where Should We Begin? (Ester Perel): Real-life couples therapy sessions; www.estherperel.com/podcast

Sex-Positive Retail and Educational Websites

Agreeable Agony (agreeableagony.com): Kink toys, such as ropes for bondage, and so on

Goodvibes.com (sex toys AND feminist-oriented information): Good Vibes began in 1977 when feminist sex activist Joani Blank opened her first sex toy store in San Francisco to provide high quality products, originally geared toward women's bodies. I remember receiving their catalogues in the mail in the 90s, examining with delight all the types of toys and props solely made for pleasure! They have online ordering plus 9 physical locations (mostly in California plus two in the Boston area). Their San Francisco Polk Street location features the Vibrator Museum. Good Vibes was a worker-owned co-op for about 14 years, later becoming a corporation in 2006. In 1995, they declared May International Masturbation Month, as a "sex-positive response to the firing of then-Surgeon General Dr. Joycelyn Elders." If you search through their website, you can investigate the categories of toys for sale (gender play, vibrators, bondage, etc.), plus a variety of free information, and sex tips and tricks. Good Vibes also carries many erotic fiction and nonfiction books for your inspiration (e.g., best women's erotica, best lesbian erotica, books on orgasm, feminist porn, polyamory).

Babeland (www.babeland.com): This sex toy store opened in 1993 in response to the lack of female-centered sex toy stores in the Seattle area. They have an additional store in the New York City area. All of their inventory is available via its website, which also contains sexual health information.

Smitten Kitten (www.smittenkittenonline.com): This newer, progressive sex toy store and website opened in 2003 to promote and facilitate nontoxic sex toy use for everyone. While based in Minneapolis (hosting local events), everything can be ordered online. They also started the website Badvibes.org in 2004 to help combat toxic materials used in sex toys and promote transparency in the sex toy industry.

LGBTQ Educational and Information Websites

Advocates for Trans Equality (transequality.org)
Bisexuality (bi.org)
Bisexual Resource Center (biresource.org)
Diverse Elders Coalition (diverseelders.org)
Human Rights Campaign (hrc.org)
Lesbian Herstory Archives (lesbianherstoryarchives.org)
LGBTQ student resources (glsen.org)
Making Gay History (makinggayhistory.com)
National Black Justice Collective (nbjc.org)
National LGBTQ Task Force (thetaskforce.org)

National Resource Center on LGBTQ+ Aging (lgbtagingcenter.org)
Old Lesbian Oral Herstory Project (olohp.org)
Older Lesbians Organizing for Change (oloc.org)
PFLAG (formerly known as Parents, Families, and Friends of Lesbians and Gays) (pflag.org)
Sage: Advocacy and Services for LGBTQ+ Elders (sageusa.org)
Stonewall Veterans' Association (stonewallvets.org)
The Trevor Project (thetrevorproject.org): "saving young LGBT lives"

Gender, Transgender, Intersex Educational and Information Resources

Cisgender Privilege Checklist (projecthumanities.asu.edu/cisgender-privilege-checklist)
Montañez, A. (2017, September 1). Beyond XX and XY: The extraordinary complexity of sex determination. *Scientific American.* https://www.scientificamerican.com/article/beyond-xx-and-xy-the-extraordinary-complexity-of-sex-determination
Emily Quinn (www.emilord.com): Intersex activist
Gender neutral terms (https://nonbinary.wiki/wiki/Gender_neutral_language_in_English)
Intersex (isna.org/faq/what_is_intersex)
Judith Butler: Your Behavior Creates Your Gender (www.youtube.com/watch?v=Bo7o2LYATDc&t=28s)
Nationwide Childrens' THRIVE Program (www.nationwidechildrens.org/specialties/behavioral-health/outpatient-services)
National Queer and Transgender Therapists of Color Network (www.nqttcn.com)
National resource for transgender equality (transequality.org)
Philadelphia Trans Wellness Conference (www.mazzonicenter.org/trans-wellness)
Sex Down South Conference (www.sexdownsouth.com): Annual conference exploring sexuality, women of color, transgender and gender diverse (TGD) people, sex workers, people with disabilities, etc.
Transgender Gender-Variant & Intersex Justice Project (tgijp.org)
Transhealth (transhealth.org)
Translate Gender (www.translategender.org)
TransProud (transproud.com)
Trans Student Educational Resources (www.transstudent.org)
Why Pronouns Matter for Trans People (www.youtube.com/watch?v=N_yBGQqg7kM&feature=youtu.be)
World Professional Association for Transgender Health: "Standards of care for the health of transgender and gender diverse people, version 8 (www.tandfonline.com/doi/pdf/10.1080/26895269.2022.2100644): "The overall goal of the ... Standards of Care ... is to provide clinical guidance to health care professionals to assist transgender and gender diverse [TGD] people in accessing safe and effective pathways to achieving lasting personal comfort with their gendered selves."

LBGTQ and Spirituality Websites

Baptist: Association of Welcoming and Affirming Baptists (awab.org)
Faithfully LGBT (www.believeoutloud.com/voices/article/i-am-faithfullylgbt): Testimonies of LGBTQ Christians
Judaism (reformjudaism.org): Has LGBTQ resources such as LGBTQ equality and gender expression.
Muslims for Progressive Values (mpvusa.org)
Roman Catholic (dignityusa.org)

Fidelity and Affairs

Many of us will work with clients recovering from being on either end of an affair.

- *Rethinking Infidelity ... a Talk for Anyone Who Has Ever Loved* by Esther Perel (www.youtube.com/watch?v=P2AUat93a8Q): This TED Talk covers questions folks may have about how this could have happened to them.

- *The Secret of Desire in a Long-Term Relationship*: TED Talk by Esther Perel (www.ted.com/talks/esther_perel_the_secret_to_desire_in_a_long_term_relationship?language=en)
- *Where Should We Begin* podcast by Esther Perel (www.estherperel.com/podcast): This podcast focuses on couples and sexuality, featuring a diversity of couples presenting their sexual concerns (each couple receiving one session of help) for Ester Perel's piercing explorations.

Consensual NonMonogamy and/or Polyamory Websites

Polyamory glossary (www.morethantwo.com/polyglossary.html)
Loving More (www.lovingmorenonprofit.org)

Bondage, Domination, Sadism, and Masochism/Kink Websites, Including Resources for Clinicians

FetLife.com: This is a social media website for kink-interested individuals. Not all individual profiles are "vetted." There are many instructional and educational events listed as well.

kinkacademy.com: Website with 2000+ videos plus experts on kink topics ranging from bondage to wrestling

slutphd.com/archives-2: The writer of this blog is an active kinkster AND studies kink (etc.) for a living.

National Coalition for Sexual Freedom (www.ncsfreedom.org): Protects rights of erotically marginalized people; includes the Kink Aware Professionals Directory

The Eulenspiegel Society (TES; www.tes.org): Nonprofit BDSM/leather fetish group

transweek.org: Annual transgender week in Cape Cod, oriented to kink/BDSM.

Sex-Positive (Including LGBTQ+ Positive) Television Series

Awkwafina is Nora from Queens (HBO, 2020–2023): Hilarious comedy with vagina- and vibrator-friendly scenes, diverse racial casting (including LGBTQ).

The Bisexual (Hulu, 2018): Comedy/drama that explores one woman coming to terms with her bisexuality.

Bridgerton (Netflix, 2020–2024): Romance series with diverse racial casting and fairly realistic erotic scenes.

Broad City (Comedy Central, Hulu, 2014–2019): Hilarious comedy, very vagina and queer friendly.

Dying for Sex (Hulu, 2025): A woman with a terminal cancer diagnosis follows her sexual and arousal bliss, and in the process, learns to heal her past childhood sexual trauma.

Grace and Frankie (Netflix, 2015–2022): Hilarious comedy depicting two older ciswomen who make lube, vibrators, and other inventions for the aging population. Great role modeling of elders and positive sexuality. Positive LGBT depictions. A+ casting: Jane Fonda, Lily Tomlin, Sam Waterson, Martin Sheen.

Heartbreak High (Netflix, 2022–). Dramedy set in an Australia high school with diverse depictions of race, gender, and neurodiversity.

Heartstopper (Netflix, 2022–): Super adorable comedy following the relationship of an out-gay high schooler and his romantic interest

Insecure (HBO, 2015–2021): Comedy produced and created by co-star Issa Rae as a follow-up to her original YouTube series *Awkward Black Girl*. *Insecure* authentically explores the insecurities, friendships, and dating/sexual/romantic experiences of two Black women, with realistic and positive depictions of sexuality.

Interview with the Vampire (AMC+, 2022–): Very close adaption of the book series of the same name, without LGBTQ main characters Lestat (pansexual) and Louis.

L Word: Generation Q (Showtime, 2019–2023): Modern drama, realistic depiction of lesbians.

Master of None (Netflix, 2021, Season 3): Dramedy. This season nearly exclusively focuses on the sexual and emotional relationship between two Black lesbians.

Motherland: Fort Salem (Freeform, 2020–2022): Diverse, mostly female casting depicting empowered ciswomen; LGBT friendly.

Mrs. Fletcher (HBO, 2019): Positive exploration of middle-aged mother finally exploring her sexuality.

Queer as Folk (Showtime, 2000–2005): Comedy following the lives of gay men and lesbian couples. Both a British and American version were produced.

Sens8 (Netflix, 2015–2018): Sci-fi thriller by the Wachowski siblings. Positive depictions of LGBTQ sexuality, diverse cast.

Sex and the City (HBO, 1998–2004)/*And Just Like That* (Max, 2021–): Often referenced early cable TV show prominently centering the sexual and romantic pleasure and priorities of four iconic thirtysomething feminist cisgender women.

Sex Education (Netflix, 2019–2023): Comedy series where the son of a sex therapist ends up providing his high school peers with proxy sex therapy.

Shrill (Hulu, 2019–2021): Body positive dramedy with BIPOC (Black, Indigenous, and people of color) and LGBTQ casting.

The Sex Lives of College Girls (HBO, 2021–): Mindy Kaling and Co. hilarious comedy series following the sexual and romantic escapades of four cisgender female college roommates at a fictional private Vermont liberal arts college.

Tales of the City (Netflix 2019 reboot): Serial drama with diverse LGBTQ casting.

Transparent (Amazon Prime, 2014–2019): Beloved dramedy series about a family learning their father is transgender.

Warrior Nun (Netflix, 2020–2022): Fun action show, positive LGBTQ characters.

We Are Who We Are (HBO, 2020): Incredibly well-done drama set in Italy on an American military base depicting the teen children of military exploring gender and sexuality.

Welcome to Chippendales (Hulu, 2022–2023): Very well done series depicting the rise and fall of the famous male review company.

Sex-Positive (Recent) Films[1]

Disappearance of Shere Hite (2023): This poignant documentary traces the rise and fall of the acceptance of Shere Hite's research on female sexuality and pleasure, locating the acceptance and rejection within continued erotophobic and anti-feminist U.S. culture.

Poor Things (2023): Incredibly, this unusual fiction film features a woman's pleasure front and center. Feminist and sex-positive, including self-pleasure.

Pornography Resources

Some clients will present with complaints of feeing like they watch too much porn or that their partner watches too much porn. Research is showing both some very specific benefits (couples who openly discuss porn likes and dislikes correlate with better overall sexual communication and satisfaction) as well as detriments for many (losing self-esteem due to comparing oneself to unrealistic standards, activities, adaptation to "super stimulus," etc.). Here are resources that can help provide clarity and perspective on the influence of porn on our clients' sexual health.

- *Porn Sex vs. Real Sex* video (www.youtube.com/watch?v=q64hTNEj6KQ)
- Corinna, H. (2023). "Making sense of sexual media." (www.scarleteen.com/article/politics_sexuality_etc/making_sense_of_sexual_media)
- Gottman, J., & Gottman, J. (2024). "An open letter on porn." (www.gottman.com/blog/an-open-letter-on-porn): In this letter, pre-eminent relationship researchers discuss their concerns and the research related to porn viewing, read all the way through to their update.
- Yourbrainonporn.com: This website advertises itself as a clearinghouse of scientific research and information regarding the impact of porn on the brain, originally developed by Gary Wilson. While AASECT denounces the pathologizing of porn use and states there is no scientific evidence for "porn addiction," clients with "out of control" usage have reported feeling helped by this website.

1 This is a very short list of recent positive films, a more comprehensive list is beyond the scope of this book.

- *Make Love Not Porn* (http://makelovenotporn.com): This website features real world folks sharing their sexual selves and interactions, often in very different ways from the porn industry. This site is a membership site and viewers pay the participants with membership and fees.
- *Feminist-approved porn list* (www.reddit.com/r/chickflixxx): This Reddit page is for women-identified folks to post links to their favorite feminist erotica and porn. This running list helps to normalize female-bodied pleasure and desire among "regular" (non-porn industry) folk, showing female pleasure as hot, crucial, and beautiful. One caveat—sex educators often emphasize the importance of paying for porn in order to honor and pay the sex worker for the time and effort they put into putting themselves out there.
- erikalust.com: This website promotes feminist ethical porn. Erika Lust made her first indie erotic short film in 2004 (*The Good Girl,* ironically) and hasn't looked back. She promotes ethics, cinematic quality, and empowerment of women in her erotic films. Her website contains her own film catalogue, plus other directors' films she has selected for their ethical and artistic sensibilities. This is porn your clients can feel very good about paying for and watching.

Sexual Health Phone Apps

Bwom: Assists with pelvic health, oriented toward those with uteruses. (Android only)

Clue Period and Health Tracker: Awesome menstruation and health tracker app that has many categories folks can respond to each day, including unprotected sex, high sex interest, mood-related, bowel movement, and so on. Many options are free.

Eve: "Savvy period and sex tracker."

Gottman Card Decks: "Helpful questions, statements, and ideas for improving your relationship." Gottman Card Decks App - Couples | The Gottman Institute

My Sex Doctor: "Targeted at young adults, this app wants to 'start a welcome and long-due revolution, one where you no longer have to risk embarrassment.'"

OkaySo phone app (https://okayso.org): App where people can ask questions about sex, relationships, and identity.

SEXUAL HEALTH BOOKS

Professional Therapy/Clinical Resources

Baird, S. (2023). *EMDR therapy and sexual Health: A clinician's guide.* Springer Publishing Company.

Betchen, S., & Davidson, H. (2018). *Master conflict therapy: A new model for practicing couples and sex therapy.* Routledge.

Bruess, C. E., & Schroeder, E. (2018). *Sexuality education: Theory and practice* (7th ed.). ETR.

Buehler, S. (2022). *What every mental health professional needs to know about sex* (3rd ed.). Springer Publishing Company.

Chang, S. C., Singh, A. A., & Dickey, L M. (2018). *A clinician's guide to gender-affirming care.* Context Press. (First in-depth book for therapists who work with transgender clients.)

Constantinides, D. M., Sennott, S. L., & Chandler, D. (2019). *Sex therapy with erotically marginalized clients: Nine principles of clinical support.* Routledge.

Davis, M. (2019). *Our whole lives: Sexuality education for older adults.* Unitarian Universalist Association.

DeFur, K., & Johnson, A. (2017). *Our whole lives: Sexuality education for grades 4–6* (2nd ed.). Unitarian Universalist Association.

Gambescia, A., Weeks, G., & Hertlein, K. (2021). *A clinician's guide to systemic sex therapy* (3rd ed.). Routledge. (AASECT award-winning book.)

Hall, K., & Binik, Y. (2020). *Principles and practice of sex therapy* (6th ed.). Guilford Press.

Kleinplatz, P. (2012). *New directions in sex therapy: Innovations and alternatives.* Routledge. (AASECT award-winning book.)

Lev, A. (2013). *Transgender emergence: Therapeutic guidelines for working with gender-variant people and their families.* Taylor & Francis.

Levine, S. B. (Ed.). (2015). *Handbook of clinical sexuality for mental health professionals.* Brunner-Routledge.

Nelson, T. (2019). *Integrative sex & couples therapy: A therapist's guide to new and innovative approaches.* Pesi Publishing and Media.

Ogden, G. (2018). *Expanding the practice of sex therapy: The neuro update edition.* Routledge. (Ogden's book expands upon her 4-D Wheel of Sex Therapy, with this edition bringing relevant neuropsychological developments including the mention of EMDR.)

Shahbaz, C. (2017). *Becoming a kink aware therapist.* Routledge.

Weiner, L., & Avery-Clark, C. (2017). *Sensate focus in sex therapy: The illustrated manual.* Routledge.

Wilson, P. (2014). *Our whole lives: Sexual education for grades 7–9* (2nd ed.). Unitarian Universalist Area Church.

General Sex-Positive/Sexuality Information, Essays, Memoir[2]

Auteri, S. (2018). *A dirty word: How a sex writer reclaimed her sexuality.* Cleis Press. (Excellent memoir of a woman who discloses reduced sexual interest and how she particularly resonated with the Dual Control brake/accelerator model to increase her sexual interest).

Bader, M. (2003). *Arousal: The secret logic of sexual fantasies.* St. Martin's Griffin.

Blank, J. (1997). *First person sexual: Women and men write about self-pleasuring.* Down There Press.

brown, a. m. (2019). *Pleasure activism: The politics of feeling good.* AK Press. (This is an extraordinary recent release that looks at the intersection of pleasure, sexuality, race [a construct], and activism.)

Dischiavo, R. (2016). *The deep yes: The lost art of true receiving.* Spanda Press. (This is a great book to refer clients to, particularly your clients that have trouble "receiving" and enjoying pleasure.)

Dodson, B. (1996). *Sex for one: The joy of self-loving.* Random House. (Betty Dodson, the "mother of masturbation," wrote the first edition of this sentinel book "Sex for One" in 1987 and it has been a game-changer for the orgasm-challenged, helping many folks [mostly with clitorises and vulvas] learn to have orgasms.)

Hirsch, J. & Khan, S. (2021). *Sexual citizens: Sex, power, and assault on campus.* W. W. Norton.

Janssen, E., & Bancroft, J. (2007). The dual control model: The role of sexual inhibition and excitation in sexual arousal and behavior. In E. Janssen (Ed.), *The psychophysiology of sex* (pp. 197–222). Indiana University Press.

Joannides, P. (2017). *Guide to getting it on,* unzipped *V.9.0.* Goofy Foot Press. (Revised and updated illustrated editions are published nearly every year. Consider it a modern bible on everything sexuality-related. Comprehensive reference book for clients and offices.)

Klein, M., & Robbins, R. (1999). *Let me count the ways.* Jeremy P. Tarcher. (Explains how to make sex more enjoyable focusing on sensuality and *outercourse* [not intercourse].)

Kleinplatz, P. J. & Menard, A. D. (2020). *Magnificent sex: Lessons from extraordinary lovers.* Routledge.

Komisaruk, B., Whipple., B., Nasserzadeh, S., & Beyer-Flores, C. (2010). *The orgasm answer guide.* Johns Hopkins University Press.

Kort, J. (2019). *Erotic orientation: Helping couples and individuals understand their sexual lives.* Smart Sex, Smart Love Books.

Lehmiller, J. (2018). *Tell me what you want: The science of sexual desire and how it can help improve your sex life.* Da Capo Lifelong Books.

Moen, E., & Nolan, M. (2018). *Drawn to sex, volume 1: The basics.* Erika Moen Comics and Illustration.

Moen, E., & Nolan, M. (2020). *Drawn to sex, volume 2: Our bodies and health.* Erika Moen Comics and Illustration. (These illustrated guides can be helpful sex educational resources for our more intellectually challenged clients.)

2 Favorite and most helpful books have descriptions in parentheses.

Moon, A. (2020). *Getting it: A guide to hot, healthy hookups and shame-free sex.* Clarkson Potter/ Ten Speed. (Modern very inclusive guide book on navigating romance and sex.)
Morin, J. (1996). *The erotic mind: Unlocking the inner sources of passion and fulfillment.* Harper Perennial. (A seminal and revolutionary book changing the way people think about sex.)
Morin, J. (1998). *Anal pleasure and health: A Guide for men and women.* Down There Press.
Nagoski, E. (2024). *Come together: The science (and art!) of creating lasting sexual connections.* Ballantine Books. (Nagoski expounds on info from *Come as You Are* to help long-term partners retain and enjoy their sexual relationship.)
Ogden, G. (2008). *The return of desire: A guide to rediscovering your sexual passion.* Trumpeter.
Perry, F. (2019). *How to have feminist sex: A fairly graphic guide.* Penguin Random House. (This is my favorite go-to illustrated book for feminist-oriented sexual pleasure.)
Queen, C., & Rednour, S. (2015). *The sex & pleasure book: Good vibrations guide to great sex for everyone.* Barnaby.
Tallon-Hicks, Y. (2022). *Hot and inbothered: How to think about, talk about, and have the sex you really want.* Harper Paperbacks.
Taormino, T. (2010). *The big book of sex toys.* Quiver Books.
Yeshe, L. T. (2010). *Introduction to tantra: The transformation of desire.* Readhowyouwant.com.

General Sexuality History and/or Science

D'Emilio, J., & Freedman, E. B. (2012). *Intimate matters: A history of sexuality in America* (3rd ed.). University of Chicago Press.
Foucault, M. (1980). *The history of sexuality* (Vol. I). Vintage.
Roach, M. (2009). *Bonk: The curious coupling of sex and science.* Canongate Books.

Healing From Sexual Trauma

Bass, E. (2008). *The courage to heal: A guide for women survivors of child sexual abuse* (20th anniversary ed.). Harper Collins.
Cohn, R. (2011). *Coming home to passion: Restoring loving sexuality in couples with histories of childhood trauma and neglect* (1st ed.). Praeger.
Levine, P. (2010). *In an unspoken voice: How the body releases trauma and restores goodness.* North Atlantic Books.
Lew, M. (2004). *Victims no longer: The classic guide for men recovering from sexual child abuse.* Harper Perennial.
Porges, S. (2011). *The polyvagal theory: Neurophysiological foundations of emotions, attachments, communication, and self-regulation.* W. W. Norton.
Maltz, W. (2012). *The Sexual healing journey: A guide for survivors of sexual abuse* (3rd ed. revised and updated). William Morrow Paperbacks.
Saakvitne, K., Gamble, S. J., Pearlman, L., & Lev, B. T. (2000). *Risking connection: A curriculum for working with survivors of childhood abuse.* Sidran Press.
Shapiro, F. (2013). *Getting past your past: Take control of your life with self-help techniques from EMDR therapy.* Rodale Books.
Van der kolk, B. (2015). *The body keeps the score: Brain, mind, and body in the healing of trauma.* Penguin Books.

Clitoris, Vulva, Vagina, and/or Woman-Identified Related Sexual Health

Brotto, L. (2018). *Better sex through mindfulness: How women can cultivate desire.* Greystone Books.
Cass, V. (2007). *The elusive orgasm: A woman's guide to why she can't and how she can orgasm.* DeCapo Press.
Diamond, L. (2009). *Sexual fluidity: Understanding women's love and desires.* Harvard University Press.
Enright, L. (2019). *The vagina: A reeducation.* Allen and Unwin.
Ensler, E. (2001). *The vagina monologues.* Villiard.

Goldstein, A., Pukall, C. F., & Goldstein, I. (2011). *When sex hurts: A woman's guide to banishing sexual pain*. De Capo Press.
Gross, R. E. (2022). *Vagina obscura: An anatomical voyage*. W. W. Norton.
Hite, S. (1976). *The Hite report: A nationwide study of female sexuality*. Macmillan.
Kinsey, A. C., Pomeroy, W., Baxter, M., Clyde, E., & Gebhard, P. H. (1953). *Sexual behavior in the human female*. W.B. Saunders.
Mintz, L. (2009). *A tired woman's guide to passionate sex*. Adams Media.
Moon, A. (2015). *Girl Sex 101*. Lunatic Ink.
Lister, L. (2015). *Code red: Know your flow, unlock your monthly superpowers and create an amazing bloody life*. SHE Press UK.
Mintz, L. (2018). *Becoming cliterate: Why orgasm equality matters and how to get it*. HarperOne.
Nagoski, E. (2019). *Come as you are workbook: A practical guide to the science of sex*. Simon & Schuster. (This is the companion workbook to *Come as You Are*, with handy worksheets, questionnaires, and suggested assignments.)
Nagoski, E. (2021). *Come as you are: Revised and updated*. Simon & Schuster. (This book has some of the best current information on how to help people with clitorises, vulvas, and vaginas experience orgasm and pleasure [and to help those that care about clitorises and vaginas, etc.].)
Newman, F. (2012). *The whole lesbian sex book: A passionate guide for all of us*. Cleis Press. (Covers bisexual and transwomen; has detailed drawings.)
Resh, E. (2013). *Women, sex, power, and pleasure*. Hay House.
Stendhal, R. (2011). *True secrets of lesbian desire: Keeping sex alive in long-term relationships*. North Atlantic Books.
Sugrue, D., Foley, S., & Kope, S. (2012). *Sex matters for women: A complete guide to taking care of your sexual self*. Guilford Press.
Taormino, T. (2011). *The secrets of great g-spot orgasms and female ejaculation*. Quiver Books.
Tumbarello, L. (2018). *The heart of self-care: A woman's guide to joyful living and well-being*. Joyful Living Press.
Thomashauer, R. (2018). *Pussy: A reclamation*. Hay House.
Wolf, N. (2012). *Vagina: A new biography, revised and updated*. Harper Collins.

Pregnancy and Birth-Related Sex-Positive[3]

Young, M. (2016). *The ultimate guide to sex through pregnancy and motherhood*. Cleis Press.

Penis and/or Man-Identified Sexual Health

Chia, M., Abrams, A., & Douglas, A. (2001). *The multi-orgasmic man: Sexual secrets every man should know*. Harper Collins.
Danoff, D. (2015). *The ultimate guide to male sexual health: How to stay vital at any age*. Beyond Words. (This book is especially helpful for our aging clients who may be struggling with physical changes.)
Glickman, C., & Emirzian, A. (2013). *The ultimate guide to prostrate pleasure: Erotic exploration for men and their partners*. Cleis Press.
Haberman, H. (2001). *The family jewels: A guide to male genital play and torment*. Greenery Press.
Kinsey, A., Charles, P., Wardell, B., & Martin, C. E. (1948). *Sexual behavior in the human male*. W.B. Saunders.
McCarthy, B., & Metz, M. (2004) *Coping with erectile dysfunction*. New Harbinger Publications. (This classic book is often recommended to clients struggling with erections.)
Metz, M., & McCarthy, B. (2004). *Coping with premature ejaculation: How to overcome PE, please your partner and have great sex*. New Harbinger Publications.
Spitz, A. (2018). *The penis book: A doctor's complete guide to the penis—from size to function and everything in between*. Rodale.

3 While endless titles exist focusing on pregnancy and birth, this section focuses on sex-related titles.

Lesbian and Gay Specific Resources, Memoirs, History and Activism

Acquaviva, K. (2017). *LGBTQ-inclusive hospice and palliative care: A practical guide to transforming professional practice*. Harrington Park Press.
Andrews, M. (1996). *The preacher's son*. Window Books.
Baker, M.-J., & Scheele, J. (2016). *Queer: A graphic history*. Icon Books.
Bechdel, A. (2006). *Fun home: A family tragicomic*. Mariner Books.
Bronski, M. (2011). *A queer history of the United States*. Beacon Press.
Carter, D. (2010). *Stonewall: The riots that sparked the gay revolution*. Griffin.
Faderman, L. (1991). *Odd girls and twilight lovers: A history of lesbian life in twentieth-century America*. Columbia University Press.
Fleishman, J. (2020). *The stonewall generation: LGBTQ elders on sex, activism, and aging*. Unitarian Universalist Area Church. (This recently published book interviews LGBTQ elders "who came of age around the time of the Stonewall Riots" and is a treasure-trove of LGBTQ liberation history.)
Frank, N. (2009). *Unfriendly fire: How the gay ban undermines the military and weakens America*. Thomas Dunne Books.
Johnson, E. P. (Ed.). (2016). *No tea, no shade: New writings in black queer studies*. Duke University Press.
Kort, J. (2018). *Cracking the erotic code: Helping gay men understand their sexual fantasies*. Smart Sex, Smart Love Books.
Kort, J. (2018). *LGBTQ clients in therapy: Clinical issues and treatment strategies*. W. W. Norton.
Marcus, E. (2002). *Making gay history: The half-century fight for lesbian and gay equal rights*. Harper Perennial.
Mogul, J. L., Ritchie, A. J., & Whitlock, K. (2012). *Queer (in)justice: The criminalization of LGBT people in the United States*. Beacon Press.
New York Library. (2019). *The Stonewall reader*. Penguin Classics.
Roughgarden, J. (2004). *Evolution's rainbow: Diversity, gender, and sexuality in nature and people*. University of California Press.
Shilts, R. (2007). *And the band played on: Politics, people and the AIDS epidemic, twentieth anniversary edition*. St. Martin's Press.
Vaid, U. (2013). *Irresistible revolution: Confronting race class and the assumptions of LGBT politics*. Magnus Books.
Williams, W. (1992). *The spirit and the flesh: Sexual diversity in American Indian culture*. Beacon Press.

Bisexuality Specific Resources, Memoirs, History, and Activism

Andrew, E. (2000). *Swinging on the garden gate*. Skinner House Books.
Beauchemin, F. (Ed.). (2016). *How queer!: Personal narratives from bisexual, pansexual, polysexual, sexually-fluid, and other non-monosexual perspectives*. Our Own Authority.
Bisexual Anthology Collective. (1998). *Plural desires: Writing bisexual women's realities*. Sister Vision Press.
Burleson, W. (2005). *Bi America: Myths, truths, and struggles of an invisible community*. Routledge.
Eisner, S. (2013). *Bi: Notes for a bisexual revolution*. Seal Press.
Harrad, K. (Ed.). (2018). *Claiming the b in LGBT*. Thorntree Press.
Hutchins, L., & Ka'ahumanu, L. (Eds.). (1994) *Bi any other name: Bisexual people speak out*. Alyson Books.
Kolodny, D. (Ed.). (2000). *Blessed by spirit: Bisexual people of faith*. Bloomsbury Academic.
Ochs, R. (2001). *Bisexual resource guide*. Bisexual Resource Center.
Ochs, R., & Rowley, S. L. (2005). *Getting bi*. Bisexual Resource Center.
Ochs, R., & Williams, S. (2014). *RECOGNIZE: The voices of bisexual men*. Bisexual Resource Center.
Orndorff, K. (Ed.). (1999). *Bi lives: Bisexual women tell their stories*. See Sharp Press.

Transgender Specific Resources, Memoirs, History, Activism, and Education

Bornstein, K. (2013). *My new gender workbook: A step-by-step guide to achieving world peace through gender anarchy and sex positivity* (2nd ed.). Routledge.

Bornstein, K., & Bergman, S. B. (2010). *Gender outlaws: The next generation.* Seal Press.

Califia, P. (2003). *Sex changes: Transgender politics.* Cleis Press.

Chang, S. C., Singh, A. A., & Dickey, L. M. (2018). *A clinician's guide to gender-affirming care.* Context Press. (First in-depth book for therapists who work with transgender clients.)

Duron, L. (2013). *Raising my rainbow: Adventures in raising a fabulous, gender creative son.* Broadway Books.

Erickson-Schroth, L. (Ed.). (2022). *Trans bodies, trans selves: A resource by and for transgender communities.* Oxford University Press.

Fielding, L. (2021). *Trans sex: Clinical approaches to trans sexualities and erotic embodiments.* Routledge.

Feinberg, L. (1996). *Transgender warriors: Making history from Joan of Arc to Rupaul.* Beacon Press.

Feinberg, L. (1999). *Trans liberation: Beyond pink or blue.* Beacon Press.

Feinberg, L. (2004). *Stone butch blues* (3rd printing). Alyson Publications. (Categorized as "fiction," reads like a memoir.)

Green, E., & Maurer, L. (2015). *The teaching transgender toolkit.* Planned Parenthood of the Southern Finger Lakes.

Iantaffi, A. (2017). *How to understand your gender: A practical guide for exploring who you are.* Jessica Kingsley Publishers.

Lev, A. I., & Gottlieb, A. R. (2019). *Families in transition: Parent perspectives on raising gender diverse children, adolescents, and young adults.* Harrington Park Press

Maynard, D. M. (2019). *The reflective workbook for partners of transgender people: Your transition as your partner transitions.* Jessica Kingsley Publishers.

Pfeffer, C. A. (2017). *Queering families: The postmodern partnerships of cisgender women and tansgender men.* Oxford University Press.

Rajunov, M., & Duane, A. S. (2019). *Nonbinary: Memoirs of gender and identity.* Columbia University Press.

Shlasko, D. (2017). *Trans allyship workbook: Building skills to support trans people in our lives.* Think Again Training.

Singh, A. A., & Dickey, L. M. (2017). *Affirmative counseling with transgender and gender nonconforming clients.* In K. A. DeBord, A. R. Fischer, K. J. Bieschke, & R. M. Perez (Eds.), *Handbook of sexual orientation and gender diversity in counseling and psychotherapy* (pp. 157–182). American Psychological Association. https://doi.org/10.1037/15959-007

Snorton, C. R. (2017). *Black on both sides: A racial history of trans identity.* University of Minnesota Press.

Stryker, S. (2017). *Transgender history: The roots of today's revolution.* Seal Press.

Wilchins, R. (2017). *TRANS/gressive: How transgender activists took on gay rights, feminism, the media, congress ... and won!* Riverdale Avenue Books.

Body Image

Bacon, L. (2010). *Health at every size: The surprising truth about your weight, revised and updated.* Benbella Books. (My "go to" book for clients struggling with weight-related, self-esteem issues.)

Queen, C. (2013). *Exhibitionism for the shy* (2nd ed.). Down There Press. (First edition published 1995)

Age-Appropriate Sex and Sexuality Development Books for Children

Harris, R., & Emberley, M. (1999, 2014). *It's so amazing!: A book about eggs, sperm, birth, babies, and families.* Candlewick Press.

Hindman, J. (1983). *A very touching book: For little people and for big people.* Alexandria.

Saltz, G., & Cravath, L. A. (2008). *Amazing you: Getting smart about your private parts.* Puffin Books.

Sanders, J. (2016). *My body! What I say goes!: A book to empower and teach children about personal body safety, feelings, safe and unsafe touch, private parts, secrets and surprises, consent, and respectful relationships.* Educate2Empower Publishing.

Silverberg, C. (2016). *Sex is a funny word: A book about bodies, feelings, and YOU.* Triangle Square.

Silverberg, C., & Smyth, F. (2018). *What makes a baby.* Triangle Square.

Spelman, C. M., & Weidner, T. (1997). *Your body belongs to you.* Albert Whitman.

Age-Appropriate Sex and Sexuality Development Books for Teens

Corinna, H. (2016). *S.E.X.: The all-you-need-to-know sexuality guide to get you through your teens and twenties* (2nd ed.). De Capo Lifelong Books.

Hasler, N. (2010). *SEX: A book for teens.* Zest Books.

Lang, J. (2018). *Consent: The new rules of sex education: Every teen's guide to healthy sexual relationships.* Althea Press.

Planned Parenthood. (2019). *In case you're curious: Questions about sex from young people with answers from the experts.* Viva Editions.

Sex Education Resource Books for Parents and Caregivers

Brand, A. (2021). *Stop sweating and start talking: How to make sex chats with your kids easier than you think.* Wise Ink Creative Publishing.

Levine, J. (2002). *Harmful to minors: The perils of protecting our children.* Da Capo Lifelong Books.

Roffman, D. M. (2001). *Sex and sensibility: The thinking parents' guide to talking to sense about sex.* Da Capo Lifelong Books.

Roffman, D. M. (2012). *Talk to me first: Everything you need to know to become your kids 'go-to' person about sex.* Da Capo Lifelong Books.

Sex and Aging

Brick, P., Lunquist, J., Sandak, A., & Taverner, B. (2009). *Older, wiser, sexually smarter: 30 sex ed lessons for adults only.* Planned Parenthood of Greater Northern New Jersey.

Doll, G. A. (2012). *Sexuality and long-term care: Understanding and supporting the needs of older adults.* Health Professions Press.

Price, J. (2006). *Better than I ever expected: Straight talk about sex after sixty.* Seal Press.

Price, J. (2011). *Naked at our age: Talking out loud about senior sex.* Seal Press.

Price, J. (2014). *The ultimate guide to sex after 50.* Cleis Press.

Sex and Aging: Menopause Specific

Dunn, J. (2023). *Hot and bothered: What no one tells you about menopause.* Penguin Random House. (New book by journalist Jancee, who turned her investigative powers to menopause as she entered this time for herself.)

Gilberg-Lenz, S., & Korn, M. (2022). *Menopause boot camp: Optimize your health, empower your self, and flourish as you age.* Harper.

Mosconi, L. (2024). *The menopause brain: New science empowers women to navigate the pivotal transition with knowledge and confidence.* Avery.

Sex and Cultural and Racial Diversity

Boykin, K. (2005). *Beyond the down-low: Sex, lies, and denial in black America.* Carroll & Graff.

Carol, J. (2009). *Sexuality now: Embracing diversity.* Cengage Learning.

King, J. L. (2004). *On the down low: A journey into the lives of straight Black men who sleep with men.* Broadway Books.

Moultrie, M. (2017). *Passionate and pious: Religious media and black women's sexuality.* Duke University Press.

Myers, N. J. (2003). *Black hearts: The development of black sexuality in America.* Trafford Publishing.

Staples, R. (2006). *Exploring black sexuality.* Rowman & Littlefield.

Sue, D. W. (2010). *Microaggressions in everyday life: Race, gender, and sexual orientation.* Wiley.

Sex and Disabilities

Andrews, A. (2020). *A quick and easy guide to sex and disability*. Limerence Press.
Buehler, S. (2011). *Sex, love, and mental illness: A couple's guide to staying connected*. Praeger.
Katz, A. (2009). *Sex when you're sick: Reclaiming sexual health after illness or injury*. Praeger.
Kaufman, M., Silverberg, C., & Odette, F. (2007). *The ultimate guide to sex and disability*. Cleis Press.
Kroll, K., & Klein, E. L. (2001). *Enabling romance: A guide to love, sex, and relationships for people with disabilities (and the people who care about them)*. United Spinal Association.
McRuer, R., & Mollow, A. (Eds.). 2012. *Sex and disability*. Duke University Press.
Schovr, L., & Jensen, S. (1988). *Sexuality and chronic illness: A comprehensive approach*. Guilford Press.

Sex and Spirituality

Bolz-Weber, N. (2019). *Shameless: A sexual reformation*. Convergent Books.
Brownson, J. V. (2015). *Reframing the church's debate of same sex relationships*. Erdmanns.
Klein, L. K. (2018). *Pure: Inside the evangelical movement that shamed generations of young women and how I broke free*. Atria Books and Simon & Shuster.
Seller, T. (2017). *Sex, god, and the conservative church: Erasing shame from sexual intimacy*. Routledge.
Stayton, W. (2020). *Sinless sex: A challenge to religions*. Luminare Press.

Committed (Mostly Monogamous) Relationships, Affairs, and Sexual Health

Perel, E. (2009). *Mating in captivity: Unlocking erotic intelligence*. Harper Collins.
Perel, E. (2017). *The state of affairs: Rethinking infidelity*. Harper Collins.
Schnarch, D. (2011). *Intimacy and desire: Awaken the passion in your relationship*. Beaufort Books.
Schnarch, D. (2011). *Passionate marriage: Keeping love and intimacy alive in committed relationships*. Beaufort Books.

Polyamory, Open Relationships, and Consensual Non-Monogamy

Easton, D. (2009). *The ethical slut: A practical guide to polyamory, open relationships, and other adventures*. Celestial Arts.
Fern, J. (2020). *Polysecure: Attachment, trauma and consensual nonmonogamy*. Thorntree Press.
Labriola, K. (2013). *The jealousy workbook: Exercises and insights for managing open relationships*. Greenery Press.
Sheff, E. (2013). *The polyamorists next door*. Rowman & Littlefield.
Sheff, E., & Wolf, T. (2015). *Stories from the polycule*. Thorntree Press.
Taormino, T. (2008). *Opening up: A guide to creating and sustaining open relationships*. Cleis Press.
Veaux, F., & Rickert, E. (2014). *More than two: A practical guide to ethical polyamory*. Thorntree Press.
Wolf, T. (2016). *Ask me about polyamory: The best of kimchi cuddles*. Thorntree Press.

Bondage, Domination, Sadism and Masochism/Kink-Related Lay and Professional Books

Bader, M. J. (2002). *Arousal: The secret logic of sexual fantasies*. Thomas Dunne Books.
Baldwin, G. (2003). *Ties that bind: SM/leather/fetish/erotic style: Issues, commentary, and advice* (2nd ed.). Daedalus.
Beckmann, A. (2009). *The social construction of sexuality and perversion: Deconstructing sadomasochism*. Palgrave Macmillan.
Brame, G. G., Brame, W. D., & Jacobs, J. (1993). *Different loving: The world of sexual dominance and submission*. Villard Books.
Easton, D., & Liszt, C. A. (1997). *The topping book, or getting good at getting bad*. Greenery Press.
Easton, D., & Liszt, C. A. (1997). *The bottoming book, or how to get terrible things done to you by wonderful people*. Greenery Press.
Easton, D., & Liszt, C. A. (2000). *When someone you love is kinky*. Greenery Press.

Harrington, L. (2009). *Sacred kink*. Mystic Productions.

Kaldrea, R., & Tenpenny, J. (2009). *Dear Raven and Joshua: Questions and answers about master/slave relationships*. Alfred Press.

Kleinplatz, P., & Moser, C. (Eds.). (2006). *Sadomasochism: Powerful pleasures*. Harrington Park Press.

Langdridge, D., & Marker, M. (Eds.). (2007). *Safe, sane, and consensual: Contemporary perspectives on sadomasochism*. Palgrave Macmillan.

Midori. (2005). *Wild side sex: The book of kink: Educational, sensual, and entertaining essays*. Daedalus.

Newmahr, S. (2011). *Playing on the edge: Sadomasochism, risk, and intimacy*. Indiana University Press.

Sadie, S. (Ed.). (2007) *Spiritual transformation through BDSM: Stories and submissions from fellow travellers*. Ephemera Bound.

Stein, D., & Schachter, D. (2009). *Ask the man who owns him: The real lives of gay masters and slaves*. Perfectbound Press.

Thompson, M. (Ed.). (2004). *Leatherfolk: Radical sex, people, politics, and practice* (3rd ed.). Daedalus.

Bondage, Domination, Sadism and Masochism/KINK Beginner's Manuals

Bannon, R. (1993). *Learning the ropes: A basic guide to safe and fun S/M lovemaking*. Daedalus.

Califia, P. (2001). *Sensuous magic: A guide to S/M for adventurous couples* (2nd ed.). Cleis Press.

Easton, D., & Hardy, J. W. (2001). *The new bottoming book*. Greenery Press.

Easton, D., & Hardy, J. W. (2003). *The new topping book*. Greenery Press.

Green, L. (1998). *The sexually dominant woman: A workbook for nervous beginners* (2nd ed.). Greenery Press.

Henkin, W. A., & Holiday, S. (2003). *Consensual sadomasochism: How to talk about it & how to do it safely* (2nd ed.). Daedalus.

Jacques, T., Dale, D., Hamilton, M., & Sniffer. (1993). *On the safe edge: A manual for SM play*. Whole SM.

Ortman, D. M., & Sprott, R. A. (2013). *Sexual outsiders: Understanding BDSM sexualities and communities*. Rowman & Littlefield.

Rinella, J. (2004). *The complete slave: Creating and living an erotic dominant/submissive lifestyle* (2nd ed.). Daedalus.

Taormino, T. (2012). *The ultimate guide to kink*. Cleis Press.

Taormino, T. (2013). *50 shades of kink: An introduction to BDSM*. Cleis Press.

Varrin, C. (2004). *Female dominance: Rituals and practice*. Citadel Publishing.

Warren, J. (2000). *The loving dominant* (2nd ed.). Greenery Press.

Out of Control Sexual Behavior

Braun-Harvey, D., & Vigorito, M. (2016). *Treating out of control sexual behavior: Rethinking sex addiction*. Springer Publishing Company.

Pornography and Sex-Work History and Activism

Delacoste, F. (1998). *Sex work: Writings by women in the sex industry* (2nd ed.). Cleis Press.

Ley, D. (2016). *Ethical porn for dicks: A man s guide to responsible viewing pleasure*. ThreeL Media.

Rogers, V. (2016). *We need to talk about pornography: A resource to educate young people about the potential impact of pornography and sexualized images on relationships body image and self-esteem*. Jessica Kingsley Publishers.

Smith, M., & Mac, J. (2018). *Revolting prostitutes: The fight for sex workers' rights*. Verso.

Taormino, T. (2002). *True lust: Adventures in sex, porn, and perversion*. Cleis Press.

Taormino, T., Perrenas-Shimzu, C. Penley, C., & Miller-Young, M. (Eds.). (2013). *The feminist porn book: The politics of producing pleasure*. The Feminist Press.

Sex-Positive Erotic Books

Anderson, G. (2024). *Want: Sexual fantasies by anonymous*. Henry N. Abrams.

Brent, B., & Queen, C. (2000). *Best bisexual erotica*. Black Books.

Bright, S. (1997–2003). *Best American erotica* (Annual Series). Touchstone.

Califa, P. (1988). *Macho sluts*. Alyson Publications.

Foster, E. (2016). *How not to fall* (Belhaven series). Kensington. (These are written by a sex educator ["Emily Foster" is the author's nom de plume for this series] and portray sex-positive hot depictions of feminist cis-gender heterosexual erotic interactions, from accurate naming of body parts, to realistic descriptions of the nuances of sexual desire and interest. Anyone with a geeky bent will also enjoy the neurophysiological terms scattered throughout. This series deliberately counteracts the misinformation and harmful stereotype perpetuations in the *50 Shades of Grey* series.)

Herotica series (feminist erotica series from 1993 to 2003), often edited by Susie Bright or Marcy Sheiner. Down There Press.

Kwon, R. O., & Greenwell, G. (2021). *Kink stories*. Simon & Shuster.

Queen, C., & Schimel, L. (1996). *Switch hitters: Lesbians write gay erotica and gay men write lesbian erotica*. Cleis Press.

Rosen, R. (2018). *Best gay erotica of the year* (Vol. 4). Down There Press.

Sexsmith, S. (2021). *Best lesbian erotica of the year* (Vol. 6). Cleis Press.

Taormino, T. (2011). *Sometimes she lets me: Best butch/femme erotica*. Cleis Press.

Taormino, T. (2011). *Take me there: Trans and genderqueer erotica*. Cleis Press.

SEXUAL HEALTH TRAINING PROGRAMS

Organizations Offering Sexual Health and Sexuality-Related Memberships, Workshops, Continuing Education Units, and Professional Training

- American Association of Sexuality Educators, Counselors, and Therapists (AASECT; www.aasect.org): Annual conference, trainings.
- Institute for Sexuality Education and Enlightenment (ISEE; instituteforsexuality.com): Offers dozens of webinars related to a multitude of sexuality and sexual health topics. In-person trainings are generally offered a couple times of year in Massachusetts and Oregon. ISEE offers the mandatory Sexual Attitude Reassessment (SAR) class for proceeding with any kind of sex educator or counselor certification.
- Integrative Psychiatry and Sexuality Counseling Associates (www.thriveintegrativepsych.com): Evelyn Resh, CSC, CNM, MPH, MSN, and associates provide medical and psychiatric consultation, treatment, and trainings.
- International Society for Sexual Medicine (ISSM; www.issm.info): Mission is to become the leading and most trusted authority in human sexual health by providing high-quality publications, research, and global opportunities for education, professional development, and the exchange of knowledge.
- International Society for the Study of Women's Sexual health (ISSWSH; www.isswsh.org): ISSWSH is a multidisciplinary, academic, and scientific organization that provides communication among scholars, researchers, and practitioners, supports ethics and professionalism, and educates the public about womens' sexuality and health.
- New England Sex Therapy (newenglandsextherapy.com): Jassy Casella Timberlake, LMFT provides sex therapy and supervision and has a wealth of experience informed by decades of work.
- Safer Society (safersocietypress.org): Mission is to provide services and resources for preventative and restorative responses to sexual and social violence.
- Sexual Medicine Society of North America (SMSNA; www.smsna.org): Objective is to advance, foster, and uphold excellence in practice, research, education, and ethical standards related to the "study of human sexual function and dysfunction."

- Society for Sex Therapy and Research (www.sstarnet.org): International organization lists sex therapists, sex researchers, and has an annual conference.
- Stop it now! (stopitnow.org): Offers child sexual abuse prevention trainings.
- Shine (www.ourshine.org): Ashley Mader, PhD provides consultation, trainings, and workshops related to aging and sexuality. She is a sex therapist specializing in older adults and aging. She provides consultation and general sex therapy and education trainings and consultation. Former co-host of podcast on sex and aging *Our Better Half.*

Sexuality-Related Educational Certificates and Programs

Institute for Sexuality Education and Enlightenment (ISEE; instituteforsexuality.com): Certification Programs in Sex Educator, Sex Counselor, AASECT-Approved Sex Therapist, and an ACES certificate (Advancing Clinical Excellence in Sexuality)

Institute of Somatic Sexology (https://instituteofsomaticsexology.com/courses/certificate-in-sexological-bodywork)

Robert Wood Johnson Medical School, Piscataway, New Jersey: Post-graduate training in relationship and sex therapy. Offers a week-long sexuality course (40 hours) that's not offered by any other program (counts as graduate credit if individual writes a paper).

Sex Educator Training Programs

Institute for Sexuality Education and Enlightenment (ISEE; instituteforsexuality.com): Certification program in xex educator.

Our Whole Lives (OWL) Sexuality Education Curricula (uua.org/re/owl): "Honest, accurate information about sexuality changes lives. It dismantles stereotypes and assumptions, builds self-acceptance and self-esteem, fosters healthy relationships, improves decision-making, and has the potential to save lives. For these reasons and more, we are proud to offer Our Whole Lives (OWL), a comprehensive, lifespan sexuality education curricula for use in both secular settings and faith communities." Curricula covers grades K-1, 4–6, 7–9, 10–12, Young Adult, Adult, and Older Adult. Most recent publications includes: Davis, Melanie (2019). *Our whole lives: Sexuality education for older adults*. Unitarian Universalist Association and deFur, K., & Johnson, A. (2017). *Our whole lives, second edition: Sexuality education for grades 4–6.* Unitarian Universalist Association.

Planned Parenthood (www.plannedparenthood.org/learn/for-educators): Planned Parenthood is the largest provider of sex education in the United States. Each state-affiliated Planned Parenthood offers various trainings for professionals and sex educators. For example, information on training in Massachusetts can be found at www.plannedparenthood.org/planned-parenthood-massachusetts/local-training-education/professionals.

Graduate Level Sexuality Programs

American Academy of Clinical Sexology,[5] Maimonides University, North Miami, Florida: PhD in pastoral clinical sexology. Prepares students for sex therapy certification in Florida (a requirement in Florida if wanting to practice in this state). Emphasizes the importance of religion in providing therapy.

California Institute of Integral Studies,[4–6] San Francisco, California: Masters and PhD in human xexuality

Columbia University Mailman School of Public Health,[4] New York, New York: MPH in sexuality and health. Equips students with skills needed to address health issues (e.g., reproductive health, and child and adolescent health) related to sexuality through interdepartmental studies. (Note: Students applying for the program are expected to have worked for 2 years in the field of public health, which can include undergraduate volunteer/practicum experiences.)

4 Program reflecting training primarily as a researcher.

5 Program reflecting a practitioner model/clinical skills.

6 Program reflecting general sexology.

Hofstra University, Interdisciplinary Studies/Marriage & Family Therapy,[5] New York, New York: MA in interdisciplinary studies/marriage and family therapy (plus family counseling certification). Provides skills needed for marriage/family counseling and introduces students to sexuality education, counseling, and research.

Institute for Advanced Study of Human Sexuality,[6] San Francisco, California: MA, MPH, EdD, PhD, DHS (Doctor of Human Sexuality), plus certification options—human sexuality. Seeks to train sexologists. Offers long-distance learning. Certificate programs are unique to the Institute (e.g., erotology). The master's program also allows students to travel to Paris or China for a cultural perspective on public health.

Kinsey Institute at *Indiana University,*[4] Bloomington, Indiana: PhD minor in human sexuality; majors include counseling, education, health behavior, psychology, and sociology. Offers research programs investigating a variety of sex topics and a summer institute for students who are not involved with the university. Houses one of the largest library holdings on human sexuality, as well as a sexuality art museum. Hosts seminars on sexuality and holds special events.

San Francisco State University Program in Sexuality Studies,[4] San Francisco, California: MA in human sexuality. Provides a foundation for sex counseling, teaching, and research. Specializes in gay, lesbian, and bisexual studies. Houses the Institute on Sexuality, Social Inequality, and Health; the National Sexuality Resource Center; and the Center for Research on Gender and Sexuality; it also has a summer institute.

University of Connecticut, Social Processes of HIV/AIDS Training Program, Storrs, Connecticut: MA, PhD in social psychology with a specialization in HIV prevention. Conducts HIV risk dynamics and prevention research.

University of Guelph, Department of Family Relations & Applied Nutrition,[4,5] Guelph, Ontario, Canada: MSc in couple and family therapy; PhD in family relations and human development. Emphasizes child/adolescent development, social/personality development, parent–child relations, social gerontology, human sexuality, and marriage/family therapy.

University of Hawaii, Human Sexuality Program, Department of Social Work; Pacific Center for Sex and Society, Department of Anatomy and Reproductive Biology,[4,5] Honolulu, Hawaii: MA, PhD specializes in human sexuality counseling. Houses the Pacific Center for Sex and Society, which provides research opportunities.

University of Minnesota, Department of Family Social Science,[4,5] St. Paul, Minnesota: MA, PhD in family social science; MFT certification for clinical track. Specializes in marriage/family and sex therapy.

University of New Brunswick, Department of Psychology,[4,5] Fredericton, New Brunswick, Canada: PhD in psychology. Prepares students for clinical or experimental psychology involving human sexuality.

University of Quebec, Department of Sexology,[5] Montreal, Quebec, Canada: BA, MA in sexology. Focuses on sex education. Master's level encompasses sex therapy and research, plus more advanced sex education.

University of Utah, Department of Psychology,[4,5] Salt Lake City, Utah: PhD in clinical psychology. Emphasizes human sexuality in research and clinical work.

University of Wisconsin, Departments of Social Psychology & Microsociology,[4] Madison, Wisconsin: PhD in psychology or sociology. Focuses on human sexuality, especially sex research. Part of a consortium where a student may study at the University of Chicago, University of Minnesota, or Wisconsin.

Widener University, Human Sexuality Program,[5] Wayne, Pennsylvania: MEd, EdD in human sexuality education/clinical sexuality. Prepares professionals for sex education, consulting, research, and counseling. Also offers joint degree programs with social work or clinical psychology. Program is both distance and work friendly in that human sexuality courses are offered on weekends. One semester course is generally two weekends. Also provides opportunity to study abroad.

Internship and Post-Doctoral Programs

University of California, Center for AIDS Prevention Studies, San Francisco, California: Grants traineeships in AIDS Prevention Studies.

University of Minnesota, Department of Family Practice & Community Health, Minneapolis, Minnesota: Fellowships in human sexuality, dysfunction, and disease prevention for post-doctorates in clinical psychology. Conducts sexuality research, provides sex education, offers clinical services for sexual and relationship problems, and promotes community sexual health via community health initiatives. Houses the Center for Sexual Health and the Center for HIV/STI Intervention & Prevention Studies.

ASSESSMENT TOOLS

This is a short list of sexuality-related assessment tools that may be helpful to you and your clients. Note that several are gendered in a binary manner.

- Clayton, A., Segraves, R. T., Leiblum, S., Basson, R., Pyke, R., Cotton, D., Lewis-D'Agostino, D., Evans, K., Sills, T., & Wunderlich, G. (2006). Reliability and validity of the Sexual Interest and Desire Inventory–Female (SIDI-F), a scale designed to measure severity of female hypoactive sexual desire disorder. *Journal of Sex & Marital Therapy, 32*(2), 115–135. https://doi.org/10.1080/00926230500442300
- Cooper, E. B., Fenigstein, A., & Fauber, R. L. (2014). Faking orgasm scale for women. *PsycTESTS*. https://doi.org/10.1037/t72337-000
- Decreased Sexual Desire Screener (DSDS): 5 questions screen for decreased sexual desire, a common issue in sex therapy
- Dennerstein, L., Lehert, P., & Dudley, E. (2001). Short scale to measure female sexuality: Adapted from McCoy Female Sexuality Questionnaire. *Journal of Sex & Marital Therapy, 27*(4), 339–351. https://doi.org/10.1080/009262301317081098
- Female Sexual Function Index (FSFI): 19 questions assess female sexuality and screen for sexual dysfunction
- Gordon, B. L. (2018). *Development and validation of a Tantric Sex Scale: Sexual-mindfulness, spiritual purpose, and genital/orgasm de-emphasis* [Master's thesis, Bowling Green State University]. OhioLINK Electronic Theses and Dissertations Center. http://rave.ohiolink.edu/etdc/view?acc_num=bgsu154203013060414
- Hasson, R., & Ginzburg, K. (2024). The development and psychometric evaluation of the Sexual Fantasy Experience Scale. *Archives of Sexual Behavior, 53*(3), 1015–1030. https://doi.org/10.1007/s10508-023-02794-1
- Janssen, E., Vorst, H., Finn, P., & Bancroft, J. (2002). The Sexual Inhibition (SIS) and Sexual Excitation (SES) scales. I. Measuring sexual inhibition and excitation proneness in men. *The Journal of Sex Research, 39*(2), 114–126. https://doi.org/10.1080/00224490209552130
- Meston, C. M., Freihart, B. K., Crosby, C. L., Stephenson, K. R., & Trapnell, P. D. (2024). Psychometric evaluation and adaptation of the five-factor Sexual Satisfaction Scale (SSS-W) for use in men: The Sexual Satisfaction Scale (SSS). *Journal of Sex & Marital Therapy, 50*(2), 216–229. https://doi.org/10.1080/0092623X.2023.2270205
- Sexual Function Questionnaire (Part A): binary gender focused, short questionnaire assessing for impact of medication on sexual functioning
- Turning on/Turning off: Individual Differences in Sexual Inhibition and Excitation (part of an ongoing research study) https://iu.co1.qualtrics.com/jfe/form/SV_9LBtS5dal6c37Rr?survey_id=9dff4e9a3dd78f2c4cfb
- Webb, A. E., Reissing, E. D., & Huta, V. (2022). Orgasm Rating Scale and Bodily Sensations of Orgasm Scale: Validation for use with pre, peri, and post-menopausal women. *Journal of Sexual Medicine, 19*(7), 1156–1172. https://doi.org/10.1016/j.jsxm.2022.03.621

SUMMARY

Thank you for showing curiosity, courage, intention, and personal, educational, and professional growth in the face of our continuing erotophobic culture, by obtaining and reading this book. If this is your first educational/professional foray into increasing sexual health knowledge and competence, then we thank you deeply for choosing this book as your jumping off point. If this is not your first rodeo in this arena, then we welcome any and all feedback to improve this book as a whole (including this chapter).

We sincerely hope that all the material encountered in this book satisfies immediate questions and clinical dilemmas, and leaves you with an overwhelming thirst and hunger for the continued pursuit, digestion, and application of positive sexual health, sexual pleasure principles, and inalienable sexual rights. If this book has indeed properly done its job to wet your whistle, then may this last resource chapter encourage a fun, dynamic, and pleasurable lifelong sexual health knowledge acquisition. Engaging and positive resources for everyone (and just about every kind of learner) under the sun is listed in this chapter. May these recommended podcasts, TED Talks, websites, books, and educational programs bring hope and clarity to you and your clients.

Lastly, as mentioned in the chapter introduction, sexual health information can change quickly. Always strive to find the most updated website, book, TED Talk, and so on, to share with clients.

Now, boldly go forth armed and ready to assist clients presenting with sexual health concerns, and share more sexual health knowledge than 99% of the U.S. population!

DISCUSSION QUESTIONS

- What are some similarities and differences between work-related stress, BO, and VT?
- What are some positive and proactive self-care practices clinicians can engage in, to reduce the risk of BO (and VT, if applicable)?
- What is a sex-positive activist strategy you might feel comfortable trying out?
- How can a clinician continue to remain sex-positive despite existing in the same erotophobic society that surround clients?
- What are the top one to three books a clinician might recommend to clients?
- What top one or two assessment tools mentioned in this chapter might provide quick and helpful snapshot regarding a client's current sexual functioning?

LEARNING ACTIVITIES

CourseConnect

To access self-assessment questions and interactive, competency-based learning activities for this chapter, visit www.springerpub.com/courseconnect. See inside front cover and tear-out card for CourseConnect details.

ADDITIONAL RESOURCES

Additional resources are online and available at www.springerpub.com/courseconnect.

REFERENCES

Baird, S. (2021, December). *Burnout, vicarious trauma, and self-care for clinical staff* (online webinar). Smith College.

brown, a. m. (2019). *Pleasure activism: The politics of feeling good.* AK Press.

Freudenberger, H. J. (1974), Staff burn-out. *Journal of Social Issues, 30*, 159–165. https://doi.org/10.1111/j.1540-4560.1974.tb00706.x

Maslach, C. (1982). *Burnout: The cost of caring.* Prentice-Hall.

McCann, I. L., & Pearlman, L. A. (1990). Vicarious traumatization: A framework for understanding the psychological effects of working with victims. *Journal of Traumatic Stress, 3*(1), 131–149. https://doi.org/10.1007/BF00975140

Pearlman, L. A., & Saakvitne, K. W. (1995). *Trauma and the therapist: Countertransference and vicarious traumatization in psychotherapy with incest survivors.* W. W. Norton.

Saakvitne, K. W., & Pearlman, L. A. (1996). *Transforming the pain: A workbook on vicarious traumatization.* W. W. Norton.

Index